Geriatric Psychiatry

Editor

SOO BORSON

CLINICS IN
GERIATRIC MEDICINE

www.geriatric.theclinics.com

August 2014 • Volume 30 • Number 3

ELSEVIER

1600 John F. Kennedy Boulevard • Suite 1800 • Philadelphia, Pennsylvania, 19103-2899

http://www.theclinics.com

CLINICS IN GERIATRIC MEDICINE Volume 30, Number 3
August 2014 ISSN 0749–0690, ISBN-13: 978-0-323-32012-2

Editor: Jessica McCool
Developmental Editor: Yonah Korngold

Clinics in Geriatric Medicine (ISSN 0749-0690) is published quarterly by Elsevier Inc., 360 Park Avenue South, New York, NY 10010-1710. Months of issue are February, May, August, and November. Business and Editorial Offices: 1600 John F. Kennedy Blvd., Suite 1800, Philadelphia, PA 191023-2899. Periodicals postage paid at New York, NY, and additional mailing offices. Subscription prices are $280.00 per year (US individuals), $498.00 per year (US institutions), $145.00 per year (US student/resident), $370.00 per year (Canadian individuals), $632.00 per year (Canadian institutions), $195.00 per year (Canadian student/resident), $390.00 per year (foreign individuals), $632.00 per year (foreign institutions), and $195.00 per year (foreign student/resident). Foreign air speed delivery is included in all *Clinics* subscription prices. All prices are subject to change without notice. POSTMASTER: Send address changes to *Clinics in Geriatric Medicine*, Elsevier Health Sciences Division, Subscription Customer Service, 3251 Riverport Lane, Maryland Heights, MO 63043. Telephone: 1-800-654-2452 (U.S. and Canada); 314-447-8871 (outside U.S. and Canada). Fax: 314-447-8029. E-mail: journalscustomerservice-usa@elsevier.com (for print support) or journalsonlinesupport-usa@elsevier.com (for online support).

Reprints. For copies of 100 or more, of articles in this publication, please contact the Commercial Reprints Department, Elsevier Inc., 360 Park Avenue South, New York, New York 10010-1710. Tel.: 212-633-3874; Fax: 212-633-3820, E-mail: reprints@elsevier.com.

Clinics in Geriatric Medicine is covered in *MEDLINE/PubMed (Index Medicus), EMBASE/Excerpta Medica, Current Contents/Clinical Medicine (CC/CM),* and the *Cumulative Index to Nursing & Allied Health Literature.*

Contributors

EDITOR

SOO BORSON, MD
Professor Emerita, Department of Psychiatry and Behavioral Sciences, University of Washington School of Medicine; Affiliate Professor, Department of Psychosocial and Community Health, University of Washington School of Nursing, Seattle, Washington

AUTHORS

PATRICIA A. AREAN, PhD
Professor, Department of Psychiatry, University of California, San Francisco, San Francisco, California

DAN G. BLAZER, MD, PhD
JP Gibbons Professor of Psychiatry and Behavioral Sciences, Duke University School of Medicine, Durham, North Carolina

DANIEL M. BLUMBERGER, MD, MSc
Clinician Scientist and Medical Head, Temerty Centre for Therapeutic Brain Intervention, Centre for Addiction and Mental Health; Assistant Professor, Department of Psychiatry, Faculty of Medicine, University of Toronto, Toronto, Ontario, Canada

ANNA BORISOVSKAYA, MD
Acting Assistant Professor, Mental Health Service, VA Puget Sound Healthcare System; Department of Psychiatry and Behavioral Sciences, University of Washington, Seattle, Washington

SOO BORSON, MD
Professor Emerita, Department of Psychiatry and Behavioral Sciences, University of Washington School of Medicine; Affiliate Professor, Department of Psychosocial and Community Health, University of Washington School of Nursing, Seattle, Washington

WHITNEY L. CARLSON, MD
Clinical Assistant Professor, Department of Psychiatry and Behavioral Services, University of Washington School of Medicine, Seattle, Washington

JOSHUA CHODOSH, MD, MSHS
Professor of Medicine, David Geffen School of Medicine at University of California, Los Angeles; Director, Veterans' Cognitive Assessment and Management Program (V-CAMP); Assistant Chief of Staff, VA Greater Los Angeles Healthcare System, Los Angeles, California

SHAUNE DEMERS, MD
Assistant Professor, Department of Psychiatry and Behavioral Sciences, University of Washington, Seattle, Washington

MARY GANGULI, MD, MPH
Professor of Psychiatry, Neurology, and Epidemiology, University of Pittsburgh School of Medicine, Western Psychiatric Institute and Clinic, Pittsburgh, Pennsylvania

JOSEPH E. GAUGLER, BA, MS, PhD
Associate Professor, McKnight Presidential Fellow, Center on Aging, School of Nursing, University of Minnesota, Minneapolis, Minnesota

NALAKA S. GOONERATNE, MD, MSc
Associate Professor, Division of Geriatric Medicine, Department of Medicine; Division of Sleep Medicine, Center for Sleep and Circadian Neurobiology, School of Medicine, University of Pennsylvania, Philadelphia, Pennsylvania

JULIE HUGO, MD
Assistant Professor of Psychiatry, University of Pittsburgh School of Medicine, Western Psychiatric Institute and Clinic, Pittsburgh, Pennsylvania

ZAHINOOR ISMAIL, MD
Clinical Associate Professor of Psychiatry and Neurology, University of Calgary and Hotchkiss Brain Institute, Calgary, Alberta, Canada

ALEXIS KUERBIS, LCSW, PhD
Clinical Director and Assistant Professor, Research Foundation for Mental Hygiene, Inc. and Columbia University Medical Center, New York, New York

ANDREA L. MAXWELL, MD
Acting Assistant Professor, Mental Health Service, VA Puget Sound Healthcare System; Department of Psychiatry and Behavioral Sciences, University of Washington, Seattle, Washington

SUSAN MEREL, MD
Assistant Professor, Division of General Internal Medicine, Department of Medicine, University of Washington, Seattle, Washington

ALISON A. MOORE, MD, MPH
Professor of Medicine and Psychiatry, Division of Geriatric Medicine, David Geffen School of Medicine at University of California, Los Angeles, Los Angeles, California

JENNIFER MOYE, PhD
VA Boston Health Care System; Department of Psychiatry, Harvard Medical School, Boston, Massachusetts

BENOIT H. MULSANT, MD, MS
Physician in Chief, Centre for Addiction and Mental Health; Professor and Vice-Chair, Department of Psychiatry, Faculty of Medicine, University of Toronto, Toronto, Ontario, Canada

GRACE NIU, PhD
National Institute of Mental Health Post Doctoral Fellow, Department of Psychiatry, University of California, San Francisco, San Francisco, California

THUAN D. ONG, MD, MPH
Assistant Professor, Division of Gerontology and Geriatric Medicine, Department of Medicine, University of Washington School of Medicine, Seattle, Washington

MARCELLA PASCUALY, MD
Associate Professor, Mental Health Service, VA Puget Sound Healthcare System;
Department of Psychiatry and Behavioral Sciences, University of Washington,
Seattle, Washington

TEDDIE POTTER, PhD, RN
Clinical Associate Professor, School of Nursing, University of Minnesota, Minneapolis,
Minnesota

LISIANE PRUINELLI, RN, MSN
School of Nursing, University of Minnesota, Minneapolis, Minnesota

KIRAN RABHERU, MD
Professor, Department of Psychiatry, University of Ottawa; Medical Director, Geriatric
Psychiatry and Electroconvulsive Therapy Program, The Ottawa Hospital, Ottawa,
Ontario, Canada

MARK J. RAPOPORT, MD
Staff Psychiatrist, Sunnybrook Health Sciences Centre; Associate Professor, Department
of Psychiatry, Faculty of Medicine, University of Toronto, Toronto, Ontario, Canada

SUSAN J. ROUSE, PMH-CNS-BC
VA Boston Health Care System, Boston, Massachusetts

PAUL SACCO, PhD, LCSW
Assistant Professor, University of Maryland School of Social Work, Baltimore, Maryland

MARK SNOWDEN, MD, MPH
Associate Professor, Department of Psychiatry and Behavioral Sciences, University of
Washington School of Medicine, Seattle, Washington

ELIZABETH VIG, MD, MPH
Staff Physician, Geriatrics and Extended Care, VA Puget Sound Health Care System,
University of Washington; Associate Professor, Division of Gerontology and Geriatric
Medicine, Department of Medicine, University of Washington, Seattle, Washington

MICHAEL V. VITIELLO, PhD
Department of Psychiatry and Behavioral Sciences, School of Medicine, University of
Washington, Seattle, Washington

LUCY Y. WANG, MD
Acting Assistant Professor, Mental Health Service, VA Puget Sound Healthcare System;
Department of Psychiatry and Behavioral Sciences, University of Washington, Seattle,
Washington

Contents

> Because neurodegenerative dementias are progressive and ultimately fatal, a palliative approach focusing on comfort, quality of life, and family support can have benefits for patients, families, and the health system. Elements of a palliative approach include discussion of prognosis and goals of care, completion of advance directives, and a thoughtful approach to common complications of advanced dementia. Physicians caring for patients with dementia should formulate a plan for end-of-life care in partnership with patients, families, and caregivers, and be prepared to manage common symptoms at the end of life in dementia, including pain and delirium.

> Family caregiving is nonroutine help that is provided to a relative in need. On average, family caregivers have provided assistance for about 5 years, and close to half help their relatives with 1 or more activities of daily living in the United States. Family caregivers' unmet needs and the negative health outcomes they may experience demand effective, sustained clinical engagement. Clinical interventions that are intensive, individualized, and delivered over time to parallel chronic disease trajectories seem most effective. Principles of clinical assessment, tenets of a partnership-based health care framework, and newly emerging resources are presented to help guide clinicians' efforts to partner with family caregivers.

Other Mental Health Problems in Older Adults

> The broadening use of antidepressants among older Americans has not been associated with a notable decrease in the burden of geriatric depression. This article, based on a selective review of the literature, explores several explanations for this paradox. The authors propose that the effectiveness of antidepressants depends in large part on the way they are used. Evidence supports that antidepressant pharmacotherapy leads to better outcomes when guided by a treatment algorithm as opposed to attempting to individualize treatment. Several published guidelines and pharmacotherapy algorithms developed for the treatment of geriatric depression are reviewed, and an updated algorithm proposed.

> An update is provided on the current information regarding late life depression with regard to assessment, clinical implications, and treatment recommendations. Several treatments are considered evidence-based, but when deployed into field trials, the efficacy of these treatments falls short.

It is thought that the lower impact in community trials is due in large part to patient, clinical, environmental, socio-economic, and cognitive correlates that influence treatment response. The aim is to assist providers in making decisions about what type of treatment to recommend based on a sound assessment of these clinical correlates.

Suicide is the deliberate act of causing death by self-directed injurious behavior with intent to die. Assisted dying, also known as assisted suicide, involves others to help hasten death. Physician-assisted dying specifically refers to the participation of a physician in facilitating one's death by providing a lethal means. Any decision to actively end a life has profound emotional and psychological effects on survivors. This article discusses the effects that older adults' deaths through suicide, assisted dying, and physician-assisted dying have on survivors and the implications for clinical practice.

Most older patients adapt after catastrophic medical diagnoses and treatments, but a significant number may develop posttraumatic stress disorder (PTSD) symptoms. PTSD symptoms create added burden for the individual, family, and health care system for the patient's recovery. Medical-related PTSD may be underdiagnosed by providers who may be unaware that these health problems can lead to PTSD symptoms. Treatment research is lacking, but pharmacologic and nonpharmacologic approaches to treatment may be extrapolated and adjusted from the literature focusing on younger adults. Additional study is needed.

Approximately 5% of older adults meet criteria for clinically significant insomnia disorders and 20% for sleep apnea syndromes. It is important to distinguish age-appropriate changes in sleep from clinically significant insomnia, with the latter having associated daytime impairments. Non-pharmacologic therapies, such as cognitive-behavioral therapy for insomnia, can be highly effective with sustained benefit. Pharmacologic therapies are also available, but may be associated with psychomotor effects. A high index of suspicion is crucial for effective diagnosis of sleep apnea because symptoms commonly noted in younger patients, such as obesity or loud snoring, may not be present in older patients.

Although the myth that older adults do not use mood-altering substances persists, evidence suggests that substance use among older adults has been underidentified for decades. The baby boom generation is unique in its exposure to, attitudes toward, and prevalence of substance use—causing projected rates of substance use to increase over the next twenty years. Given their unique biological vulnerabilities and life stage, older adults who misuse substances require special attention. Prevalence rates of substance use and misuse among older adults, methods of screening and assessment unique to older adults, and treatment options for older adults are reviewed.

Health care systems are evolving toward population-based approaches to managing disease, including mental and behavioral health problems. This article describes population-based care management for treatment of geriatric patients in primary care and the challenges of implementation. The article addresses the issues of program fidelity and real-world treatment of those who do not fit the model or do not respond as hoped. It also discusses the special obstacles facing efforts to apply population-based principles of mental health care in nursing homes, where regulatory requirements, more than evidence about effective treatment, drive what interventions are provided.

CLINICS IN GERIATRIC MEDICINE

Preface

Update in Geriatric Psychiatry

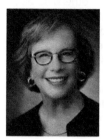

Soo Borson, MD
Editor

This issue of *Clinics in Geriatric Medicine* provides a comprehensive update for clinicians and health care decision-makers who are charged, as never before, with a mandate to collaborate in bringing evidence-based mental health care to older adults. These twelve articles together comprise a practice manual, a teaching text, and a springboard for health system reform in the care of patients with the most common—and among the most difficult—mental health problems in geriatrics. They provide state-of-the-science overviews of the prevalence, etiology, risk factors, diagnosis, assessment, and evidence-based care of patients with depression, traumatic medical experiences, substance abuse, sleep disorders, and dementia through all of its stages and complications.

The articles by Hugo and Ganguli ("Dementia and Cognitive Impairment: Epidemiology, Diagnosis, and Treatment"), Merel, DeMers, and Vig ("Palliative Care in Advanced Dementia"), Gooneratne and Vitiello ("Sleep in Older Adults: Normative Changes, Sleep Disorders, and Treatment Options"), and Kuerbis, Sacco, Blazer, and Moore ("Substance Abuse Among Older Adults") stand as individual reference manuals for clinicians dealing with these specific issues and for students and scholars seeking the most up-to-date evidence.

Depression is the primary focus of three articles in this set. Mulsant, Blumberger, Ismail, Rabheru, and Rapoport ("A Systematic Approach to Pharmacotherapy for Geriatric Major Depression") provide a clear, usable, and evidence-based synthesis of outcome studies of drug therapies for depression in older adults, show that the popular practice of choosing antidepressants based on patients' clinical features is not supported by data, and offer a stepped-care approach that is simple and safe for patients across the spectrum of illness and easily implemented by nonspecialist as well as psychiatric physicians. Arean and Niu ("Choosing Treatment for Depression in Older Adults and Evaluating Response") provide evidence that executive dysfunction, easily measured in any clinical setting, impedes response to antidepressant medication and show that problem-solving psychotherapy can overcome this source

Clin Geriatr Med 30 (2014) xiii–xv
http://dx.doi.org/10.1016/j.cger.2014.06.001
0749-0690/14/$ – see front matter © 2014 Published by Elsevier Inc.

of treatment resistance. Their thoughtful piece on nonpharmacologic treatment of late life depression summarizes evidence about efficacy of this and other psychotherapeuties and highlights social factors that interfere with access and response to conventional depression treatment. They show that the addition of social case management for individuals living in poverty can reverse what would otherwise be a failure of treatment. Carlson and Snowden ("Community Treatment of Older Adults: Principles and Evidence Supporting Mental Health Service Interventions") describe progress toward implementing population-based depression care in both clinical and nontraditional settings and illustrate how the same principles can be effective when applied to other psychiatric illnesses in older people.

Carlson and Ong ("Suicide in Later Life: Failed Treatment or Rational Choice?") face, head on, what happens when treatment fails—through missed opportunities in depression treatment or the futility inherent in incurable, severe medical illness. In addition to summarizing data on suicide in late life and the movement toward broader legal access to choice and physician assistance in dying for the terminally ill, the authors provide highly personal accounts of the emotional, existential, and moral impact on clinicians of their patients' decisions to die and call for open dialogue among physicians, care teams, and health care administrators to promote the healing process.

Dementia is the focus of four of the twelve articles in this series, five if we count Gaugler, Potter, and Pruinelli's article on partnering with caregivers (although their article deals with caregiving in the context of late-life disability more broadly), which provides a usable and complete resource for families and other caregivers. Our emphasis on dementia in this issue reflects the new diagnostic thinking and criteria embodied in DSM-5, the new federal priorities for better patient and family care established by the National Alzheimer's Plan of 2010, and the new opportunities for clinicians, patients, and families created by the Affordable Care Act. A new Medicare benefit, the Annual Wellness Visit, mandates detection of cognitive impairment in clinical settings, with a focus on primary care, and Centers for Medicare and Medicaid Services (CMS) has authorized incentive payments to physicians who adhere to a specific set of dementia care quality measures. Hugo and Ganguli ("Dementia and Cognitive Impairment: Epidemiology, Diagnosis, and Treatment") describe the new DSM-5 nomenclature and standards for diagnosis of dementia and mild cognitive impairment, summarize recent epidemiologic findings and clinical features of the recognized dementia subtypes, identify appropriate roles for specialists, and address initial therapeutic interventions. Wang, Borisovskaya, Maxwell, and Pascualy ("Common Psychiatric Problems in Cognitively Impaired Older Patients: Causes and Management") emphasize the multifactorial causation of behavioral and psychological symptoms of dementia, provide an up-to-date review of evidence regarding psychotropic drug therapies, and show how a thorough evaluation of the origin of symptoms can be used effectively to organize treatment. Managing the end of life in dementia, to comfort patients and families and avoid burdensome treatments and transitions, concludes the article by Merel and colleagues ("Palliative Care in Advanced Dementia") and follows their useful review of stage-specific goals and processes of care for clinicians and caregivers. Borson and Chodosh ("Developing Dementia Capable Health Care Systems: A 12-Step Program") offer a blueprint for overcoming our health systems' "addiction" to acute care for dementia, perhaps the quintessential chronic disease that influences outcomes of all the others, and achieving the high-quality health care for patients and families that are primary goals of the National Alzheimer's Plan. Each of the 12 steps toward dementia-capable health care systems is built on evidence of how health care currently fails patients and families, of what works in randomized trials of care management, and of what health care systems can do to maximize the value of their clinicians to the patients they serve. Partnership with care-givers, articulated here as a transformational model for health care by Gaugler and colleagues, is a theme that runs through all of the articles on dementia in this collection, but also sets a tone and a focus for doing better in everything we do to care for older people.

Soo Borson, MD
University of Washington School of Medicine
2375 South Toledo Avenue
Palm Springs, CA 92264, USA

E-mail address:
soob@uw.edu

Dementia and Cognitive Impairment

Developing Dementia-Capable Health Care Systems: A 12-Step Program

Soo Borson, MD[a,b,*], Joshua Chodosh, MD, MSHS[c]

KEYWORDS

- Dementia • Alzheimer disease • Primary care • Comprehensive management
- Care coordination • Partnership • Quality measurement • Annual wellness visit

KEY POINTS

- Increasing detection of dementia through routine cognitive assessment is the first step toward improving care at the population level.
- Key goals of population-based health care for dementia are to reduce excess morbidity, poor health outcomes, and preventable emergencies for both patients and their family caregivers.
- The main components of high-quality dementia care are known and can be implemented and measured in primary care settings.
- Delivering those components requires transforming the culture and processes of health care into a sustainable, dementia-capable structure.
- Dementia-capable health care systems are those that provide individualized, coordinated, and integrated medical and psychosocial care for patients and their care partners, delivered by cohesive teams of clinicians, staff, and health care administrators.
- Many steps toward dementia-capable systems can be implemented now, supported by new national policies favoring early detection, care planning, and coordination, support for caregivers, and measurement of care quality.

THE PROBLEM

Alzheimer disease (AD), the most common cause of dementia in later life, affects nearly 5 million people in the United States.[1] But for patients and families, finding clinicians prepared to navigate the diagnostic process, offer treatment, and provide

---

[a] Department of Psychiatry and Behavioral Sciences, University of Washington School of Medicine, Seattle, WA, USA; [b] Department of Psychosocial and Community Health, University of Washington School of Nursing, Seattle, WA, USA; [c] David Geffen School of Medicine at UCLA, Veterans' Cognitive Assessment and Management Program (V-CAMP), VA Greater Los Angeles Healthcare System, 11301 Wilshire Boulevard (11G), Los Angeles, CA 90073, USA
* Corresponding author. 2375 South Toledo Avenue, Palm Springs, CA 92264.
E-mail address: soob@uw.edu

Clin Geriatr Med 30 (2014) 395–420
http://dx.doi.org/10.1016/j.cger.2014.05.001
0749-0690/14/$ – see front matter © 2014 Elsevier Inc. All rights reserved.

geriatric.theclinics.com

knowledgeable and compassionate long-term management, remains a matter of luck. Physicians, other primary care providers (PCPs), and health care systems in the United States do not adhere to uniform expectations or evidence-based approaches to recognizing dementia, or to providing long-term health management and support for dementia patients and their caregivers. Compounding this problem are the limited access to dementia specialist consultations and the absence of quality monitoring to evaluate the care that patients receive, leaving little practical opportunity to achieve real-time improvement.

The mood in health care at the national level is one of energetic innovation, giving rise to a wealth of chronic disease management programs, a rapidly evolving science of implementation, and broad engagement of many stakeholders in improving chronic care. The health care and societal costs of dementia care are high (at least comparable with those of heart disease and cancer),[2] and many thoughtfully conducted clinical demonstrations and intervention trials have identified where gaps exist in health services and defined what works in dementia care. However, health care systems have been slow to translate the evidence into practice; barriers to change, such as entrenched attitudes and the costs inherent in innovation, are substantial. Our aim is to help bring solutions within reach by outlining steps to promote implementation of sustainable systems of dementia care. We term such health care systems "dementia-capable".

PCPs (who may be physicians, nurse practitioners, or physician assistants) play an essential role in implementation of dementia-capable health systems, but they vary broadly in knowledge, skill set, and system resources,[3] all of which affect their level of engagement in managing patients with dementia. It is useful to consider how professionals and health systems respond to heart failure, another similarly complex challenge in chronic disease care. Some PCPs diagnose heart failure themselves, obtain the necessary diagnostic tests, prescribe medical and lifestyle interventions, schedule regular follow-up, and make adjustments in the treatment plan as clinical changes warrant. Some PCPs may prefer that the patient be managed by a cardiologist from diagnosis onward. In the second scenario, the PCP mainly acts as a monitor: on observing a new symptom, the PCP encourages an earlier-than-planned visit to the cardiologist. If lack of PCP capability and heart failure prevalence overwhelm the supply of cardiologists within a health care system, an administrator can choose to hire more, and solve the problem of clinical capacity at the system level. Similarly, in dementia, some PCPs take on all aspects of diagnosis and management, whereas others would, if they could, refer even the most straightforward patients to a specialist (geriatrician, geriatric psychiatrist, or neurologist). However, the specialty-trained physician workforce is too small to care for the large and increasing numbers of patients with dementia, and it is decreasing (**Fig. 1**). Hiring more specialists to manage the need is not a viable health system response, nor is simply expecting PCPs to do more without structural changes in the delivery of care.

A recent modeling study[4] estimated that a typical PCP can manage between ~1300 and 2000 patients, varying with the level of task delegation that is built into the practice structure. If the age distribution of primary care patients reflects national demographics,[5] about 13% of a typical 2000-patient panel (260 patients) are older than 65 years. Of these patients, 5% to 10% (13–26 patients) have AD and perhaps 3 to 10 more have other dementias, but only half are recognized. However, the numbers of older adults with some cognitive disability are potentially larger, reflecting the wide spectrum of systemic and cerebral conditions that are associated with cognitive impairment. Moreover, the disproportionate use of health care by older patients means that a still larger percentage of clinical encounters involve individuals with cognitive impairment, but much of that impairment goes either unnoticed or

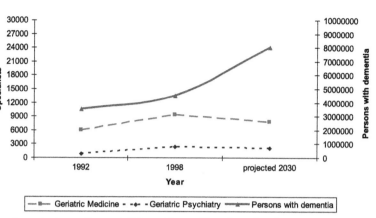

US Geriatric Specialist Workforce v. Persons with Alzheimer Dementia

Geriatric Medicine · ◆ · Geriatric Psychiatry ▲ Persons with dementia

Fig. 1. Inadequate dementia specialist workforce. (*Data from* Brookmeyer R, Gray S, Kawas C. Projections of Alzheimer's disease in the United States and the public health impact of delaying disease onset. Am J Public Health 1998;88(9):1337–42; and Geriatric specialists. Available at: http://www.eldercareworkforce.org/research/issue-briefs/research:geriatrics-workforce-shortage-a-looming-crisis-for-our-families/#_edn10. Accessed May 29, 2014. Copyright S.M. DeMers and S. Borson.)

unremarked,[6] never becoming a focus of clinical care. The combination of low frequency of frank dementia and low rates of provider recognition means that on-the-job experience by itself does not materially improve clinicians' ability to provide high-quality care for affected patients.

THE SOLUTION

In this article, we outline an incremental approach to health care redesign to achieve high-quality dementia management in health care systems. This approach includes what PCPs can accomplish now, the additional resources they require, how nonphysician staff can be used, retrained, or added to support PCP time and effort, and what clinical and institutional intelligence must be cultivated for sustainable improvements in care. Despite the shortage of providers with dementia expertise, smarter, dementia-capable health care systems can use their precious specialist resources more effectively by establishing coordinated systems that are supported by well-designed electronic health records (EHRs), tailored to assist in dementia care.[7] Our goal is to show how redesign can be achieved in 12 steps linked to focused strategies that address each of the major deficiencies in health care for dementia and to show the ways that patients and their caregivers benefit through prevention or resolution of dementia-driven health care complications. Steps 1 to 3 deal with preparation for improving dementia management by increasing recognition, diagnosis, and clinician engagement; steps 4 to 7 address the 4 distinct domains that comprise high-quality clinical care; and steps 8 to 12 address health system changes needed to support this care and measure its quality (**Box 1**).

Step 1: Think Differently About Dementia

Many clinicians think of dementia as an abstract disease state caused by specific disorders[8,9] and one that is mainly a problem for families and social workers. However,

---

Box 1
Twelve steps to dementia-capable health care systems

Increase recognition and engagement

   Step 1: think differently about dementia

   Step 2: focus on detection in primary care settings

   Step 3: engage care partners early

Organize comprehensive clinical care

   Step 4: treat the disease process

   Step 5: screen for and manage behavioral and psychological problems

   Step 6: account for dementia in all clinical decisions

   Step 7: make caregivers health care partners

Make necessary health system changes

   Step 8: specify quality goals and organize care to meet them

   Step 9: plan for complexity

   Step 10: formalize care coordination

   Step 11: make information accessible

   Step 12: make job satisfaction a priority

---

2 other crucial aspects of dementia emerge from the vantage point of patient care: (1) it creates hidden vulnerability and (2) it acts as an organizing principle. As a hidden vulnerability, dementia (brain failure) can be invisible to clinicians until it is relatively advanced or unmasked by acute illness or another condition such as depression[10] or adverse effects of medications.[11] As a condition that undermines autonomy, dementia becomes an organizing principle[12] in health care, changing the context, the participants, the methods, and the outcomes of clinical decision making. These important characteristics of dementia have had little or no influence on health care delivery systems.

Valid and reliable diagnostic standards exist for most causes of dementia (see the article by Hugo and Ganguli elsewhere in this issue), but physicians often do not diagnose it[13] or document it when they do,[14] and they find no clear pathways for organizing comprehensive patient care or support within their own clinical systems to encourage them to make, record, and use a diagnosis in planning care.[15] This situation leaves health systems without accurate data on the prevalence and care of patients with dementia in their populations and unable to plan rationally for improvements in care. It also leaves many patients and families uncertain about what help they can or should expect from clinicians. Personal communications from physicians echo these themes:

"I'm not sure why I should diagnose dementia; I don't really know what to do after that." "I might see something (cognitive impairment), but I wait until the family brings it up or asks for a referral." "I don't have enough time to deal with it." "The pills we have…well, I just don't see them working that well." "What if I told the patient he had Alzheimer's and it wasn't that?" "I'm afraid she'd get depressed if I told her she had Alzheimer's." "It's just too complicated – not like most of the other problems I see in my older patients." "It's hard – it's emotional for me too.

Physicians can learn to diagnose and manage dementia comfortably when supported by well-prepared clinical and administrative health care teams. Peer-to-peer physician education and federally supported workforce education can increase awareness and skills.[16,17]

Focused strategy

Provide a variety of educational approaches (e.g., newsletter bulletins, text messages, email announcements, and formal programs) to teach physicians and other health care professionals about dementia diagnosis and its effects on clinical care.

Step 2: Increase Recognition of Dementia in Primary Care Settings

The first goal of dementia detection is to find patients whose cognitive deficits have gone unnoticed in routine clinical encounters but are severe enough to interfere with patient self-care and medical management. Dementia experts and specialty organizations universally recommend identification of dementia when it is present[18] and agree that recognition can be substantially improved with simple assessments.[6,19,20] Several brief tools are effective, practical, and easily incorporated into routine clinical visits as well as the Medicare annual wellness visit, which requires objective cognitive assessment,[21,22] and some have been validated for administration by nonphysician staff[23,24] as a cognitive vital sign.[25]

Focused strategy

Train office staff to conduct short cognitive assessments such as the Mini-Cog. This can be performed when vital signs are checked and medications are reconciled. Incorporate cognitive assessments into EHR templates that populate encounter forms, triggered by preassigned patient age and other characteristics.

Step 3: Engage Family Members as Soon as Cognitive Impairment Is Suspected

A colleague tells this story: "A physician presents to the memory clinic with her spouse (also a physician). Notes from the referring provider document concerns about her memory. At her last visit, she told her PCP her memory was better, so he changed the diagnosis from possible dementia to mild cognitive impairment. At our first visit, she is so obviously impaired I attempt only a Mini-Cog, but she cannot register 3 words. I try a clock drawing test, drawing a circle to get her started. She draws several smaller circles in and around mine. I ask her husband what her doctors have previously told them; he says this is the first time he (or anyone else) has ever come with her to an appointment. There is no indication that the PCP ever tried to speak to a family member."
—Courtesy of J.R. McCarten, MD

Detecting cognitive impairment in primary care does not automatically improve dementia diagnosis, disclosure, and treatment planning. The recent systematic evidence review conducted for the US Preventive Services Task Force concluded (as did the first such review published in 2003)[26] that detection alone has not been shown to improve decision making.[19] A randomized trial of simple cognitive assessment by medical assistants in primary care[24] found a positive and specific impact on dementia-relevant physician actions, but in only about 20% of patients who screened positive. When cognitive impairment is suspected based on screening or other indicators, family members must be engaged to provide essential information about a patient's everyday cognition and function to help direct further evaluation. Family engagement also sets the stage for development of an ongoing partnership, which, for patients with dementia, becomes the foundation of their health care into the future.

Mrs Murley, age 79 years, was anticoagulated with warfarin for atrial fibrillation. Her attentive children were aware that she needed regular INR monitoring but were uncomfortable "butting in". When they reminded her about an upcoming appointment, she cheerfully responded, "I'll have your father take me tomorrow." When she died several months later of a cerebral hemorrhage with an INR 3.5 times the upper target limit, her dementia had not been formally diagnosed and no plan was in place to help her and her family safely manage and monitor her medication.

Focused strategy

Schedule a visit with the patient and a care partner when cognitive impairment is first suspected (or shown). Consider ordering a home visit if no care partner can be found. Insist on having a variable field added to the EHR that identifies and locates the patient's key care partners.

Step 4: Diagnose and Manage Dementia as a Disease Process

For most patients, primary care clinicians can, with appropriate guidance, work up, diagnose, and disclose the presence of dementia to patients and family members. The guidance they need includes which tests to consider and which diagnoses to exclude; signs and symptoms that distinguish AD from rarer dementias; the role of cognition-enhancing medications in management; what initial steps to take to address problems in behavior and mood; and how to talk about the problem with caregivers.[27] Dementias with features unfamiliar to most generalist clinicians, such as early age of onset, rapid progression, or association with neurologic signs, are more difficult to diagnose without specialized assistance.

A previously healthy 42-year-old man brought shame to his prominent family when he was prosecuted for sexual abuse of a teenaged niece and fired from his job. Depressed, he had to move back in with his parents. A general psychiatrist treated him with a selective serotonin reuptake inhibitor and counseling without improvement. Within a few months, he had become aggressive and delusional, and his psychiatric diagnosis was changed to schizophrenia. Shortly thereafter, he lost the ability to speak. Eighteen months after his first behavioral symptom, he was diagnosed with frontotemporal dementia. He died 3 years later, strangulated in his bedclothes. Autopsy confirmed the diagnosis.

Earlier recognition of the real nature of this patient's illness might have fostered easier acceptance by his family and community, fewer futile treatments, and a less traumatic death.

As part of characterizing dementia, staging is important in primary care because of its correlations with caregiver burden, mood and behavioral problems, need for supportive services or residential care, and long-term prognosis. Staging is based on the severity of cognitive and functional deficits caused by dementia and is most clearly defined for AD.[28] A clinical rule of thumb is that mild dementia impairs 1 or more independent activities of daily living, such as working, socializing, taking medications, managing money, and organizing activities and transportation. Loss of independence in 1 basic activity of daily living (e.g., bathing, dressing) signifies moderate stage, and dementia is severe when the patient can no longer function autonomously in any sphere of life (see the article by Merel and colleagues elsewhere in this issue for further discussion of how dementia stage influences clinical care). The most widely studied functional staging instruments are the Clinical Dementia Rating, which has not been adapted for rapid administration in nonspecialist settings, and the Global Deterioration Scale/Functional Assessment Staging (GDS/FAST) procedures.[28] The 7 GDS/FAST stages are based on readily observed changes in cognition and function, from stage 1 (no impairment) to stage 7 (advanced, preterminal dementia). Staging can help clinicians and families to plan ahead for increases in everyday support, structure, and supervision and the possibility that important neuropsychiatric problems may arise and require treatment. The GDS/FAST system was based on clinical observations of patients with AD but may still provide broad guidance in other dementia types, and clinical support staff can use it. The following vignette shows the relevance of staging:

Mr Traylor, 69 years old when first diagnosed with mild cognitive impairment (GDS stage 3), improved to near-normal (stage 2) after burr hole evacuation of bilateral nontraumatic subdural hematomas discovered during a workup for cognitive symptoms. A year later, he showed unmistakable signs of AD dementia and brightened with treatment with a cholinesterase inhibitor (stage 4). Five years after his first symptoms, his wife was now managing all aspects of his everyday well-being, activities, and health care (moderate dementia, GDS stage 5), and he was finally willing to attend an adult day program, providing her with important time for herself. At 8 years, he could not talk about recent key events in the family's life, had become severely agitated and overactive (GDS stage 6, moderately severe dementia) and could no longer be cared for at home, because of his wife's exhaustion. His agitation was partially eased by judicious use of low-dose antipsychotic medication and a move to a small dementia care home. Ten years after first symptoms, he could not speak, walk, or recognize his wife of nearly 60 years, and frequently resisted personal care (very severe dementia, stage 7). He fell, broke a hip, and was transferred to a hospital, where he seemed comfortable if unaware of his circumstances. His wife, who had been prepared for this eventuality by a series of previous conversations with his physician and was now supported by the hospital palliative care team, was able to resist pressures to authorize a futile surgical procedure. He was transferred back to his care home, where he died without signs of distress, surrounded by his family.

Focused strategy

Provide primary care clinicians with straightforward guidelines for evaluating cognitive impairment and dementia, and train support staff to use simple staging tools in diagnosed patients.

Step 5: Screen for and Manage Mood and Behavioral Problems

Changes in personality, mood, and behavior are inherent in the dementia syndrome, and, when severe, take precedence in health care until improved or resolved. (See the article by Wang and colleagues elsewhere in this issue for a detailed discussion of pathogenesis and management.) Practical guidance for generalists in assessment and management of mood and behavior problems is available on websites (e.g., actonalz.org and alz.org) and in documents[27] that are easy to access at the point of care. Because dementia impairs self-reporting and self-management, caregivers become clinicians' primary source of information about patient mood and behavior problems, and the primary recipients of interventions to help manage them. All but the most severe problems are likely to improve with nonpharmacologic interventions,[27] such as activity planning, pleasant events scheduling, support and stress reduction for caregivers, and changes in routines and environmental stimulation matched to the patient's needs. Although PCPs can and should understand the general principles and primary role of nonpharmacologic management, nonphysician clinicians (social workers and nurses who specialize in psychosocial assessment, intervention, and referral to community educational and support resources) can offer a more complete array of choices tailored to each family's needs.

Focused strategy

Train social workers or nurses already working in your health care system to help caregivers manage and monitor mood and behavior at home. The Alzheimer's Association is 1 source of such training.

Step 6: Account for Dementia in Clinical Decisions Regarding Evaluation and Treatment of Comorbid Conditions, Patient Safety, and Life Expectancy

Life expectancy
Survival after a diagnosis of AD is affected by many factors; key examples are shown in **Table 1**.

Comparable mortality data are difficult to find for dementias less prevalent than AD, but in dementia with Lewy bodies, prominent autonomic dysfunction is associated with lower survival.[31] Recognizing that dementia shortens life beyond expectations for common causes of death alone should help clinicians decide whether to recommend interventions with significant test or treatment burden, or long lag times to observed benefit.[32]

Focused strategy

Use scripted statements to help manage the mutual discomfort of clinicians, patients, and family members when planning for health care that is influenced by life expectancy. For example, "No one can know for sure how long people will live. My predictions may well be wrong, but best estimates would tell me that your husband's dementia is likely to shorten his life; 5 years would not be an unreasonable estimate. We should think about what medical care is likely to be helpful. Some treatments take much longer than 5 years before there is any benefit."

Table 1
Factors influencing survival after a diagnosis of AD

Source	Variable	Survival (Mean [y]) (Standard Deviation)
MoVIES Study[29]	Age	
	<75 y	8.3 (4.6)
	≥85 y	3.8 (1.9)
ADPR/ACT Study[30]	Stage (MMSE)	
	Mild[25–30]	7
	Moderate[18–24]	5
	Severe (≤17)	<4
	Clinical features	
	Rapid cognitive decline (>5 MMSE points in first year after diagnosis)	
	Gait impairment, falls, incontinence	
	Wandering, getting lost	
	Frontal release signs	
	Comorbidities	
	Ischemic heart disease, congestive heart failure, diabetes	

Abbreviations: ADPR/ACT, Alzheimer's Disease Patient Registry/Adult Changes in Thought; MMSE, Mini-Mental State Examination; MoVIES, Monongahela Valley Independent Elders Study; scored 0–30, with higher scores indicating better cognitive function.

Interactions of dementia with comorbid conditions

Brain dysfunction, comorbid conditions, and medical treatments may interact along unidirectional, bidirectional, or circular pathways. Although the principle applies to all chronic conditions, diabetes offers a clear example. Brain dysfunction is present in twice as many older diabetics as nondiabetics[33] and increases the risk of frequent hypoglycemic events.[34] Moreover, serious hypoglycemic events are associated with future dementia in nondemented individuals.[35,36] Because hypoglycemia imposes a potentially preventable risk for onset or worsening of cognitive impairment, liberalization of diabetes treatment targets should be considered, as recommended in a recent consensus report from the American Diabetes Association and American Geriatrics Society.[37] Similarly, for hypertension in patients older than 60 years, new management guidelines recommend treating to a target of less than 150 mm Hg systolic and less than 90 mm Hg diastolic (lower only if well tolerated),[38] based on updated evidence relating blood pressure to risk of and time to vascular events; overtreatment increases risk for hypotension and potentially deleterious effects on the brain. Hypotension may go unrecognized as a cause of falls and injuries, ischemic cardiac, cerebral, or renal events (weak spells, confusional episodes, ministrokes, and worsening of preexisting renal insufficiency). Impaired central regulation of blood pressure, inadvertent overuse or overprescribing of medications (cardiac, antihypertensive, anticoagulant, or antidiabetic drugs), a noncompliant vascular system, physiologic increases in insensible fluid loss, low fluid intake because of impaired perception or fear of incontinence, and intentional underuse of medication because of poor understanding or side effects unrecognized by the physician: all may contribute to potentially preventable bad outcomes of chronic disease management in demented patients.

> *Mr Newhouse was an 83-year-old man with vascular dementia, congestive heart failure (CHF), and gait apraxia, who was started on twice-daily furosemide as part of his CHF therapy. He saw his cardiologist 2 months later who noted, in addition to dyspnea and marginal oxygen saturations, lower extremity edema and an 11.3-kg (25-pound) weight gain. A medication review showed that Mr Newhouse was taking furosemide once in the morning, at most. "Once a day is good enough." It was only after further discussion and personal engagement with the patient's daughter that the provider learned that Mr Newhouse does not like taking the medication, especially at night, because it causes nocturia: he struggles to get out of bed and get to the bathroom (gait apraxia). Sometimes, he does not make it in time and ends up urinating on the floor. Once, he slipped and fell, injuring his knee. Neither the patient nor his caregiver understood that the medication was necessary to maintain comfortable breathing. The provider had to adjust his original assumption that the patient simply did not like taking medications and "knew better than the doctor" (which, in some ways, of course, he did). Learning the reasons for the patient's behavior changed the care plan: a bedside commode, mobility aids, and more suitable medication schedule were patient-centered adjustments that increased the likelihood of success in his CHF care.*

Focused strategy

Use checklists to monitor and update comorbid medical conditions, track treatments, and specify the added risks that they may pose in the presence of dementia. Spell out what caregivers need to do to manage the patient's health at home, and assess their understanding and ability to take on these tasks. You can start this as part of the health risk assessment in the annual wellness visit, which also calls for identifying all providers involved in the patient's care to promote collaboration and coordination. All of these elements can be incorporated into the EHR.

Everyday safety

Driving A recently updated American Academy of Neurology practice parameter[39] cited evidence that up to 75% of individuals with mild dementia can pass an on-road driving test, although some states mandate reporting of suspected unsafe driving or any dementia diagnosis. Tips for evaluating driving risk[39] are shown in **Box 2**.

Box 2
Factors associated with unsafe driving in dementia

More advanced dementia stage

History of citations or crashes

Family reports of unsafe driving

Self-reported driving restrictions

Impulsive or aggressive personality characteristics

Focused strategy

Ask about driving in any patient with cognitive impairment. Recommend behind-the-wheel testing and say, "I know that you have been an excellent driver but sometimes people with memory or other problems with thinking are not aware of limitations that put them at serious risk for a car accident. It would be good for you to know. I want you and your family to be safe."

Injuries Each year, more than half of individuals with AD sustain injuries requiring medical treatment[40] (about half because of falls), and in a series of 139 patients living alone,[41] 31 potentially preventable emergencies occurred over a follow-up period of 18 months. Among these emergencies were serious medical illness caused by failure to obtain treatment of a mild problem; a house fire caused by an unattended stove; injuries caused by forgetting to use mobility assistive devices; dehydration; infection; and hip fractures.

Medication problems

Misadherence Problems with knowledge, reporting, management, and mechanics of using medications are commonplace in individuals with cognitive impairment.[42–44]

Misprescribing The negative impact of anticholinergic medications in patients with dementia has been widely publicized, although discontinuing any but the most potent agents does not necessarily benefit patients. General guidance to help providers evaluate risks associated with specific drugs and drug classes in older adults is now widely disseminated.[45]

Unusual but serious medication side effects The common side effects of cholinesterase inhibitors used to treat AD and some other dementias are well known, but other potential hazards are not; analysis of more than 80,000 patients with a dementia diagnosis showed that patients receiving a cholinesterase inhibitor had nearly twice the rate of hospital visits for syncope as untreated individuals, more visits for bradycardia, and more permanent pacemaker placements and hip fractures.[46]

Mr Xavier was an 87-year-old with moderate AD who was started on a cholinesterase inhibitor for worsening memory impairment. He had periodic medical evaluations with his PCP since starting this medication. His physician had noted resting heart rates in the low 50s but no related symptoms. Three months later, after 2 falls and episodes of agitated behavior, Mr Xavier returned to the office, at which time his resting heart rate was 38. The cholinesterase inhibitor was stopped, and there were no subsequent falls or agitated behavior over the next 6 months. His resting heart rate increased to 58 off medication.

> **Focused strategy**
>
> Train social workers or nurses to talk with family caregivers about injury risk and safety strategies. Ask patients to tell you what medications they take, and show you how they use them; if they cannot do this accurately, involve the caregiver. Use Web resources (such as actonalz.org) to find suitable safety checklists. Request EHR tools that list potentially harmful medications and flag any that appear in your patient's medication profile. Be alert to unusual side effects.

Potentially avoidable acute care

Patients with dementia have higher (in some cases, 5-fold) rates of potentially preventable hospitalizations for both medical and psychiatric diagnoses than other older adults.[47–49] In a study that used epidemiologically sound ascertainment of incident cases,[48] stringent adjustment for multiple confounders, and a follow-up period of up to 8 years, rates of avoidable hospitalizations were still nearly 80% higher in dementia, yet reasons for admission, such as CHF and pneumonia, were similar to those for non-demented individuals. Some causes are more directly traceable to the effects of cognitive impairment,[47] including injuries linked to inattentiveness, poor motor control, or unnoticed environmental hazards, neurobehavioral problems and delirium, delayed recognition of an emerging acute medical problem, errors in medication management (too much or too little), and failures of homeostasis (e.g., dehydration). Similar effects are seen for emergency department visits.

Integrating awareness of dementia into medical care for comorbid diseases may reduce the need for acute care. In a recent study of patients hospitalized for CHF,[50] documentation of cognitive impairment by the clinician was associated with lower 6-month mortality and readmission rates. In another study of older adults,[51] a standard index of comorbidity computed from prescription records underestimated disease burden relative to a comprehensive clinical assessment; dementia (even when mild) exaggerated the discrepancy, suggesting that common chronic conditions may be undertreated in cognitively impaired patients.

> **Focused strategy**
>
> Teach providers in the clinic, emergency department, and hospital about interactions between dementia and general medical conditions. Use brief clinically relevant checklists, integrated into the EHR, to track potential problems and identify patients who need complex care management.

Step 7: Make Caregivers Your Clinical Partners. Assess Their Information, Health, and Care Needs

Things change so much with (my husband with dementia), and with me…and the kids, too. I want to know my doctor will try to understand what's going on and answer my questions, help me know how to deal with things and what to expect. It's not just about the Alzheimer's – it's his heart problems too, and he gets upset by things so easily. He takes so many medications. How can I know if they're the right ones? He sees 5 different doctors. I'm never sure they talk to each other. And even if my doctor doesn't always know all the answers, I need to know s/he will guide me to someone who can help. But just being there for us makes a big difference. I guess I want a doctor who will "have my back" – one I can count on to be there for us all the way through.

Caregivers as people, proxies, and partners

Patients and family members seeking explanations for a cognitive problem want to know about the process and results of the diagnostic evaluation but feel overwhelmed when information is provided as a "crash course" at the end of a diagnostic process.[52] For those fortunate to receive diagnostic and treatment information, many do not experience the process as patient-centered[53] or as leading toward clear definitions of the roles and responsibilities of family caregivers, clinicians, and other members of the care team, or to a cohesive plan of care. It is not surprising that a plan rarely follows a diagnosis, given that clinicians lack guidance on how best to manage dementia.

Focused strategy

Use talking points to increase provider comfort with difficult conversations and find ways to ask questions that create meaningful dialogue. Example: "Before we go over the results of our tests, it is helpful for me to hear your concerns and to know what you understand about all of this." Do this first to ground the subsequent discussion in awareness of the patient's and caregiver's present knowledge and fears. "From what I understand about what has been happening this past year and the tests we have done, your/your wife's thinking problems are likely due to a condition known as Alzheimer's disease. This must be difficult to hear right now... but there is much to be done that can be very helpful to both of you. We'll talk about that."

Patient centeredness: application to dementia caregiving networks Patient-centered care focuses on negotiating between medical priorities and patient/family preferences and choice, and balancing the burdens of illness and treatments through effective relationships and communication between providers and patients. Three helpful constructs have recently been articulated,[54] each imposing a distinctive demand on the physician: (1) to understand the relevant biopsychosocial context in which the clinical problem is occurring; (2) to actively cultivate a shared understanding of the problem and the patient's (and caregiver's) experience of it; and (3) to be willing to share responsibility (and power) for what and how care is provided. In dementia, patients communicate with variable clarity about their experience, understanding of their condition, and wishes for care (relatively well in the early stages, but less well as dementia progresses). Clinicians, then, need to rely more on their skills in observing and interpreting nonverbal communication, and on working with caregivers and helping them function effectively as reporters, advocates, and mediators of patient centeredness in care. Clinicians' readiness to share responsibility and power, without abrogating their professional responsibility to guide clinical care, is the foundation of collaboration: finding common ground, creating a therapeutic alliance, and accepting the affective and relational aspects of clinical care[55] as assets that facilitate, rather than impede, the achievement of therapeutic goals (**Box 3**).

Box 3
The main goals of dementia care

1. Intervening to improve patients' and families' ability to live with the day-to-day effects of dementia

2. Seeking to anticipate, prevent, or mitigate its medical and psychosocial complications

Patient centeredness is key to guiding effective clinical encounters, planning care, and creating an effective, enduring interactional structure for clinicians, patients, and families within a health care system.

Being a caregiver Effective communication in the interest of dementia care requires an understanding of the lived experience of caregiving. This experience, which includes becoming a caregiver (a person who provides for another what would normatively be done by the person for themselves) is a developmental process that is charted along a mostly slow, almost imperceptibly undulating path, punctuated by nodes (periods at which change comes rapidly or decisively, and reality seems altogether different). The point of formal medical diagnosis can be 1 such node, triggering a sense of a new reality, regardless of how much care might have been provided beforehand.[56] Caregivers who receive education and support soon after diagnosis experience substantial immediate benefits in self-confidence[57]; the Alzheimer's Association provides such assistance through its early stage groups for patients and caregivers. Clinicians who recognize the dynamic course of dementia and the parallel trajectory of the caregiving career find it easier to provide excellent care to patients and families.

Turning points in the lives of caregivers occur predictably with progression of dementia to the next stage of functional dependency but also after catastrophic medical or behavioral events or changes in the caregiver's own health. Most often, gradual, subtle shifts of autonomous functions from the patient to the caregiver produce only incremental increases in the burden of care, resulting in a lag between what other family members (and perceptive clinicians) see and what the primary caregiver is able to acknowledge. Caregiver burden and stress have become a permanent part of the Alzheimer caregiving lexicon and a primary or secondary measure of the efficacy of many types of interventions. The Alzheimer's Association[58] reported that 60% of dementia caregivers experience moderate to severe stress, and, in elderly spouses, high, unmitigated caregiving stress can be lethal.[59] However, research on predictors, correlates, and interventions to manage stress and burden in dementia caregivers shows the complexity of these phenomena.

Managing the problems of caregiving The perceived burden of caregiving is associated with specific exposures (e.g., to the patient's unexpected outbursts of anger), caregiver vulnerabilities (personal health problems, anger, and anxiety), and specific caregiver resources (coping style, outlook on life, and social supports).[60] A recent twin study found that both genetic factors and early environment influence the relationship between later caregiving and anxiety, depression, and stress.[61]

Several experimental interventions have been shown in randomized trials to help caregivers manage specific behavioral and functional problems in patients and reduce their own feelings of stress and depression,[62] but not all caregivers need the same kinds of help. In REACH II (Resources for Enhancing Alzheimer's Caregiver Health),[63] one of the few studies to examine variation in caregiver response to an intervention, only those with the highest depressive symptom scores improved; results were similar for self-rated stress. In general, the strongest overall evidence supporting the efficacy of caregiver interventions is for multicomponent approaches, which closely resemble the care provided in specialized, multidisciplinary dementia clinics or as part of collaborative care management paradigms. Key factors in their success are active engagement of patients (as appropriate), caregivers, and families; individual tailoring; and flexible long-term access to management support and assistance, which begins soon after diagnosis/disclosure and continues or resumes as needed.[64] Other interventions showing some efficacy combine information and individualized processing of problems in care, but peer support, referral to support groups, or self-help materials as the sole intervention are not effective.[64] (See the articles by Gaugler and colleagues, Merel and colleagues, and Wang and colleagues elsewhere in this issue for more discussion of caregiving.)

Focused strategy

Train social workers or nurses working within health care systems in dementia care management. The Alzheimer's Association and other organizations provide a variety of resources for such training. Provide opportunities to increase care management skills by participating in clinical case conferences with others from their discipline.

Caregivers as patients

Dementia caregivers are also, of course, patients with their own health concerns and needs. As patients, their health and health care utilization and costs are affected by caregiving stresses and burdens. A recent large study of caregivers enrolled in a Medicare Advantage plan found substantially higher odds of being treated for a wide range of symptoms and conditions (both medical and emotional) and greater use of outpatient, emergency, and home health care, relative to matched noncaregivers, resulting in an average of $867 higher per-patient cost over 36 months.[65]

The dementia caregiving network as the unit of health care

Most health care systems have no way to identify caregivers in either the patient's or the caregiver's EHR. However, the needs of patients and caregivers are widely acknowledged by dementia clinicians and researchers as intimately interlinked. A new instrument distills this principle into a simple tool to identify unmet needs. The Dementia Services Mini-Screen,[66] consisting of a single-item caregiver stress question and a short list of high-impact patient behavior problems, is a powerful predictor of medical and psychosocial needs for both patients and caregivers.

Focused strategy

Make the health and well-being of your patient's caregiver your priority. Spend time with the caregiver alone as part of the patient's visit to assess their level of stress and need for assistance. If you are not their PCP, request permission to share information with that provider. Refer to your health system social worker to provide additional support and assistance and follow up to be sure the connection is made.

Step 8. Set Specific Quality Goals for Care of Patients with Dementia, and Organize Clinical Information Gathering, Decision Making, and Care Tracking to Help Achieve Them

Understanding the interrelated components of health care for people with dementia, and knowing how to work with and help family members who care for patients at home, are skills that must become routine in clinical practice; they are an essential part of the culture of dementia-capable health care systems. The current physician-centric structure of most health care systems, the emphasis on episodic care delivered to 1 patient by 1 or a series of individual providers, and the sizable financial incentives favoring procedure-based over cognitive activities of providers[67] work poorly for chronic disease care in general and worse for dementia. In dementia, although we know what processes are needed, we have yet to structure our systems to provide them. Older[68] and newer[69] indicators of dementia care quality synthesize data on evidence-based care processes into a set of measures that can be tested with providers and used to assess the performance of health care systems. These measures can be easily incorporated into an organized, domain-based, dyadic approach to health care for patients with dementia (**Fig. 2**).

The previous sections provide the rationale for dividing dementia care into 4 core domains: dementia as a disease state; associated mood and behavioral problems; medical comorbidities and safety risks; and caregiver and family issues and concerns.

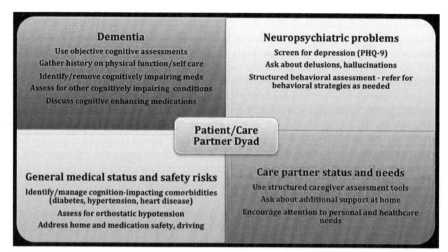

Fig. 2. Four-part model for dementia care assessment, tracking, and quality management. (*Data from* Lessig M, Farrell J, Madhavan E, et al. Cooperative dementia care clinics: a new model for managing cognitively impaired patients. J Am Geriatr Soc 2006;54:1937–42.)

Organizing clinical assessment around these 4 domains should start soon after the initial dementia diagnosis and disclosure, processes that set the stage for long-term partnership among patient, caregiver, and clinician. A domain-based assessment maintains a structured format and coherent framework for patient care, helps identify problems in caregiving and needs for caregiver education and assistance, and supports clinical improvement by tracking patient and caregiver responses to interventions. **Fig. 2** shows a simple assessment grid for primary care; the level of detail can be expanded for more specialized applications, and aggregated data from multiple providers can be used to identify system-level gaps and facilitate formation of more efficient team-based care.

Using the 4-part model is helpful in managing the complexity of dementia care. During the evaluation phase, a clinician can, if needed, conduct 4 visits: 1 for each of the 4 domains and each reimbursable by Medicare. Depending on findings, 1 or more of these domains of care may require active, focused follow-up, and the comprehensive assessment as a whole can be repeated as clinical change occurs. Documented assessment of each domain of care (and its associated processes and goals), at least once a year, can be used as a measure of health care quality in its own right. Repeated measurement is required by the predictably changing problems and needs of dementia dyads over time[69]; annual reassessment is not sufficient for clinical management of most patients, and frequency must be dictated by active problem domains at any given point in time. A useful rule of thumb is every 6 months for mild dementia and every 4 months thereafter, with the expectation that interval problems are actively tracked and managed using communication tools made available by health care systems as part of their dementia care packages.

Focused strategy

Teach clinicians to use a 4-part approach to assessment and care of dementia patients. Develop EHR templates to simplify the assessment and documentation process. Use the annual wellness visit to help anchor clinical care, and make families aware of this copay-free Medicare benefit. Negotiate visit frequency according to the activity of clinical problems and caregivers' need for support.

Step 9. Plan for Complexity (and Measure It)

Managing complex care calls for systematic, planned actions that simplify goals and promote a sense of coherence for both patient/caregiver networks and clinicians. Three complementary approaches are especially promising: taking patient-centered care seriously; making care coordinators members of the clinical team[70,71]; and developing quantitative methods to deal pragmatically with the joint effects of multimorbidity, demographic influences on health and health care, and features of health care organizations, to name a few of the sources of complexity. One new quantitative method, the Geriatric Complexity of Care Index (GXI),[72] groups patients with dissimilar clinical problems by indexing the expected intensity of primary care management. In an initial study,[72] the GXI was superior to conventional comorbidity measures in predicting ambulatory care visit numbers, exposure to polypharmacy, and total number of quality measures that would apply to each patient, but not other outcomes, and the conditions it measures are not all found in clinical or health systems data. However, the principles of measuring disease complexity are important for future development of guidelines for managing complexity in practice.[73,74]

Patient-centered care aims to extend care beyond disease management to incorporate its lived reality and the goals, values, and priorities of patients and families. Organizational innovations such as patient-centered medical homes can improve patient experience and reduce clinician burnout.[75,76] Medical home–like concepts specific for dementia care (specialty-led medical neighborhoods[77]) have been described in both geriatric[78] and geropsychiatric outpatient[79] settings. Models like these bring specialist expertise to the diagnostic, neurobehavioral, medical, and family caregiving complexity inherent in much of dementia care and show how to operationalize the concept of dementia as an organizing principle for health care. They do not answer the undersupply of dementia specialists or the difficulties of translating multidomain care models into sustainable programs in health systems. This strategy requires solutions at higher levels of health care organization than the clinician-dyad encounter.

Focused strategy

Test the value of quantitative tools to identify groups of patients with varying needs for specialized care and meet those needs through patient-centered, coordinated, and actively managed care plans.

Step 10. Negotiate Defined Roles and Responsibilities for All Partners in Care, and Integrate Them by Care Coordination

The role of the PCP

In response to the global undersupply of specialists to care for patients with dementia, a panel of dementia specialists and PCPs in the European Union proposed modest but specific roles for the PCP in a 2009 position paper.[80] The panel assigned responsibility to the PCP for case finding, diagnosis, and management of uncomplicated dementia, including identification and monitoring of dementia-associated risks (e.g., falls, neuropsychiatric symptoms, and poor nutrition). Additional responsibilities within the scope of primary care practice are to provide up-to-date preventive and therapeutic interventions and basic counseling and education for family caregivers, with the goal of crisis prevention.

Families' needs for information, support, and referral for community-based services eventually go beyond those basic elements; many caregivers have several different unmet needs that require engagement of a mix of medical and psychosocial care providers,[66] who may not communicate effectively or coordinate care without explicit connecting steps. The expertise required to assess dyadic needs, individualize psychosocial interventions, and monitor functional risks is most readily found in specially trained nonphysician providers. Randomized trials have reported successful care management by social workers,[81] advanced practice nurses,[82] and occupational therapists,[83] working flexibly as interventionists, dementia care managers, communication specialists, and early-warning systems for emerging problems.

If these models are successful in improving quality of care, why are they not more widely implemented? One reason is financial: none has focused on reducing high-cost care (e.g., preventable hospitalizations) as an outcome, and none has shown cost savings[84,85] or cost neutrality. Care coordination models are covered inconsistently or not at all by health insurance. Medicare explicitly excludes payment for a clinician's work with family members on behalf of a patient unless the patient is present, yet much of what caregivers need in terms of information, explanation, and skills to manage a demented patient's health care is best provided in separate caregiver visits.

The role of community-based organizations

Some of the roles piloted by social workers in dementia care management trials, especially caregiver education, support, and referral for community services, can be effectively delivered through direct partnership between providers in a health care system and community-based organizations (CBOs), such as the Alzheimer's Association. Partnership is more successful when they share a common computerized record.[84] These collaborations bring value, but integration of CBO interventions and clinical care is not automatically robust.[86,87] One Alzheimer's Association chapter has built, through intensive outreach to and between physicians, a growing network of providers and clinics who refer patients by word of mouth or via Direct Connect, a fax referral program from the physician's office or clinic to chapter staff. Sixty-one percent of Direct Connect referrals resulted in successful contact with patients and caregivers. Over 3 years, the Association increased the number of physician relationships from 113 to 498; **Fig. 3** shows results of this physician outreach effort created and led by staff at the Alzheimer's Association/Minnesota-North Dakota Chapter (with funding by the GHR Foundation).

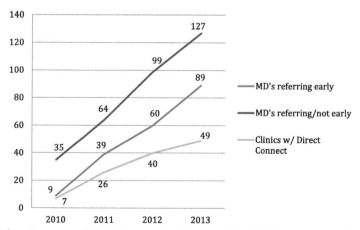

Fig. 3. Enhancing connectivity between physicians and the Alzheimer's Association. (*Courtesy of* Michelle Barclay, MA, Alyssa Aguirre, LCSW, and Maria Clarys, BA, Alzheimer's Association Minnesota/North Dakota Chapter.)

The dementia care manager within the health care system

The single most effective innovation to improve dementia care is the hiring and training of dedicated care managers who facilitate optimal use of community resources, coordinate care between CBOs and medical providers, and contribute management activities specific to their own discipline.[88] Models of dementia care with superior outcomes in randomized trials use either social workers or advanced practice nurses as care managers. Comparison of 6 randomized controlled trials using a structured case management evaluation tool[89] showed that higher intensity of care management and fuller integration of health and social care services (and in some instances, acute and long-term care settings) were common to the best-performing models.

Focused strategy

Recruit or retrain social workers or advanced practice nurses to provide dementia-specific care management and act as peer champions. This is an efficient way to rapidly increase dementia care capacity.

Step 11. Create Effective Communication Tools that Make Information Accessible to Providers, Family and Community Care Partners, and Care Managers

Health care systems face unprecedented challenges to supporting effective, sustained communication between providers and patients. How much time providers allocate (the length and focus of a visit, time spent talking vs doing) is increasingly defined and controlled by systems that use large provider panels, and by the payment arrangements they make with providers and insurers, although independent office practices struggle with the same issues. Short, single-problem visits, still driven by traditional views of the medical encounter as a 1-way transaction focused on bodily injuries and short-term ills, leave little room for complexity. Complexity (in age, functional status, comorbid disease, emotional and behavioral influences, and social-relational qualities that have much to do with chronic disease management) calls on clinicians to use excellent cognitive skills. These skills embody the ability and willingness to think through and integrate complex information into a coherent approach to the patient, preferably one that is contextual, social, and relational in addition to disease focused, to communicate clear and manageable goals and recommendations for care, and to acknowledge the potential burden of care and negotiate around it.

At the process level, dementia care exaggerates the divide between the improvements in organizational efficiency and factual accuracy expected from burgeoning communication and medical record technologies, and the homely virtues of learning about and attending to the patient's and family's needs, wants, and preferences over time, which are core tenets of high-quality care and care that is patient centered.[90] Nevertheless, high-quality communication is an indispensable feature of a dementia-capable health care system. Its content includes gathering accurate and meaningful information from patients and families; delivering health care information in understandable ways at the right time and to the right people; detecting communication barriers and correcting miscommunication; and having time to ensure sufficient opportunity and access to channels of communication. These elements build and strengthen relationships, and strong relationships between providers and dyads are the basis of effective long-term management. Responsibility for effective communication resides within the human interaction that occurs during the clinical encounter, but health care systems can facilitate or impede the process by the way they craft and deploy new communication tools.

Focused strategy
Use easy to understand patient/caregiver questionnaires, problem-based information sheets, and EHR-based patient portals for information transfer. Narrow the focus of the clinical visit to a specific dementia-related problem, and conclude with an action plan. Follow up on the plan. Make it easy to access the PCP's assistant by telephone, email, and fax. Consider individual patient information clearinghouses that exploit EHR capabilities to support multidirectional communication.

Step 12. Make PCP Job Satisfaction a Priority

Large health systems have many patients with dementia, but individual PCPs typically have few. Providers would understandably be reluctant to take on greater numbers, anticipating the higher intensity that can be associated with seeing and managing dementia differently, unless health systems embrace new tools to manage this intensity. Relatively simple changes at the level of the clinical encounter and the health care organization could speed improvements in care. At the encounter level, changes include: (1) focused previsit assessments delegated to other members of the primary care team (medical assistants, nurses); (2) brief assessment instruments that are relevant to the goals of care and patient/family needs and are easily accessible in the EHR; (3) communication protocols for managing between-visit questions and needs; (4) medical assistants as scribes (or more user-friendly EHR interfaces and templates) for medical record documentation during the office visit; and (5) brief EHR-accessible, problem-specific management "pearls" to reinforce on-the-spot education. Providers who are better informed find it easier to address dementia-related issues and can use their time more efficiently and effectively. Spending more time face to face with patients and families (and less time managing the administrative aspects of care) improves both physician and patient satisfaction and can even return joy to the physician's practice life.[91] This situation results in more meaningful relationships between patients, families, and physicians, greater professional satisfaction and sense of accomplishment, and more sustainable care.

At the organizational level, planning for dementia care improvement relies on acquiring better data about the scope and nature of the need. Using the annual wellness visit as a practice standard to estimate the prevalence of cognitive impairment and associated medical complexity, identify actual or potential caregivers in the lives of affected patients, and evaluate urgent needs for dementia-specific care[66] would streamline estimation of how many, and where, staff need to be prepared to deliver it.

SUMMARY

Development of dementia-capable health systems requires simpler, yet broader, clinical paradigms than those used by dementia specialists in their own practices, and whose work has provided most of what we know about caring for patients with dementia. Methods and models can be friendly to primary care clinicians and to systems concerned about improving patient experience and quality of care without incurring large excess costs. Much of the work to improve care focuses first on highly symptomatic patients and burdened caregivers; this care can be well managed by social work or nursing disciplines, in close, team-based coordination with PCPs. Such collaborative models have shown improved care quality and psychosocial outcomes.[81,88] Implementing proven models of care and improving general health outcomes and utilization profiles for patients and caregivers are the next thresholds.

Given the small numbers of patients with dementia seen by most PCPs, a dementia care management system that is shared among several PCPs is sensible and can be activated through enhanced communication systems for patient/caregiver dyads, physicians, and care managers that are supported by EHR packages. However, no care management system works without dementia-capable PCPs who manage patients' chronic diseases and who understand that the psychosocial care provided by care managers is integral to patients' health care. Nor does a care management system work without health systems that place high priority on relationships between providers and patient/caregiver dyads. With engaged PCPs and care managers, the clinical efforts of dementia specialists (in short supply) can then be selectively directed toward complicated diagnostic and management issues and to supporting and overseeing several dementia care management teams within the same primary care system.

The 12-step program we propose in this article is designed to support clinicians and health care systems in a phased process of becoming dementia capable. The steps are conceptually linked (each contributes a key component), but not all must be implemented at once. Some steps, such as timely recognition of cognitive impairment, can be quickly accomplished (and are already financially incentivized under Medicare) through implementation of the annual wellness visit within a practice or system. Others, such as modifications to the EHR to facilitate accurate dementia diagnosis, quality management, and communication, require more investment of time and resources. Care management training for a limited group of staff, social work, or nursing professionals requires an intermediate, but still small, level of organizational commitment.

Any proposal for health care redesign for a specific condition begs the question of how priorities are set. Is dementia care of high enough priority to justify the necessary investment? National initiatives argue 'yes': the National Alzheimer's Plan calls for substantive improvements in health care quality for patients with dementia and in support and assistance for family caregivers.[92] New dementia care quality measures[69] have been authorized for physician incentive payments under the Physician Quality Reporting System. Do all patients with dementia and all caregivers require the full scope or intensity of services possible within the structure shown in **Fig. 4**? Clearly not,[66] or not all at the same time, but when they need it, all deserve access to the best that health care can provide: multicomponent services, flexibly combined, that can be quickly engaged when needed and stand ready until they are.

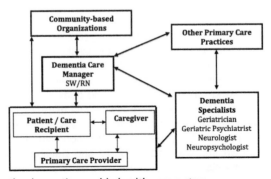

Fig. 4. Structuring the dementia-capable health care system.

ACKNOWLEDGMENTS

The term "dementia capable" was first developed for a 1990 study conducted by the US Office of Technology Assessment (US Congress, Office of Technology Assessment, *Confused Minds, Burdened Families: Finding Help for People with Alzheimer's and Other Dementias*, OTA-13A-403. Washington DC: US Government Printing Office, July 1990). Thanks to Katie Maslow for this citation, and to Drs Tatiana Sadak, J. Riley McCarten, Wayne Flicker, and David Netboy for helpful comments that improved the article.

REFERENCES

1. Hebert LE, Weuve J, Scherr PA, et al. Alzheimer disease in the United States (2010-2050) estimated using the 2010 census. Neurology 2013;80:1778–83.
2. Hurd MD, Martorell P, Delavande A, et al. Monetary costs of dementia in the United States. N Engl J Med 2013;368:1326–34.
3. Fortinsky RH, Zlateva I, Delaney C, et al. Primary care physicians' dementia care practices: evidence of geographic variation. Gerontologist 2010;50:179–91.
4. Altschuler J, Margolius D, Bodenheimer T, et al. Estimating a reasonable patient panel size for primary care physicians with team-based task delegation. Ann Fam Med 2012;10:396–400.
5. US Bureau of the Census: The Older Population: 2010. US Government 2011. https://www.census.gov/compendia/statab/2012/tables/12s0007.pdf. Accessed February 1, 2014.
6. Borson S, Scanlan JM, Watanabe J, et al. Improving identification of cognitive impairment in primary care. Int J Geriatr Psychiatry 2006;21:349–55.
7. Purvis S, Brenny-Fitzpatrick M. Innovative use of electronic health record reports by clinical nurse specialists. Clin Nurse Spec 2010;24:289–94.
8. Wilcock J, Iliffe S, Griffin M, et al. Tailored educational intervention for primary care to improve the management of dementia: the EVIDEM-ED cluster randomized controlled trial. Trials 2013;14:397–406.
9. Elsawy B, Higgins KE. The geriatric assessment. Am Fam Physician 2011;83: 48–56.
10. Pfennig A, Littmann E, Bauer M. Neurocognitive impairment and dementia in mood disorders. J Neuropsychiatry Clin Neurosci 2007;19:373–82.
11. Pugh MJ, Marcum ZA, Copeland LA, et al. The quality of quality measures: HEDIS(R) quality measures for medication management in the elderly and outcomes associated with new exposure. Drugs Aging 2013;30:645–54.
12. Lazaroff A, Morishita L, Schoephoerster G, et al. Using dementia as the organizing principle when caring for patients with dementia and comorbidities. Minn Med 2013;96:41–6.
13. van den Dungen P, van Marwijk HW, van der Horst HE, et al. The accuracy of family physicians' dementia diagnoses at different stages of dementia: a systematic review. Int J Geriatr Psychiatry 2012;27:342–54.
14. Chodosh J, Petitti DB, Elliott M, et al. Physician recognition of cognitive impairment: evaluating the need for improvement. J Am Geriatr Soc 2004;52:1051–9.
15. Harris DP, Chodosh J, Vassar SD, et al. Primary care providers' views of challenges and rewards of dementia care relative to other conditions. J Am Geriatr Soc 2009;57:2209–16.
16. Cameron MJ, Horst M, Lawhorne LW, et al. Evaluation of academic detailing for primary care physician dementia education. Am J Alzheimers Dis Other Demen 2010;25:333–9.

17. Health Resources and Services Administration (HRSA). Geriatrics and allied health: comprehensive geriatric education programs. Available at: http://bhpr. hrsa.gov/grants/geriatrics. Accessed November 9, 2009.
18. Ashford JW, Borson S, O'Hara R, et al. Should older adults be screened for dementia? Alzheimers Dement 2006;2:76–85.
19. Lin JS, O'Connor E, Rossom RC, et al. Screening for cognitive impairment in older adults: a systematic review for the US Preventive Services Task Force. Ann Intern Med 2013;159:601–12.
20. McCarten JR, Anderson P, Kuskowski MA, et al. Finding dementia in primary care: the results of a clinical demonstration project. J Am Geriatr Soc 2012;60:210–7.
21. Cordell CB, Borson S, Boustani M, et al, Medicare Detection of Cognitive Impairment Workgroup. Alzheimer's Association recommendations for operationalizing the detection of cognitive impairment during the Medicare Annual Wellness Visit in a primary care setting. Alzheimers Dement 2013;9:141–50.
22. Holsinger T, Plassman BL, Stechuchak KM, et al. Screening for cognitive impairment: comparing the performance of four instruments in primary care. J Am Geriatr Soc 2012;60:1027–36.
23. Scanlan J, Borson S. The Mini-Cog: receiver operating characteristics with expert and naive raters. Int J Geriatr Psychiatry 2001;16:216–22.
24. Borson S, Scanlan J, Hummel J, et al. Implementing routine cognitive screening of older adults in primary care: process and impact on physician behavior. J Gen Intern Med 2007;22:811–7.
25. Borson S, Scanlan J, Brush M, et al. The Mini-Cog: a cognitive 'vital signs' measure for dementia screening in multi-lingual elderly. Int J Geriatr Psychiatry 2000; 15:1021–7.
26. Boustani M, Peterson B, Hanson L, et al. Screening for dementia in primary care: a summary of the evidence for the US Preventive Services Task Force. Ann Intern Med 2003;138:927–37.
27. Group Health Cooperative. Dementia and cognitive impairment: diagnosis and treatment guideline. 2009. Available at: http://www.ghc.org/all-sites/guidelines/dementia.pdf. Accessed January 8, 2013, 2013.
28. Rikkert MG, Tona KD, Janssen L, et al. Validity, reliability, and feasibility of clinical staging scales in dementia: a systematic review. Am J Alzheimers Dis Other Demen 2011;26:357–65.
29. Ganguli M, Dodge HH, Shen C, et al. Alzheimer disease and mortality: a 15-year epidemiological study. Arch Neurol 2005;62:779–84.
30. Larson EB, Shadlen MF, Wang L, et al. Survival after initial diagnosis of Alzheimer disease. Ann Intern Med 2004;140:501–9.
31. Stubendorff K, Aarsland D, Minthon L, et al. The impact of autonomic dysfunction on survival in patients with dementia with Lewy bodies and Parkinson's disease with dementia. PLoS One 2012;7:e45451.
32. Lee SJ, Leipzig RM, Walter LC. Incorporating lag time to benefit into prevention decisions for older adults. JAMA 2013;310:2609–10.
33. Lu FP, Lin KP, Kuo HK. Diabetes and the risk of multi-system aging phenotypes: a systematic review and meta-analysis. PLoS One 2009;4:e4144.
34. Punthakee Z, Miller ME, Launer LJ, et al, ACCORD Group of Investigators, ACCORD-MIND Investigators. Poor cognitive function and risk of severe hypoglycemia in type 2 diabetes: post hoc epidemiologic analysis of the ACCORD trial. Diabetes Care 2012;35:787–93.
35. Whitmer RA, Karter AJ, Yaffe K, et al. Hypoglycemic episodes and risk of dementia in older patients with type 2 diabetes mellitus. JAMA 2009;301:1565–72.

36. Yaffe K, Falvey CM, Hamilton N, et al, Health ABC Study. Association between hypoglycemia and dementia in a biracial cohort of older adults with diabetes mellitus. JAMA Intern Med 2013;173:1300–6.

37. Sue Kirkman M, Briscoe VJ, Clark N, et al, Consensus Development Conference on Diabetes and Older Adults. Diabetes in older adults: a consensus report. J Am Geriatr Soc 2012;60:2342–56.

38. James PA, Oparil S, Carter BL, et al. 2014 evidence-based guideline for the management of high blood pressure in adults: report from the Panel Members Appointed to the Eighth Joint National Committee (JNC 8). JAMA 2013;311:507–20.

39. Iverson DJ, Gronseth GS, Reger MA, et al. Practice parameter update: evaluation and management of driving risk in dementia: report of the Quality Standards Subcommittee of the American Academy of Neurology. Neurology 2010;74:1316–24.

40. Oleske DM, Wilson RS, Bernard BA, et al. Epidemiology of injury in people with Alzheimer's disease. J Am Geriatr Soc 1995;43:741–6.

41. Tierney MC, Charles J, Naglie G, et al. Risk factors for harm in cognitively impaired seniors who live alone: a prospective study. J Am Geriatr Soc 2004;52:1435–41.

42. Lakey SL, Gray SL, Borson S. Assessment of older adults' knowledge of and preferences for medication management tools and support systems. Ann Pharmacother 2009;43:1011–9.

43. Sela-Katz P, Rabinowitz I, Shugaev I, et al. Basic knowledge of the medication regimen correlates with performance on cognitive function tests and diagnosis of dementia in elderly patients referred to a geriatric assessment unit. Gerontol 2010;56:491–5.

44. Allen SC, Jain M, Ragab S, et al. Acquisition and short-term retention of inhaler techniques require intact executive function in elderly subjects. Age Ageing 2003;32:299–302.

45. American Geriatrics Society Beers Criteria Update Expert Panel. Updated Beers Criteria for potentially inappropriate medication use in older adults. J Am Geriatr Soc 2012;60:616–31.

46. Gill SS, Anderson GM, Fischer HD, et al. Syncope and its consequences in patients with dementia receiving cholinesterase inhibitors: a population-based cohort study. Arch Intern Med 2009;169:867–73.

47. Bynum JP, Rabins PV, Weller W, et al. The relationship between a dementia diagnosis, chronic illness, Medicare expenditures, and hospital use. J Am Geriatr Soc 2004;52:187–94.

48. Phelan EA, Borson S, Grothaus L, et al. Association of incident dementia with hospitalizations. JAMA 2012;307:165–72.

49. Lin PJ, Fillit HM, Cohen JT, et al. Potentially avoidable hospitalizations among Medicare beneficiaries with Alzheimer's disease and related disorders. Alzheimers Dement 2013;9:30–8.

50. Dodson JA, Truong TT, Towle VR, et al. Cognitive impairment in older adults with heart failure: prevalence, documentation, and impact on outcomes. Am J Med 2013;126:120–6.

51. Borson S, Scanlan JM, Lessig M, et al. Comorbidity in aging and dementia: scales differ, and the difference matters. Am J Geriatr Psychiat 2010;18:999–1006.

52. Abley C, Manthorpe J, Bond J, et al. Patients' and carers' views on communication and information provision when undergoing assessments in memory services. J Health Serv Res Policy 2013;18:167–73.

53. Manthorpe J, Samsi K, Campbell S, et al. From forgetfulness to dementia: clinical and commissioning implications of diagnostic experiences. Br J Gen Pract 2013;63:e69–75.

54. Dubbin LA, Chang JS, Shim JK. Cultural health capital and the interactional dynamics of patient-centered care. Soc Sci Med 2013;93:113–20.

55. Epstein RM. Whole mind and shared mind in clinical decision-making. Patient Educ Couns 2013;90:200–6.

56. Ducharme F, Levesque L, Lachance L, et al. Challenges associated with transition to caregiver role following diagnostic disclosure of Alzheimer disease: a descriptive study. Int J Nurs Stud 2011;48:1109–19.

57. Ducharme FC, Levesque LL, Lachance LM, et al. "Learning to become a family caregiver" efficacy of an intervention program for caregivers following diagnosis of dementia in a relative. Gerontologist 2011;51:484–94.

58. Alzheimer's Association Facts and Figures 2013. Available at: http://www.alz.org/downloads/facts_figures_2013.pdf. Accessed February 9, 2014.

59. Schulz R, Beach SR. Caregiving as a risk factor for mortality: the Caregiver Health Effects Study. JAMA 1999;282:2215–9.

60. Vitaliano PP, Russo J, Young HM, et al. Predictors of burden in spouse caregivers of individuals with Alzheimer's disease. Psychol Aging 1991;6:392–402.

61. Vitaliano P, Strachan E, Dansie E, et al. Does caregiving cause psychological distress? The case for familial and genetic vulnerabilities in female twins. Ann Behav Med 2014;47(2):198–207.

62. Brodaty H, Arasaratnam C. Meta-analysis of nonpharmacological interventions for neuropsychiatric symptoms of dementia. Am J Psychiatry 2012;169:946–53.

63. Hatch DJ, Dehart WB, Norton MC. Subjective stressors moderate effectiveness of a multi-component, multi-site intervention on caregiver depression and burden. Int J Geriatr Psychiatry 2014;29(4):406–13. http://dx.doi.org/10.1002/gps.4019.

64. Parker D, Mills S, Abbey J. Effectiveness of interventions that assist caregivers to support people with dementia living in the community: a systematic review. Int J Evid Based Healthc 2008;6:137–72.

65. Suehs B, Shah S, Davis C, et al. Household members of persons with Alzheimer's disease: health conditions, healthcare resource utilization, and healthcare costs. J Am Geriatr Soc 2014;62(3):435–41.

66. Borson S, Scanlan JM, Sadak T, et al. Dementia services mini-screen: a simple method to identify patients and caregivers in need of enhanced dementia care services. Am J Geriatr Psychiatry 2013. http://dx.doi.org/10.1016/j.jagp.2013.11.001. pii:S1064–7481(13)00401-6.

67. Sinsky CA, Dugdale DC. Medicare payment for cognitive vs procedural care: minding the gap. JAMA Intern Med 2013;173:1733–7.

68. Feil DG, MacLean C, Sultzer D. Quality indicators for the care of dementia in vulnerable elders. J Am Geriatr Soc 2007;55(Suppl 2):S293–301.

69. Odenheimer G, Borson S, Sanders AE, et al. Quality improvement in neurology: dementia management quality measures. Neurology 2013;22(81):1545–9.

70. Smith SM, Soubhi H, Fortin M, et al. Managing patients with multimorbidity: systematic review of interventions in primary care and community settings. BMJ 2012;345:e5205.

71. American Geriatrics Society Expert Panel on the Care of Older Adults with Multimorbidity. Patient-centered care for older adults with multiple chronic conditions: a stepwise approach from the American Geriatrics Society. J Am Geriatr Soc 2012;60:1957–68.

72. Min L, Wenger N, Walling AM, et al. When comorbidity, aging, and complexity of primary care meet: development and validation of the Geriatric CompleXity of Care Index. J Am Geriatr Soc 2013;61:542–50.
73. Tinetti ME, Fried TR, Boyd CM. Designing health care for the most common chronic condition–multimorbidity. JAMA 2012;307:2493–4.
74. Fried TR, Tinetti ME, Iannone L. Primary care clinicians' experiences with treatment decision making for older persons with multiple conditions. Arch Intern Med 2011;171:75–80.
75. Liss DT, Fishman PA, Rutter CM, et al. Outcomes among chronically ill adults in a medical home prototype. Am J Manag Care 2013;19:e348–58.
76. Reid RJ, Coleman K, Johnson EA, et al. The Group Health medical home at year two: cost savings, higher patient satisfaction, and less burnout for providers. Health Aff (Millwood) 2010;29:835–43.
77. Fisher ES. Building a medical neighborhood for the medical home. N Engl J Med 2008;359:1202–5.
78. Boustani MA, Sachs GA, Alder CA, et al. Implementing innovative models of dementia care: the Healthy Aging Brain Center. Aging Ment Health 2011;15: 13–22.
79. Lessig M, Farrell J, Madhavan E, et al. Cooperative dementia care clinics: a new model for managing cognitively impaired patients. J Am Geriatr Soc 2006;54: 1937–42.
80. Villars H, Oustric S, Andrieu S, et al. The primary care physician and Alzheimer's disease: an international position paper. J Nutr Health Aging 2010;14:110–20.
81. Vickrey BG, Mittman BS, Connor KI, et al. The effect of a disease management intervention on quality and outcomes of dementia care: a randomized, controlled trial. Ann Intern Med 2006;145:713–26.
82. Callahan CM, Boustani MA, Unverzagt FW, et al. Effectiveness of collaborative care for older adults with Alzheimer disease in primary care: a randomized controlled trial. JAMA 2006;295:2148–57.
83. Gitlin LN, Winter L, Dennis MP, et al. A biobehavioral home-based intervention and the well-being of patients with dementia and their caregivers: the COPE randomized trial. JAMA 2010;304:983–91.
84. Judge KS, Bass DM, Snow AL, et al. Partners in dementia care: a care coordination intervention for individuals with dementia and their family caregivers. Gerontologist 2011;51:261–72.
85. Duru OK, Ettner SL, Vassar SD, et al. Cost evaluation of a coordinated care management intervention for dementia. Am J Manag Care 2009;15:521–8.
86. Reuben DB, Roth CP, Frank JC, et al. Assessing care of vulnerable elders–Alzheimer's disease: a pilot study of a practice redesign intervention to improve the quality of dementia care. J Am Geriatr Soc 2010;58:324–9.
87. Fortinsky RH, Kulldorff M, Kleppinger A, et al. Dementia care consultation for family caregivers: collaborative model linking an Alzheimer's association chapter with primary care physicians. Aging Ment Health 2009;13:162–70.
88. Chodosh J, Pearson ML, Connor KI, et al. A dementia care management intervention: which components improve quality? Am J Manag Care 2012;18: 85–94.
89. Somme D, Trouve H, Drame M, et al. Analysis of case management programs for patients with dementia: a systematic review. Alzheimers Dement 2012;8: 426–36.
90. Berwick DM. A user's manual for the IOM's 'Quality Chasm' report. Health Aff (Millwood) 2002;21:80–90.

91. Sinsky CA, Willard-Grace R, Schutzbank AM, et al. In search of joy in practice: a report of 23 high-functioning primary care practices. Ann Fam Med 2013;11: 272–8.
92. Alzheimer's Association Expert Advisory Workgroup on NAPA's scientific agenda for a national initiative on Alzheimer's disease. Alzheimers Dement 2012;8: 357–71.

Dementia and Cognitive Impairment
Epidemiology, Diagnosis, and Treatment

Julie Hugo, MD, Mary Ganguli, MD, MPH*

KEYWORDS

- Neurocognitive disorder • Mild cognitive impairment (MCI)
- Diagnostic and Statistical Manual of Mental Disorders, Fifth Edition (DSM-5)
- National Institute on Aging–Alzheimer's Association (NIA-AA) guidelines • Diagnosis
- Risk factors • Biomarkers • Alzheimer's disease

KEY POINTS

- Clinicians should be knowledgeable about the various neurocognitive disorders, which are common and severe in elderly adults.
- Diagnosis requires careful history taking and skilled clinical assessment, followed by appropriate laboratory investigations.
- Diagnostic imaging can be useful when interpreted by experts familiar with these conditions.
- Biomarkers for most of these disorders are still being validated and are not yet recommended for clinical use.
- Referral to specialists can be valuable for specific purposes, such as neuropsychologists for objective cognitive testing and interpretation; neurologists for diagnosis, particularly of the less common disorders; geriatric psychiatrists when there are psychological or behavioral challenges.
- Drug treatments at present provide symptomatic relief. Psychosocial and other supportive therapies are essential.

INTRODUCTION

When elderly patients and their families report symptoms of memory loss, experienced clinicians know that these concerns refer to a range of cognitive abilities or to general cognitive decline, and not just memory. However, some degree of cognitive slowing is typical of normal aging.

The clinician's first challenge is therefore to identify the cognitive changes that are clinically significant. Dementia is typically diagnosed when acquired cognitive

Department of Psychiatry, University of Pittsburgh School of Medicine, WPIC, 3811 O'Hara Street, Pittsburgh, PA 15213, USA
* Corresponding author.
E-mail address: gangulim@upmc.edu

Clin Geriatr Med 30 (2014) 421–442
http://dx.doi.org/10.1016/j.cger.2014.04.001
0749-0690/14/$ – see front matter © 2014 Elsevier Inc. All rights reserved.

geriatric.theclinics.com

impairment has become severe enough to compromise social and/or occupational functioning. Mild cognitive impairment (MCI) is a state intermediate between normal cognition and dementia, with essentially preserved functional abilities.

This article describes these entities and their diagnoses using the framework of the recently published fifth edition of the American Psychiatric Association's *Diagnostic and Statistical Manual, Fifth Edition* (DSM-5) (**Table 1**).[1] The DSM-5 diagnosis of major neurocognitive disorder, which corresponds with dementia, requires substantial impairment to be present in one or (usually) more cognitive domains. The impairment must be sufficient to interfere with independence in everyday activities. The diagnosis of mild neurocognitive disorder, corresponding with MCI, is made when there is modest impairment in one or more cognitive domains. The individual is still independent in everyday activities, albeit with greater effort. The impairment must represent a decline from a previously higher level and should be documented both by history and by objective assessment. Further, the cognitive deficits must not occur exclusively in the context of a delirium or be better explained by another mental disorder.

The clinician's second challenge is to determine the cause(s) of the cognitive impairment (ie, to identify the underlying cause). DSM-5 also provides diagnostic criteria for the most common causal subtypes of the neurocognitive disorders in all age groups. This article focuses on the neurocognitive disorders of elderly adults.

Table 1
Neurocognitive disorders as diagnosed in DSM-5

Diagnostic Criteria	Major Neurocognitive Disorder/ Dementia	Mild Neurocognitive Disorder/MCI
A	Significant cognitive decline in one or more cognitive domains, based on: 1. Concern about significant decline, expressed by individual or reliable informant, or observed by clinician 2. Substantial impairment, documented by objective cognitive assessment	Modest cognitive decline in one or more cognitive domains, based on: 1. Concern about mild decline, expressed by individual or reliable informant, or observed by clinician 2. Modest impairment, documented by objective cognitive assessment
B	Interference with independence in everyday activities	No interference with independence in everyday activities, although these activities may require more time and effort, accommodation, or compensatory strategies
C	Not exclusively during delirium	
D	Not better explained by another mental disorder	
E	Specify one or more causal subtypes, caused by: • Alzheimer's disease • Cerebrovascular disease (vascular neurocognitive disorder) • Frontotemporal lobar degeneration (frontotemporal neurocognitive disorder) • Dementia with Lewy bodies (neurocognitive disorder with Lewy bodies) • Parkinson's disease • Huntington disease • Traumatic brain injury • Human immunodeficiency virus infection • Prion disease • Another medical condition • Multiple causes	

Adapted from American Psychiatric Association. Diagnostic and statistical manual of mental disorders. 5th edition. Arlington (VA): American Psychiatric Association; 2013.

Impact of Dementia

Neurocognitive disorders, particularly major neurocognitive disorders (dementias), have severe consequences for individuals, their families, the health care system, and the economy. In the United States, Alzheimer's disease (AD) is a leading cause of death,[2] hospital admissions, skilled nursing facility admissions, and home health care. The costs of health services and the informal costs of unpaid caregiving for individuals with dementia are high and growing. Family caregivers also experience increased emotional stress, depression, and health problems.[3] In absolute numbers, 35.6 million people worldwide were estimated to be living with dementia in 2010, a number expected to reach 115.4 million people by 2050.[4]

Dementia in the Population

Prevalence, defined as the proportion of people with an illness in a given population at a given time, is an index of the burden of disease in the population. Incidence is the rate at which new disease occurs in a given population (ie, the proportion of new cases in that population over a given period of time). Incidence is therefore an index of the risk of disease in that population. Prevalence is a function of both incidence and duration. Because most dementias are not curable, their duration reflects how long individuals live with their dementia. Thus, the public health burden of dementia depends both on the development of new cases and on the survival of those cases after onset; holding incidence constant, groups with longer life expectancy have higher prevalence.

Prevalence

Prevalence of dementia increases exponentially with increasing age,[5] and doubles every 5 years after age 65 years. In high-income countries, prevalence is 5% to 10% in those aged 65 years and older, and is usually greater among women than among men, in large part because women live longer than men. Within the United States, higher prevalence has been reported in African American and Latino/Hispanic populations than in white non-Hispanic populations. Global systematic reviews and meta-analyses suggest that prevalence of dementia is lower in sub-Saharan Africa and higher in Latin America than in the rest of the world (**Table 2**). The prevalence of MCI is at present difficult to assess because it depends on the precise definitions and subtypes of MCI being studied.[15]

Life expectancy is increasing across the world, with population aging increasing the most rapidly in low-income and middle-income countries, where the prevalence of dementia is therefore expected to increase.[16] Emerging studies suggest that prevalence may be leveling off or even decreasing in high-income countries.[6,17]

Incidence

The incidence of dementia increases steadily until age 85 or 90 years, and then continues to increase but less rapidly. It is either similar in men and women or slightly higher in women. Annual age-specific rates ranged from 0.1% at age 60 to 64 years to 8.6% at age 95 years.[5,18]

Risk and Protective Factors

Risk factors are factors associated with an increased incidence rate of disease, higher odds of developing disease, or earlier onset of disease, depending on the type of statistical analysis that is performed. Protective factors represent the converse. An observed risk factor does not necessarily cause disease; a protective factor does not necessarily prevent disease and almost certainly does not treat the disease. The observed effects can potentially reflect selection or survival bias or confounding, or

Table 2
Prevalence of dementia: overall and subtypes

Investigators	Country	Study Type	Age (y)	Regions/Groups		Overall Dementia (%)	Alzheimer's Dementia (%)	Vascular Dementia (%)	Parkinson's Dementia (%)	Dementia with Lewy Bodies (%)	Frontotemporal Dementia
Prince et al,[4] 2013	Global	Meta-analysis + systematic review	≥60	Latin America		8.5	—	—	—	—	—
				Sub-Saharan Africa		5.0–7.0					
				Other world regions		2.0–4.0					
[a]Matthews et al,[6] 2013	United Kingdom	Population survey	65+	Cambridgeshire, Newcastle, and Nottingham		6.5	—	—	—	—	—
Gurland et al,[7] 1999	United States	Population survey	65+	Hispanic/Latino people	65–74	7.5	—	—	—	—	—
					75–84	27.9					
					85+	62.9					
				African Americans	65–74	9.1					
					75–84	19.9					
					85+	58.6					
				Non-Hispanic white people	65–74	2.9					
					75–84	10.9					
					85+	30.2					
[a]Hall et al,[8] 2009	United States	Population survey	70+	African Americans in Indianapolis		7.45	6.77	—	—	—	—

Study	Country	Type	Age	Sample						
Plassman et al,[9] 2007	United States	Population survey	71–79 80–89 90+	Nationally representative sample	4.97 24.19 37.36	2.32 18.1 29.7	0.98 4.09 6.19	— — —	— — —	— — —
[a]Graves et al,[10] 1996	United States	Population survey	65+	Japanese Americans	6.32	3.46	1.41	—	—	—
[a]CSHA Working Group,[11] 1994	Canada	Population survey	65+	Nationally representative sample	8	5.1	1.5	—	—	—
Aarsland et al,[12] 2005	Multinational	Systematic review	65+	—	—	—	—	0.15–0.5	—	—
Zaccai et al,[13] 2005	Multinational	Systematic review	65+	—	—	—	—	—	0–5	—
Rosso et al,[14] 2003	Netherlands	Population survey	50–59 60–69 70–79	—	—	—	—	—	—	Per 100,000 3.6 9.4 3.8

In all studies, prevalence percentage increases with age.

Abbreviation: CSHA, Canadian Study of Health and Aging.

[a] Age-specific prevalence is reported in the original articles but omitted from this table.

sometimes reverse causality. They may also depend on the timing and duration of exposure to the factor, with midlife often being the critical period.

Demographic Risk Factors

Increasing age is not only the strongest risk factor for dementia but also the only risk factor consistently identified after the eighth decade of life. Although prevalence is consistently higher among women, incidence is not; thus, the higher prevalence may largely be a function of longer life expectancy in women. Lower educational levels have been associated with higher prevalence. Within the United States, prevalence has been reported as increased in African American and Latino populations; some investigators have attributed these findings to lower education and higher cardiovascular morbidity in those populations.

Genetic Factors

Few dementias are caused by deterministic autosomal dominant genes; these are discussed later in the context of the specific disorders. Although several genes have been identified as increasing susceptibility for AD, the best-established is the apolipoprotein E (APOE) polymorphism on chromosome 19. The APOE*4 allele, associated with higher risks of hypercholesterolemia and heart disease, is also associated with dementia caused by AD, Parkinson's disease, dementia with Lewy bodies (DLB), vascular dementia, and frontotemporal dementia in men.[19–23] Individuals homozygous for APOE*4 are at greater risk of dementia than those who are heterozygous. The APOE*2 seems to have a protective effect. APOE*4 is a risk factor, not a diagnostic marker for AD. It is neither necessary nor sufficient for diagnosis, and its effect on risk seems to wear off by the eighth decade (ie, individuals who are older than 80 years, APOE*4 positive, and do not yet have dementia are at no greater risk of developing dementia than those who are APOE*4 negative).

Medical Risk Factors

Cardiovascular disease is increasingly recognized as not just a risk factor for vascular dementia but also for degenerative dementias, particularly AD. Heart disease has been associated with both dementia of the Alzheimer's type, and vascular dementia.[24] Risk factors in midlife, including hypertension, high cholesterol, high body mass index, and diabetes mellitus are associated with increased risk of dementia in late life, showing the importance of risk exposures decades earlier.[25,26] Heart failure and atrial fibrillation are risk factors for cognitive impairment and dementia.[27–29] Cardiac disease can cause or worsen cerebral hypoperfusion, creating a cellular energy crisis setting off a cascade of events leading to the production of toxic proteins.[30] In cognitively normal elderly adults, increased pulse pressure has recently been associated with alterations in biomarkers suggesting AD.[31]

Inflammation and alterations in inflammatory markers (interleukins, cytokines, C-reactive protein) have been reported in Alzheimer's and vascular dementias.[32,33] Multiple mechanisms have been proposed for the role played by inflammation in the neuropathology of AD.[34–36]

Obstructive sleep apnea, associated with hypertension, heart disease, stroke risk,[37] and white matter change,[38] is also associated with an increased risk of dementia.[39]

Stroke increases risk of dementia.[40,41]

Psychiatric Risk Factors

Depression has a complex and likely bidirectional association with dementia. Recurrent major depression in earlier adulthood seems to increase risk of dementia in later life.[42] Depression with late-life onset is thought to be an early sign of the vascular or degenerative disease causing the dementia.[43,44] Late-life anxiety is associated with cognitive impairment and decline.[45] Posttraumatic stress disorder has been reported as increasing risk of dementia.[46] Lifelong traits of harm avoidance and lesser sense of purpose have been reported as harbingers of AD.[47]

Head Injury

Head injury is associated with increased risk of dementia, in particular AD,[48] and the severity of injury seems to heighten this risk.[49,50] Neurocognitive disorders can occur immediately after a traumatic brain injury or after the recovery of consciousness at any age.[1] However, chronic traumatic encephalopathy (previously termed dementia pugilistica) is diagnosed years after repeated concussive or subconcussive blows to the head, with a clinical presentation similar to AD or frontotemporal lobar degeneration.[51]

Lifestyle and Environmental Risk Factors

Many environmental and occupational exposures have shown varying associations with neurodegenerative diseases.[52] Smoking has been associated with an increased risk of dementia[53]; although some studies have found an apparent protective effect, which could reflect survival bias (competing risks)[54] or possibly cholinergic action as also seen in Parkinson's disease.[55] Heavy consumption of alcohol increases odds of developing dementia.[56,57] Parkinson's disease risk is associated with exposure to pesticides, for which a molecular mechanism has been established.[58]

Protective Factors

Protective factors are those associated with a reduced incidence rate or reduced odds of dementia, or with delayed onset of dementia.

The concept of reserve was proposed to explain why some individuals remain cognitively intact despite the presence of neuropathology typically associated with dementia.[59] Brain reserve refers to structural capacity and integrity of the brain (eg, brain mass, preserved large neurons),[60] whereas cognitive reserve refers to its functional capacity, specifically the ability to use alternative neural networks and compensatory strategies.[61]

Education and Cognitive Activity

Where educational opportunities are universal, higher education may reflect innate reserve; the process of education may also promote the development of reserve through mechanisms such as increased dendritic branching. Education may also reflect general socioeconomic status and thus also represent quality of environmental factors like nutrition, or health care. Regardless of mechanism, higher education is associated with lower prevalence of dementia.[62]

Bilingualism has been associated with delayed onset of dementia,[63] independent of education, and may specifically protect against declines in attention and executive functioning.[64]

Cognitive activity
Lifelong occupations that do not require higher education or skilled vocational training seem to be associated with a higher risk of dementia.[65,66] Several popular leisure activities have been associated with lower risk of dementia.[67] Cognitively stimulating activities seem to have both protective and enhancing effects on cognition.[68]

Pharmacologic Factors

Several therapies for other conditions have been found in long-term observational studies to be associated with a reduced risk of dementia. However, in clinical trials, these drugs have not been found to prevent dementia. Timing and duration of the exposure might partly explain these discrepancies, because the protective effects were seen with prolonged use multiple years before dementia onset. Although some studies have found a protective relationship with the use of nonsteroidal antiinflammatory drugs,[69–71] a 2005 meta-analysis determined that many of the positive results seen in the 25 studies reviewed were caused by various forms of bias.[72] Despite mixed reports of the effects of the lipid-lowering HMG Co-A (3-hydroxy-3-methylglutaryl-coenzyme A) reductase inhibitors (statins), pooled results in a recent review as well as in a 2013 meta-analysis indicate a protective effect against dementia.[73,74]

As regards estrogen therapy, the WHIMS (Women's Health Initiative Memory Study) trial in elderly women showed no protection and possibly an increased risk from combination hormone therapy.[75,76] A 2013 meta-analysis of any use versus no use concluded that hormones had no effect on dementia.[77] However, a long-term observational study suggests that the timing of hormone therapy, at menopause, may be the critical factor.[78–80]

Lifestyle Factors

As with cardiovascular disease, population-based studies have found that mild to moderate alcohol consumption is associated with reduced risk of cognitive impairment and dementia.[56,57,81,82] Adherence to a Mediterranean diet was associated with better cognitive functioning, lower rates of cognitive decline, and a reduced risk of AD.[83] High physical activity levels are associated with reduced risk of neurodegenerative diseases.[84] Smoking shows a consistently protective effect against Parkinson's disease, potentially involving nicotine effects on cholinergic receptors.[55]

Elderly women with large social networks,[85] and who participate in mental, social, or productive activities, have shown lower incidence of dementia.[86] Social, mental, and physical lifestyle components seem important,[87] although reverse causality cannot be ruled out, given that the neuropathology often begins decades before symptom onset.

CLINICAL ASSESSMENT

Assessment is easier for the clinician when patients and/or their family members or other caregivers spontaneously express concern about cognitive difficulties. In other cases, neither patient nor caregiver report concerns but may acknowledge them if asked. Sometimes the patient denies any difficulty, and there is no reliable informant, but the clinician observes cognitive impairment, which is most likely when the clinician knows the patient well. Sometimes the clinician, or a member of the clinic staff, is tipped off by a patient forgetting to keep appointments or fill prescriptions, or being confused by simple instructions. Experienced clinicians also recognize vagueness and evasiveness in patients' responses, or catastrophizing of minor problems, as clues to failing cognition. The initial complaint may not be of cognitive loss but of changes in mood or behavior, such as apathy, anxiety, or depression.

Subjective Assessment

Whenever possible, history should be obtained both from the patient and from a family member, caregiver, or other reliable informant. In some mild cases, the patient is more aware of the deficits than the relative. The clinician should focus on changes in cognitive functioning as manifested in everyday activities. Early deficits are frequently noted in managing finances and medications. Overlearned, routine activities may be preserved but problems may be occurring in problem solving, multitasking, and dealing with new situations. **Table 3** lists the cognitive domains recognized by DSM-5 and everyday activities that involve those domains.[1]

Many patients and families accept cognitive decline as part of normal aging, and declare themselves normal on the grounds that they are no worse than others their age. Others may magnify the significance of minor changes and express fears of developing AD. Despite the value of systematic and disciplined clinical observations, clinicians' impressions can be influenced by personal expectations of what is normal for that patient. Subjective concerns alone are therefore insufficient for diagnosis.

Objective Assessment

The objective assessment requires the administration of one or more standardized tests. Neuropsychological assessment of specific cognitive domains is preferred both for detecting mild impairments and for differential diagnosis (**Table 4**). Details of such assessments are beyond the scope of this article but are readily available from other sources. If neuropsychological assessment is unavailable, objective testing can consist of a global screening scale, such as the well-known Mini-Mental State Examination (MMSE),[88] the Montreal Cognitive Assessment (MoCA),[89] or the Mini-Cog.[90] Such tests are usually sensitive enough to detect dementia but not necessarily MCI. It is critically important that a patient's test performance be interpreted in accordance with norms for that patient's age and educational level, and preferably for the relevant cultural/linguistic group and region as well.

Additional Assessments

A general physical and neurologic examination, and appropriate laboratory investigations, should be performed both to rule out treatable causes of cognitive impairment (even if they only partially explain the impairment) and to aid in differential diagnosis.

Table 3
Functional limitations associated with impairment in different cognitive domains

Cognitive Domain	Examples of Changes in Everyday Activities
Complex attention	Normal tasks take longer, especially when there are competing stimuli; easily distracted; tasks need to be simplified; difficulty holding information in mind to do mental calculations or dial a phone number
Executive functioning	Difficulty with multistage tasks, planning, organizing, multitasking, following directions, keeping up with shifting conversations
Learning and memory	Difficulty recalling recent events, repeating self, misplacing objects, losing track of actions already performed, increasing reliance on lists, reminders
Language	Word-finding difficulty, use of general phrases or wrong words, grammatical errors, difficulty with comprehension of others' language or written material
Perceptual-motor/ visuospatial function	Getting lost in familiar places, more use of notes and maps, difficulty using familiar tools and appliances
Social cognition	Disinhibition or apathy, loss of empathy, inappropriate behavior, loss of judgment

Adapted from American Psychiatric Association. Diagnostic and statistical manual of mental disorders. 5th edition. Arlington (VA): American Psychiatric Association; 2013.

Table 4
Examples of objective cognitive assessments, as noted in DSM-5

Cognitive Domains	Objective Assessment
Complex attention	Maintenance of attention: eg, press a button every time a tone is heard, over a period of time Selective attention: eg, hear numbers and letters, but count only the letters Divided attention: eg, tap rapidly while learning a story Processing speed: perform any timed task
Executive functioning	Planning: eg, maze puzzles, interpret sequential pictures or arrange objects in sequence Decision making with competing alternatives: eg, simulated gambling Working memory: hold information for a brief period and manipulate it, eg, repeat a list of numbers backward Use of feedback: use feedback on errors to infer rules to perform tasks. Inhibition: override habits; choose the correct but more complex and less obvious solution; eg, read printed names of colors rather than naming the color in which they are printed Cognitive flexibility: shift between sets, concepts, tasks, rules; eg, alternate between numbers and letters

Learning and memory	Immediate memory: repeat a list of words or digits
	Recent memory:
	  Free recall: recall as many items as possible from, eg, a list of words, or a story, or a diagram
	  Cued recall: with examiner providing cues; eg, recall as many food items as possible from the list
	  Recognition: with examiner asking, eg, whether there was there an apple on the list
	Semantic memory: recall well-known facts
	Autobiographical memory: recall personal events
	Implicit (procedural) memory: recall skills to perform procedures

Language	Expressive language: confrontation naming of, eg, objects or pictures; fluency for words in a given category (eg, animals) or beginning with a given letter, as many as possible in 1 min Grammar and syntax: omitting or incorrectly using articles, prepositions, helper verbs Receptive language: comprehend/define words, follow simple commands
Perceptuomotor functioning	Visuoconstructional: eg, draw, copy, assemble blocks Perceptuomotor: eg, insert blocks or pegs into appropriate slots Praxis: mime gestures such as saluting or actions such as using a hammer Gnosis: eg, recognize faces and colors
Social cognition	Recognize emotions: identify pictures showing, eg, happy, sad, scared, angry faces Theory of mind: consider another person's thoughts, intentions when looking at story cards; eg, why is the boy sad?

Adapted from American Psychiatric Association. Diagnostic and statistical manual of mental disorders. 5th edition. Arlington (VA): American Psychiatric Association; 2013.

This article presents the causal subtypes most likely to be seen in geriatric psychiatry settings.

Alzheimer's Disease (AD)

AD is the single most common neurodegenerative disease, characterized by progressive loss of synapses and neurons, the accumulation of amyloid plaques, neurofibrillary tangles, and prominent cholinergic deficits. It is typically diagnosed in the eighth or ninth decades of life, but early-onset forms of the disease may be diagnosed as early as the fifth decade. Average duration of survival is about 10 years after the onset of dementia, but varies widely depending on the age of onset, the severity of cognitive impairment, the presence of comorbid diseases, and other factors.[91,92]

In DSM-5,[1] AD is listed a causal subtype of both major and mild neurocognitive disorders. Criteria for this subtype harmonize with the latest expert guidelines for dementia and MCI caused by AD, as published by the National Institute on Aging/Alzheimer's Association (NIA-AA) Work Group.[93] Unlike the NIA-AA guidelines, the DSM-5 criteria are intended primarily for clinical rather than research use, and do not include preclinical AD. The diagnosis of dementia (major neurocognitive disorder) in AD requires evidence of decline to the level of substantial impairment in at least 2 cognitive domains, one of which must be memory. To diagnose MCI (mild neurocognitive disorder) in AD, decline to the level of modest impairment must be observed in memory and potentially in additional domains as well. The cognitive decline should be of insidious onset with gradual and steady progression. Impairments in memory and executive functions typically develop earlier in the disease course, whereas impairments in visuoconstructional/perceptual motor functions, language functions, and social cognition occur later. However, nonamnestic presentations also occur. Depression and apathy may occur throughout the clinical spectrum. In the middle to later stages, psychotic features, irritability, agitation, combativeness, and wandering may occur, and very late in the illness gait disturbances, dysphagia, incontinence, myoclonus, and seizures may be evident.[1]

For neurocognitive disorders to be attributed to "probable AD", there should either be evidence of autosomal dominant familial AD or no evidence of mixed cause (ie, no other contributing neurologic, psychiatric, or systemic disorder that could explain the cognitive decline). Otherwise, the diagnosis of "possible AD" is appropriate.[1]

Genetics of AD

Autosomal dominant mutations that cause rare cases of early-onset familial AD are the *amyloid precursor protein (APP)* gene on chromosome 21, the *presenilin 1 (PS1)* gene on chromosome 14, and the *presenilin 2 (PS2)* gene on chromosome 1. Individuals with Down syndrome, caused by trisomy 21, inevitably develop Alzheimer's neuropathology if they live long enough. The *APOE*4* gene, as noted earlier, increases risk of dementia but is not diagnostic.

Biomarkers for AD

Signs of cerebral amyloid deposition, such as positron emission tomography (PET) brain scans with amyloid tracers, and reduced levels of amyloid beta 42 in the cerebrospinal fluid (CSF), have been proposed as research biomarkers. Evidence of neuronal injury, such as hippocampal atrophy on magnetic resonance imaging (MRI) brain scan, temporoparietal hypometabolism on fluorodeoxyglucose PET scans, and increased total tau and phospho-tau levels in CSF, are less specific to AD but have also been proposed as research biomarkers.[1] They have not been officially validated or approved for clinical diagnostic use.

Unlike DSM-5, the NIA-AA guidelines also describe a stage of asymptomatic preclinical AD, in which the features of the disease are present as shown by biomarkers and subclinical cognitive decline detectable only by objective testing.[94]

Vascular Dementia (Vascular Neurocognitive Disorder)

In major and mild vascular neurocognitive disorders,[1] the cognitive deficits are principally attributed to cerebrovascular disease. Referred to variously as arteriosclerotic dementia, multi-infarct dementia, vascular cognitive impairment, and vascular cognitive disorder,[95] it is the second most common cause of dementia and is frequently present in combination with AD (mixed dementia). It can result from both large and small vessel disease, with the location of the lesions more important than the volume of destruction.[96] Given the variability of lesions and locations, the presenting symptoms and time course are often variable. The progression of the neurocognitive decline can be in an acute stepwise pattern, show a more gradual pattern, or can be fluctuating or rapid in its course.[1]

To diagnose vascular neurocognitive disorder, there should either be a clear history of stroke or transient ischemic attacks temporally related to the cognitive decline, or neurologic deficits consistent with sequelae of previous strokes. Cognitive decline is usually seen in the domains of complex attention and executive functions. Gait disturbance, urinary symptoms, and personality or mood changes (including emotional lability) are common.[1] The depression associated with vascular neurocognitive disorder may have a late-life presentation and be coupled with psychomotor slowing and executive dysfunction (the so-called vascular depression).[96]

Neuroimaging

Neuroimaging (computed tomography [CT] or MRI)-based evidence of significant parenchymal injury attributable to cerebrovascular disease can include one or more large vessel infarcts, a single large or strategically located infarct or hemorrhage, extensive lacunar infarcts outside the brainstem, or extensive white matter lesions.

Genetics

There are rare autosomal dominant cerebrovascular disorders, such as CADASIL (cerebral autosomal dominant arteriopathy with subcortical infarcts and leukoencephalopathy), which is a form of hereditary stroke caused by *NOTCH3* mutations on chromosome 19.

Frontotemporal Lobar Degeneration (Frontotemporal Dementia)

Frontotemporal dementia (FTD), the third most prevalent degenerative dementia, is characterized by prominent atrophy of the frontal and temporal lobes, with the predominant neuropathologic proteins containing inclusions of hyperphosphorylated tau or ubiquitin protein.

With mean onset in the sixth decade, FTD is a common cause of early-onset dementia, although 20% to 25% of individuals with this disorder are more than 65 years old.[1] The duration of survival is 6 to 11 years after symptom onset, and 3 to 4 years after diagnosis.[97] With insidious onset and gradual progression, the clinical subtypes (behavioral and language variants) of FTD correspond with specific areas of brain atrophy.

In the behavioral variant, changes in personality and behavior are most prominent, with loss of interest in personal affairs and responsibilities, social withdrawal, loss of awareness of personal hygiene, and socially disinhibited behavior.[98] Perseverative or compulsive motor behaviors, as well as hyperorality and dietary changes, may also be evident.[1] These patients are often initially seen in psychiatric settings and can be misdiagnosed as having major depressive or bipolar disorder. In addition to the behavioral variant, there are 3 language variants: (1) the semantic type, which involves a fluent aphasia with impoverished content and paraphasic errors, with intact syntax and prosody, and sometimes emotional blunting, loss of empathy, and rigid behaviors[98]; (2) progressive nonfluent aphasia; and (3) the logopenic subtype.

Genetics

In familial FTD, mutations have been associated with genes encoding proteins affecting several fundamental cellular functions, including *microtubule-associated protein tau (MAPT)*, granulin, *C9ORF72*, transactive response DNA-binding protein of 43 kDa, valosin-containing protein, chromatin-modifying protein 2B, and fused in sarcoma protein.

Neuroimaging

Structural MRI or CT can show distinct patterns of regional cortical atrophy that correlate with the clinical variants of FTD.

Dementia with Lewy Bodies (DLB)

DLB is the second most common neurodegenerative dementia. The underlying disease is primarily characterized by alpha-synuclein misfolding and aggregation within the pathognomonic Lewy bodies, which are also found in Parkinson's disease. Onset of symptoms is between the sixth and ninth decades, and average survival is 5 to 7 years.[1]

With insidious onset and gradual progression, the cognitive deficits are most prominent in the domains of attention, visuospatial functioning, and executive functioning. Additional core features include fluctuating cognition, recurrent visual hallucinations, and parkinsonism.[1] The key distinction between DLB and dementia of Parkinson's disease is based on the temporal sequence of the cognitive impairment and the movement disorder. In DLB, cognitive impairment precedes the onset of parkinsonism, whereas in Parkinson's disease the cognitive impairment occurs in the context of established Parkinson's disease.

Suggestive features of DLB include rapid eye movement (REM) sleep behavior disorder and severe neuroleptic sensitivity. Low dopamine transporter (DaT) uptake in basal ganglia shown by single-photon emission CT (SPECT) or PET imaging has been proposed as a suggestive feature. Supportive clinical features include repeated falls and syncope, transient and unexplained loss of consciousness, severe autonomic dysfunction, hallucinations in other modalities, systematized delusions, and depression.[98]

Neuroimaging

To help differentiate Lewy body–related dementias (DLB and dementia in Parkinson's disease) from other dementias, DaT PET scans may be useful. Generalized low uptake on SPECT and fluorodeoxyglucose PET with reduced occipital activity also suggests DLB. Additional testing supportive of DLB includes low-uptake metaiodobenzylguanidine (MIBG) myocardial scintigraphy, suggesting synaptic denervation, as well as prominent slow wave activity on electroencephalography with temporal lobe transient sharp waves.[99]

Neurocognitive Disorders Caused by Parkinson's Disease

These disorders are diagnosed when there is gradual cognitive decline in the presence of a well-established diagnosis of Parkinson's disease. Over the course of their disease, approximately 75% of individuals with Parkinson's disease develop a major neurocognitive disorder.[1] The pattern of cognitive deficits is variable but often affects the executive, memory, and visuospatial domains, with a slowing of information processing that suggests a subcortical picture. Associated features include psychiatric symptoms such as depressed or anxious mood, apathy, hallucinations, delusions, or personality change, as well as REM sleep behavior disorder and excessive daytime sleepiness.[1]

Neurocognitive Disorder Caused by Huntington Disease

Huntington disease is a neurodegenerative disease caused by an autosomal dominant mutation consisting of CAG repeats on chromosome 4. The neurotoxic huntingtin (HTT) protein begins by damaging the striatum of the basal ganglia but eventually affects the entire brain. Although adult-onset Huntington disease usually manifests in the fourth or fifth decades, patients have a median survival of 15 to 20 years after diagnosis, and can thus present to geriatric services. A few patients develop their first symptoms at older ages in the absence of a family history. Progressive cognitive impairment to eventual dementia is inevitable. Although cognitive deficits (executive function) and behavioral symptoms (depression, anxiety, apathy, obsessive-compulsive symptoms, and psychosis) often emerge before the motor abnormalities (bradykinesia and chorea), clinical diagnosis is rarely made from cognitive symptoms alone. A family history of the disease should alert clinicians to the possibility, and genetic testing for the *HTT* mutation is diagnostic.[1]

Neurocognitive Disorder Caused by Prion Disease

These are neurocognitive disorders caused by spongiform encephalopathies caused by transmissible misfolded protein particles called prions. The human prion disorders include kuru, sporadic Creutzfeldt-Jacob disease (CJD), familial CJD, iatrogenic CJD, Gerstmann-Sträussler-Scheinker disease, fatal insomnia, and new-variant CJD. Human transmission caused by infected growth hormone injection and corneal transplantation has been reported; cross-species transmission is exemplified by bovine spongiform encephalopathy (mad cow disease.) These illnesses progress rapidly and combine neurocognitive decline and motor features such as myoclonus and ataxia. Variant CJD may present with low mood, withdrawal, and anxiety. Individuals are typically diagnosed in their seventh and eighth decades, and the course is rapidly progressive, with survival typically less than 1 year.[99] Diagnosis can only be confirmed by biopsy or autopsy. However, MRI scanning with diffusion-weighted imaging or fluid-attenuated inversion recovery may show multifocal gray matter hyperintensities in the subcortical and cortical areas. Tau or 14-3-3 protein may be found in the cerebrospinal fluid; characteristic triphasic waves may be seen on the electroencephalogram. Genetic testing may be useful in the 15% of cases that have a family history suggesting an autosomal dominant mutation.[1]

TREATMENT
Cause-specific Treatment

If a neurocognitive disorder is diagnosed as wholly or partly caused by a treatable condition, treatment specific to that condition is the first line of defense. At this time, no disease-modifying therapies are available for any of the neurodegenerative diseases. However, symptomatic and supportive treatments are usually of value.

Symptomatic Treatment

Cholinesterase inhibitors increase cholinergic transmission at the synaptic cleft, potentially benefiting patients with cholinergic deficits as in AD. Three such drugs are currently available in the United States: donepezil, rivastigmine, and galantamine. For dementia caused by AD, a systematic review determined that all 3 drugs are comparable in efficacy and, on average, provide modest improvements in cognitive function and everyday activities and behavior in AD.[100] Although approved for use in severe dementia, many practitioners question its value in advanced disease. Evidence is mixed on the effects of these drugs on long-term outcomes, such as slowing of the rate of decline in everyday functions, and delay of institutionalization.[101]

Rivastigmine is also approved for dementia in Parkinson's disease. A large double-blind placebo-controlled trial of rivastigmine showed meaningful improvements in cognition and everyday functioning.[102,103]

Although there is expert consensus that cholinesterase inhibitors are more effective in DLB than in AD, for both cognitive and behavioral effects,[104] evidence from large controlled trials is lacking.

In vascular dementia, evidence is mixed for the cholinesterase inhibitors. They are often prescribed in vascular dementia because of the frequent co-occurrence of cerebrovascular and neurodegenerative disease.[105]

In frontotemporal dementia, there is no convincing evidence of benefits from these drugs, and there are reports that they worsen behavior symptoms.[106,107]

There is inadequate evidence on the use of cholinesterase inhibitors in other neurocognitive disorders.

In contrast, a systematic review has found minimal evidence of benefit from these drugs in MCI, either with symptom relief or delay in progression to dementia. Further, this weak evidence was overwhelmed by the risk of adverse effects, particularly gastrointestinal effects.[108]

NMDA Receptor Antagonist

One such agent, memantine, is approved for the treatment of moderate to severe dementia caused by AD. It is thought to be neuroprotective against excitotoxicity in the cortex and hippocampus. An advantage of memantine is that it is well tolerated.

A systematic review showed that memantine had a small beneficial effect on cognition at 6 months in moderate to severe AD, marginal effect on mild to moderate AD, and a small but clinically undetectable effect in mild to moderate vascular dementia.[109]

In frontotemporal dementia, memantine has shown mixed results.[107] There is preliminary evidence of benefits in DLB and dementia in Parkinson's disease; however, there have been reports of worsening delusions and hallucinations in DLB.

Serotonergic Agents

Selective serotonin reuptake inhibitor antidepressants can produce benefits for behavioral/psychiatric symptoms in frontotemporal dementia, without concomitant improvements in cognition.[110]

Dopamine Blocking Agents

Neuroleptic (antipsychotic) drugs should be prescribed in dementia with due attention to the risk of adverse cerebrovascular events.[111] They should be avoided or used with extreme caution in patients with DLB, given their sensitivity to these agents. When necessary the second-generation antipsychotics are preferred.[104] If the patient is taking a dopaminergic (antiparkinsonian) drug, lowering its dose would be the preferred first step before introducing a dopamine blocking agent.

Benzodiazepines

In general, benzodiazepines are to be avoided in the neurocognitive disorders because of the risk of paradoxic agitation as well as of falls and further diminished cognition. An exception may be the treatment of REM sleep behavior disorder in DLB.

Further discussion of the pharmacologic, psychosocial, and environmental management of neurocognitive disorders is provided elsewhere in this issue.

SUMMARY

Clinicians should be knowledgeable about the various neurocognitive disorders that are common and severe in elderly adults. Diagnosis requires careful history taking and skilled clinical assessment, followed by appropriate laboratory investigations. Diagnostic imaging can be useful when interpreted by experts familiar with these conditions. Biomarkers for most of these disorders are still being validated and are not yet recommended for clinical use. Referral to specialists can be valuable for specific purposes, such as neuropsychologists for objective cognitive testing and interpretation; neurologists for diagnosis, particularly of the less common disorders; and geriatric psychiatrists when there are psychological or behavioral challenges. Drug treatments at present provide symptomatic relief. Psychosocial and other supportive therapies are essential.

REFERENCES

1. American Psychiatric Association. Diagnostic and statistical manual of mental disorders. 5th edition. Arlington (VA): American Psychiatric Association; 2013.
2. Murphy SL, Xu J, Kochanek KD. Division of vital statistics. Deaths: final data for 2010. Natl Vital Stat Rep 2013;61(4):1. Available at: http://www.cdc.gov/nchs/data/nvsr/nvsr61/nvsr61_04.pdf. Accessed December 19, 2013.
3. Thies W, Bleiler L, Alzheimer's Association. 2013 Alzheimer's disease facts and figures. Alzheimers Dement 2013;9:208–45.
4. Prince M, Bryce R, Albanese E, et al. The global prevalence of dementia: a systematic review and metaanalysis. Alzheimers Dement 2013;9:63–75.
5. Jorm AF, Jolley D. The incidence of dementia: a meta-analysis. Neurology 1998; 51(3):728–33.
6. Matthews FE, Arthur A, Barnes LE, et al. A two-decade comparison of prevalence of dementia in individuals aged 65 years and older from three geographical areas of England: results of the cognitive function and ageing study I and II. Lancet 2013;382(9902):1405–12.
7. Gurland BJ, Wilder DE, Lantigua RF, et al. Rates of dementia in three ethnoracial groups. Int J Geriatr Psychiatry 1999;14(6):481–93.
8. Hall KS, Gao S, Baiyewu O, et al. Prevalence rates for dementia and Alzheimer's disease in African Americans: 1992 versus 2001. Alzheimers Dement 2009;5(3): 227–33.
9. Plassman BL, Langa KM, Fisher GG, et al. Prevalence of dementia in the United States: the aging, demographics and memory study. Neuroepidemiology 2007; 29:125–32.
10. Graves AB, Larson EB, Edland SD, et al. Prevalence of dementia and its subtypes in the Japanese American population of King County, Washington state. Am J Epidemiol 1996;144(8):760–71.
11. Canadian Study of Health and Aging Working Group. Canadian Study of Health and Aging: study methods and prevalence of dementia. Can Med Assoc J 1994; 150(6):899–913.

12. Aarsland D, Zaccai J, Brayne C. A symptomatic review of prevalence studies of dementia in Parkinson's disease. Mov Disord 2005;20(10):1255–63.
13. Zaccai J, McCracken C, Brayne C. A systematic review of prevalence and incidence studies of dementia with Lewy bodies. Age Ageing 2005;34(6): 561–6.
14. Rosso SM, Donker Kaat L, Baks T, et al. Frontotemporal dementia in The Netherlands: patient characteristics and prevalence estimates from a population-based study. Brain 2003;126:2016–22.
15. Ward A, Arrighi HM, Michels S, et al. Mild cognitive impairment: disparity of incidence and prevalence estimates. Alzheimers Dement 2012;8(1):14–21.
16. Prince M, Prina M, Guerchet M. World Alzheimer report 2013 journey of caring: an analysis of long term care for dementia. Alzheimer's Disease International. Available at: http://www.alz.co.uk/research/world-report-2013. Accessed December 17, 2013.
17. Rocca WA, Petersen RC, Knopman DS, et al. Trends in the incidence and prevalence of Alzheimer's disease, dementia, and cognitive impairment in the United States. Alzheimers Dement 2011;7(1):80–93.
18. Gao S, Hendrie HC, Hall KS, et al. The relationships between age, sex, and the incidence of dementia and Alzheimer disease: a meta-analysis. Arch Gen Psychiatry 1998;55(9):809–15.
19. Roses AD. Apolipoprotein E alleles as risk factors in Alzheimer's disease. Annu Rev Med 1996;47:387–400.
20. Tsuang D, Leverenz JB, Lopez OL, et al. APO ε4 increases risk for dementia in pure synucleinopathies. JAMA Neurol 2013;70(2):223–8.
21. Chuang Y, Hayden KM, Norton MC, et al. Association between APOE ε4 allele and vascular dementia: the Cache County study. Dement Geriatr Cogn Disord 2010;29:248–53.
22. Yin YW, Li JC, Wang JZ, et al. Association between apolipoprotein E gene polymorphism and the risk of vascular dementia: a meta-analysis. Neurosci Lett 2012;514(1):6–11.
23. Srinivasan R, Davidson Y, Gibbons L, et al. The apolipoprotein E ε4 allele selectively increases the risk of frontotemporal lobar degeneration in males. J Neurol Neurosurg Psychiatry 2006;77(2):154–8.
24. Justin BN, Turek M, Hakim AM. Heart disease as a risk factor for dementia. Clin Epidemiol 2013;5:135–45.
25. Kivipelto M, Ngandu T, Fratiglioni L, et al. Obesity and vascular risk factors at midlife and the risk of dementia and Alzheimer disease. Arch Neurol 2005; 62(10):1556–60.
26. Schnaider Beeri M, Goldbourt U, Silverman JM, et al. Diabetes mellitus in midlife and the risk of dementia three decades later. Neurology 2004;63(10):1902–7.
27. Tilvis RS, Kähönen-Väre MH, Jolkkonen J, et al. Predictors of cognitive decline and mortality of aged people over a 10-year period. J Gerontol A Biol Sci Med Sci 2004;59(3):268–74.
28. Qui C, Winblad B, Marengoni A, et al. Heart failure and risk of dementia and Alzheimer disease: a population-based cohort study. Arch Intern Med 2006;166(9): 1003–8.
29. Santangeli P, Di Biase L, Bai R, et al. Atrial fibrillation and the risk of incident dementia: a meta-analysis. Heart Rhythm 2012;9(11):1761–8.
30. de la Torre JC. Cardiovascular risk factors promote brain hypoperfusion leading to cognitive decline and dementia. Cardiovasc Psychiatry Neurol 2012;2012: 367516. http://dx.doi.org/10.1155/2012/367516.

31. Nation DA, Edland SD, Bond MW, et al. Pulse pressure is associated with Alzheimer biomarkers in cognitively normal older adults. Neurology 2013;81(23): 2024–7.

32. Schmidt R, Schmidt H, Curb JD, et al. Early inflammation and dementia: a 25-year follow-up of the Honolulu-Asia Aging Study. Ann Neurol 2002;52(2): 168–74.

33. Ravaglia G, Forti P, Maioli F, et al. Blood inflammatory markers and risk of dementia: the Conselice Study Of Brain Aging. Neurobiol Aging 2007;28(12): 1810–20.

34. Akiyama H, Barger S, Barnum S, et al. Inflammation and Alzheimer's disease. Neurobiol Aging 2000;21(3):383–421.

35. Schott JM, Revesz T. Inflammation in Alzheimer's disease: insights from immunotherapy. Brain 2013;136(9):2654–6.

36. Tuppo EE, Arias HR. The role of inflammation in Alzheimer's disease. Int J Biochem Cell Biol 2005;37(2):289–305.

37. Budhiraja R, Budhiraja P, Quan SF. Sleep-disordered breathing and cardiovascular disorders. Respir Care 2010;55(10):1322–32.

38. Kim H, Yun CH, Thomas RJ, et al. Obstructive sleep apnea as a risk factor for cerebral white matter change in a middle-aged and older general population. Sleep 2013;36(5):709–15.

39. Chang WP, Liu ME, Chang WC, et al. Sleep apnea and the risk of dementia: a population-based 5-year follow-up study in Taiwan. PLoS One 2013;8(10): e78655. http://dx.doi.org/10.1371/journal.pone.0078655.

40. van Kooten F, Koudstaal PJ. Epidemiology of post-stroke dementia. Haemostasis 1998;28(3–4):124–33.

41. Pendlebury ST, Rothwell PM. Prevalence, incidence, and factors associated with pre-stroke and post-stroke dementia: a systematic review and meta-analysis. Lancet Neurol 2009;8:1006–18.

42. Dotson VM, Beydoun MA, Zonderman AB. Recurrent depressive symptoms and the incidence of dementia and mild cognitive impairment. Neurology 2010; 75(1):27–34.

43. Panza F, Frisardi V, Capurso C, et al. Late-life depression, mild cognitive impairment, and dementia: possible continuum? Am J Geriatr Psychiatry 2010;18(2): 98–116.

44. Butters MA, Young JB, Lopez O, et al. Pathways linking late-life depression to persistent cognitive impairment and dementia. Dialogues Clin Neurosci 2008; 10(3):345–57.

45. Beaudreau SA, O'Hara R. Late-life anxiety and cognitive impairment: a review. Am J Geriatr Psychiatry 2008;16(10):790–803.

46. Yaffe K, Vittinghoff E, Lindquist K, et al. Posttraumatic stress disorder and risk of dementia among US veterans. Arch Gen Psychiatry 2010;67(6):608–13.

47. Wilson RS, Boyle PA, Buchman AS, et al. Harm avoidance and risk of Alzheimer's disease. Psychosom Med 2011;73(8):690–6.

48. Fleminger S, Oliver DL, Lovestone S, et al. Head injury as a risk factor for Alzheimer's disease: the evidence 10 years on; a partial replication. J Neurol Neurosurg Psychiatry 2003;74(7):857–62.

49. Guo Z, Cupples LA, Kurz A, et al. Head injury and the risk of AD in the MIRAGE study. Neurology 2000;54:1316–23.

50. Plassman BL, Havlik RJ, Steffens DC, et al. Documented head injury in early adulthood and risk of Alzheimer's disease and other dementias. Neurology 2000;55:1158–66.

51. Gavett BE, Stern RA, Cantu RD, et al. Mild traumatic brain injury: a risk factor for neurodegeneration. Alzheimers Res Ther 2010;2(3):18–21.
52. Brown RC, Lockwood AH, Sonawane BR. Neurodegenerative diseases: an overview of environmental risk factors. Environ Health Perspect 2005;113(9): 1250–6.
53. Anstey KJ, von Sanden C, Salim A, et al. Smoking as a risk factor for dementia and cognitive decline: a meta-analysis of prospective studies. Am J Epidemiol 2007;166(4):367–78.
54. Chang CC, Zhao Y, Lee CW, et al. Smoking, death, and Alzheimer disease: a case of competing risks. Alzheimer Dis Assoc Disord 2012;26(4):300–6.
55. Quik M, Perez XA, Bordia T. Nicotine as a potential neuroprotective agent for Parkinson's disease. Mov Disord 2012;27(8):947–57.
56. Anttila T, Helkala EL, Viitanen M, et al. Alcohol drinking in middle age and subsequent risk of mild cognitive impairment and dementia in old age: a prospective population based study. BMJ 2004;329(7465):539.
57. Mukamal KJ, Kuller LH, Fitzpatrick AL, et al. Prospective study of alcohol consumption and risk of dementia in older adults. JAMA 2003;289(11):1405–13.
58. Franco R, Li S, Rodriguez-Rocha H, et al. Molecular mechanisms of pesticide-induced neurotoxicity: relevance to Parkinson's disease. Chem Biol Interact 2010;188(2):289–300.
59. Fratiglioni L, Wang HX. Brain reserve hypothesis in dementia. J Alzheimers Dis 2007;12(1):11–22.
60. Katzman R, Terry R, DeTeresa R, et al. Clinical, pathological, and neurochemical changes in dementia: a subgroup with preserved mental status and numerous neocortical plaques. Ann Neurol 1988;23(2):138–44.
61. Stern Y. What is cognitive reserve? Theory and research application of the reserve concept. J Int Neuropsychol Soc 2002;8(3):448–60.
62. Meng X, D'Arcy C. Education and dementia in the context of the cognitive reserve hypothesis: a systematic review with meta-analyses and qualitative analyses. PLoS One 2012;7(6):e38268. http://dx.doi.org/10.1371/journal.pone. 0038268.
63. Alladi S, Bak T, Duggirala V, et al. Bilingualism delays age at onset of dementia, independent of education and immigrations status. Neurology 2013;81(2): 1938–44.
64. Craik FI, Bialystok E, Freedman M. Delaying the onset of Alzheimer disease: bilingualism as a form a cognitive reserve. Neurology 2010;75(19):1726–9.
65. Bonaiuto S, Rocca WA, Lippi A, et al. Education and occupation as risk factors for dementia: a population-based case control study. Neuroepidemiology 1995; 14(3):101–9.
66. Bickel H, Kurz A. Education, occupation, and dementia: the Bavarian School Sisters Study. Dement Geriatr Cogn Disord 2009;27(6):548–56.
67. Verghese J, Lipton RB, Katz MJ, et al. Leisure activities and the risk of dementia in the elderly. N Engl J Med 2003;348(25):2508–16.
68. Hughes TF. Promotion of cognitive health through activity in the aging population. Aging Health 2010;6(1):111–21.
69. Yip AG, Green RC, Huyck M, et al, MIRAGE Study Group. Nonsteroidal anti-inflammatory drug use and Alzheimer's disease risk: the MIRAGE study. BMC Geriatr 2005;5:2.
70. Szekely CA, Breitner JC, Fitzpatrick AL, et al. NSAID use and dementia risk in the Cardiovascular Health Study: role of APOE and NSAID type. Neurology 2008;70(1):17–24.

71. in 't Veld BA, Launer LJ, Hoes AW, et al. NSAIDs and incident Alzheimer's disease. The Rotterdam Study. Neurobiol Aging 1998;19(6):607–11.
72. de Craen AJ, Gussekloo J, Vrijsen B, et al. Meta-analysis of nonsteroidal anti-inflammatory drug use and risk of dementia. Am J Epidemiol 2005;161(2): 114–20.
73. Swiger KJ, Manalac RJ, Blumenthal RS, et al. Statins and cognition: a systematic review and meta-analysis of short- and long-term cognitive effects. Mayo Clin Proc 2013;88(11):1213–21.
74. Wong WB, Lin VW, Boudreau D, et al. Statins in the prevention of dementia and Alzheimer's disease: a meta-analysis of observational studies and an assessment of confounding. Pharmacoepidemiol Drug Saf 2013;22(4):345–58.
75. Shumaker SA, Legault C, Rapp SR, et al. Estrogen plus progestin and the incidence of dementia and mild cognitive impairment in postmenopausal women: the Women's Health Initiative Memory Study: a randomized controlled trial. JAMA 2003;289(20):2651–62.
76. Shumaker SA, Legault C, Kuller L, et al. Conjugated equine estrogens and incidence of probable dementia and mild cognitive impairment in postmenopausal women: Women's Health Initiative Memory Study. JAMA 2004;291(24): 2947–58.
77. O'Brien J, Jackson JW, Grodstein F, et al. Postmenopausal hormone therapy is not associated with risk of all-cause dementia and Alzheimer's disease. Epidemiol Rev 2014;36:83–103. http://dx.doi.org/10.1093/epirev/mxt008.
78. Shao H, Breitner JC, Whitmer RA, et al. Hormone therapy and Alzheimer disease dementia: new findings from the Cache County Study. Neurology 2012;79(18): 1846–52.
79. Whitmer RA, Quesenberry CP, Zhou J, et al. Timing of hormone therapy and dementia: the critical window theory revisited. Ann Neurol 2011;69(1):163–9.
80. Zandi PP, Carlson MC, Plassman BL, et al. Hormone replacement therapy and incidence of Alzheimer disease in older women: the Cache County Study. JAMA 2002;288(17):2123–9.
81. Ruitenberg A, van Swieten JC, Witteman JC, et al. Alcohol consumption and risk of dementia: the Rotterdam Study. Lancet 2002;359(9303):281–6.
82. Ganguli M, Vander Bilt J, Saxton JA, et al. Alcohol consumption and cognitive function in late life: a longitudinal community study. Neurology 2005;65(8): 1210–7.
83. Lourida I, Soni M, Thompson-Coon J, et al. Mediterranean diet, cognitive function, and dementia: a systematic review. Epidemiology 2013;24(4):479–89.
84. Hamer M, Chida Y. Physical activity and risk of neurodegenerative disease: a systematic review of prospective evidence. Psychol Med 2009;39(1):3–11.
85. Crooks VC, Lubben J, Petitti DB, et al. Social network, cognitive function, and dementia incidence among elderly women. Am J Public Health 2008;98(7): 1221–7.
86. Wang HX, Karp A, Winblad B, et al. Late-life engagement in social and leisure activities is associated with a decreased risk of dementia: a longitudinal study from The Kungsholmen Project. Am J Epidemiol 2002;155(12):1081–7.
87. Fratiglioni L, Paillard-Bog S, Winblad B. An active and socially integrated lifestyle in late life might protect against dementia. Lancet Neurol 2004;3(6): 343–53.
88. Folstein MF, Folstein SE, McHugh PR. "Mini-mental state." A practical method for grading the cognitive state of patients for the clinician. J Psychiatr Res 1975; 12(3):189–98.

89. Nasreddine ZS, Phillips NA, Bédirian V. The Montreal Cognitive Assessment, MoCA: a brief screening tool for mild cognitive impairment. J Am Geriatr Soc 2005;53(4):695–9.

90. Borson S, Scanlan J, Brush M, et al. The mini-cog: a cognitive 'vital signs' measure for dementia screening in multi-lingual elderly. Int J Geriatr Psychiatry 2000; 15(11):1021–7.

91. Brookmeyer R, Corrada MM, Curriero FC, et al. Survival following a diagnosis of Alzheimer disease. Arch Neurol 2002;59(11):1764–7.

92. Helzner EP, Scarmeas N, Cosentino S, et al. Survival in Alzheimer disease: a multiethnic, population-based study of incident cases. Neurology 2008;71(19): 1489–95.

93. McKhann GM, Knopman DS, Chertkow H, et al. The diagnosis of dementia due to Alzheimer's disease: recommendations from the National Institute on Aging–Alzheimer's Association workgroups on diagnostic guidelines for Alzheimer's disease. Alzheimers Dement 2011;7(3):263–9.

94. Sperling RA, Aisen PS, Beckett LA, et al. Toward defining the preclinical stages of Alzheimer's disease: recommendations from the National Institute on Aging–Alzheimer's Association workgroups on diagnostic guidelines for Alzheimer's disease. Alzheimers Dement 2011;7(3):280–92.

95. Jellinger KA. Morphological diagnosis of "vascular dementia"–a critical update. J Neurol Sci 2008;270(1–2):1–12.

96. Sneed JR, Culang-Reinlieb ME. The vascular depression hypothesis: an update. Am J Geriatr Psychiatry 2011;19(2):99–103.

97. Rabinovici GD, Miller BL. Frontotemporal lobar degeneration: epidemiology, pathophysiology, diagnosis and management. CNS Drugs 2010;24(5): 375–98.

98. McKeith IG, Dickson DW, Lowe J, et al. Diagnosis and management of dementia with Lewy bodies: third report of the DLB consortium. Neurology 2005;65(12): 1863–72.

99. Brown K, Mastrianni JA. The prion diseases. J Geriatr Psychiatry Neurol 2010; 23(4):277–98.

100. Birks J. Cholinesterase inhibitors for Alzheimer's disease. Cochrane Database Syst Rev 2006;(1):CD005593. http://dx.doi.org/10.1002/14651858.CD005593.

101. Press D, Alexander M. Cholinesterase inhibitors in the treatment of dementia. In: Basow DS, editor. UpToDate. Waltham (MA): UpToDate. Available at: http://www. uptodate.com/contents/cholinesterase-inhibitors-in-the-treatment-of-dementia? Accessed December 17, 2013.

102. Emre M, Aarsland D, Albanese A, et al. Rivastigmine for dementia associated with Parkinson's disease. N Engl J Med 2004;351(24):2509–18.

103. Maidment I, Fox C, Boustani M. Cholinesterase inhibitors for Parkinson's disease dementia. Cochrane Database Syst Rev 2006;(1):CD004747. http://dx.doi.org/ 10.1002/14651858.CD004747.pub2.

104. McKeith I, Mintzer J, Aarsland D, et al. Dementia with Lewy bodies. Lancet Neurol 2004;3(1):19–28.

105. Wright CB. Treatment and prevention of vascular dementia. In: Basow DS, editor. UpToDate. Waltham (MA): UpToDate. Available at: http://www.uptodate. com/contents/treatment-and-prevention-of-vascular-dementia? Accessed December 17, 2013.

106. Miller BL, Lee SE. Frontotemporal dementia: treatment. In: Basow DS, editor. UpToDate. Waltham (MA): UpToDate. Available at: http://www.uptodate.com/ contents/frontotemporal-dementia-treatment? Accessed December 17, 2013.

107. Mendez MF, Shapira JS, McMurtray A, et al. Preliminary findings: behavioral worsening on donepezil in patients with frontotemporal dementia. Am J Geriatr Psychiatry 2007;15(1):84–7.
108. Russ TC, Morling JR. Cholinesterase inhibitors for mild cognitive impairment. Cochrane Database Syst Rev 2012;(9):CD009132. http://dx.doi.org/10.1002/14651858.CD009132.pub2.
109. McShane R, Areosa Sastre A, Minakaran N. Memantine for dementia. Cochrane Database Syst Rev 2006;(2):CD003154. http://dx.doi.org/10.1002/14651858.CD003154.pub5.
110. Huey ED, Putnam KT, Grafman J. A systematic review of neurotransmitter deficits and treatments in frontotemporal dementia. Neurology 2006;66(1):17–22.
111. Gareri P, DeFazio P, Manfredi VG, et al. Use and safety of antipsychotics in behavioral disorders in elderly people with dementia. J Clin Psychopharmacol 2014;34:109–23. http://dx.doi.org/10.1097/JCP.0b013e3182a6096e.

Common Psychiatric Problems in Cognitively Impaired Older Patients

Causes and Management

Lucy Y. Wang, MD[a,b],*, Anna Borisovskaya, MD[a,b],
Andrea L. Maxwell, MD[a,b], Marcella Pascualy, MD[a,b]

KEYWORDS

- Dementia • Behavioral and psychological symptoms • Agitation • Depression
- Psychosis • Anxiety

KEY POINTS

- Psychiatric problems are common in cognitive disorders and cause distress in patients, contribute to caregiver burden, and precipitate institutionalization.
- Behavioral problems are caused by a combination in factors, including physiologic, psychological, and environmental.
- Treatment plans are more successful when they address these multiple contributing factors and, therefore, should involve both nonpharmacologic and pharmacologic therapies.
- Pharmacologic therapies are limited by side effects and, in the case of atypical antipsychotics, increased mortality risk.

INTRODUCTION

Although cognitive disorders are primarily characterized by their intellectual impairment, behavioral changes are common; most patients experience at least one of these disabling symptoms during their disease course.[1] From a patient and family perspective, problematic behaviors greatly diminish quality of life, worsen caregiver burden, and precipitate institutionalization.[2,3] Clinicians, on the other hand, find themselves in a dilemma whereby their more potentially effective pharmacologic agents are limited by significant side effects.

This work is supported by resources from the VA Puget Sound Health Care System, Seattle, Washington. Dr. Wang is supported by the VA Clinical Science Research and Development (CSR&D) Career Development Award Program (Project ID: 3125).

[a] Mental Health Service, VA Puget Sound Healthcare System, 1660 South Columbian Way, S-116, Seattle, WA 98108, USA; [b] Department of Psychiatry and Behavioral Sciences, University of Washington, 1959 NE Pacific Street, Box 356560, Seattle, WA 98108, USA
* Corresponding author.
E-mail address: lucy.wang@va.gov

The aim of this review is to provide clinicians a current conceptualization of psychiatric problems in cognitive disorders and to describe both the nonpharmacologic and pharmacologic tools available to treat them. The authors highlight the multidimensional nature of such symptoms and, likewise, the multidimensional and often multidisciplinary treatment approaches that are best able to achieve successful treatment. Although the scientific literature often presents mixed or modest results, the clinical experiences of geriatric psychiatrists has been that, with a comprehensive treatment plan as discussed later, clinicians can have optimism that treatment significantly improves the lives of our patients and their families.

Management strategies discussed here are applicable to any cognitive disorder; this review, however, is primarily based on literature relating to the major neurocognitive disorders (dementias) and Alzheimer disease in particular because it is the best studied. Pertinent differences and issues specific to other disorders are highlighted when applicable. Approaches common to all psychiatric syndromes are reviewed first, followed by sections specific to agitation, psychosis, depression, and anxiety.

GENERAL PRINCIPLES
The Initial Clinical Assessment

Psychiatric symptoms in cognitively impaired patients reflect many and varied possible underlying causes, including conditions unrelated to their cognitive disorder. Additionally, medications commonly used to treat psychiatric symptoms can impose significant side effect burdens in elderly patients. Therefore, professional guidelines universally recommend starting an assessment with a broad clinical evaluation to assess for physical illness, primary psychiatric illness, and other potentially reversible causes of psychiatric symptoms.[4–6]

The clinical assessment can be challenging, particularly because most affected individuals are unable to provide an accurate description of symptoms and the symptom course. In addition, some patients may be resistive to a physical examination and a further diagnostic work-up.[7] Assessments, therefore, often rely heavily on the caregiver report and what diagnostic testing can be obtained, although even the caregiver report can be biased because of exhaustion or burnout. With these caveats in mind, the key elements to the initial evaluation are summarized in **Box 1**.[4,6]

The differential diagnosis for psychiatric symptoms in cognitively impaired patients is broad.[4,6] Common physical conditions that contribute to psychiatric symptoms in cognitively impaired patients include undiagnosed or insufficiently treated pain, constipation, dehydration, and infections, such as urinary tract infections, dental infections, and upper respiratory illness. An exacerbation of preexisting psychiatric illness may be present in some patients, emphasizing the importance of knowing their past psychiatric histories. Other reversible physical factors that may contribute to behavioral symptoms include visual and hearing impairment, easily remediated by corrective lenses and hearing aids; medication side effects; and the effects of substances, such as alcohol, caffeine, nicotine, or illicit drugs. Even when all these factors are ruled out, it is important to keep in mind that psychiatric symptoms can be later exacerbated by such factors, so repeat evaluations after a clinical change are warranted.

Management Overview: Nonpharmacologic Approaches

After the initial clinical evaluation is complete, guidelines recommend nonpharmacologic approaches as first-line treatments.[4,6] Descriptions of nonpharmacologic treatments for specific symptoms are described in the symptom-specific sections further

---

Box 1
Key elements: initial evaluation of psychiatric symptoms in dementia

History from patients

- Can provide a picture of the patients' in-the-moment mood, discomfort, or physical symptoms

History from the caregiver

- Can provide information on the longitudinal course and severity of symptoms

Physical examination

- May be uncomfortable for cognitively impaired patients, resulting in lack of cooperation
- History from caregivers may provide information pertinent to the examination (eg, wincing in pain with transfers)

Diagnostic testing

- Strongly consider
  - Complete blood count
  - Electrolytes
  - Renal function
  - Thyroid function
  - Liver function
  - Urinalysis
  - Electrocardiogram
- If indicated
  - Neuroimaging
  - Electroencephalogram
  - Lumbar puncture

---

on in this review. Highlighted here is the key element among these approaches, which is the recognition that psychological or environmental factors need to be addressed and that caregiver support is crucial.[8,9]

For example, an unmet psychological need for increased social contact could contribute to anxiety, or an environmental exposure such as to violent images on the television can trigger agitation. Because each patient will have a different psychological, interpersonal, or environmental makeup, nonpharmacologic approaches are most successful when they are tailored to the individual patient. These approaches are varied, and several models have been proposed to conceptualize them.[1,8] These models are not mutually exclusive, with many areas of overlap. However, knowledge of one or more can be beneficial to the clinician (**Table 1**).

One intervention that is important in managing any psychiatric symptom in cognitively impaired patients is providing caregiver support. When patients are living at home, families and patients often encounter a spiraling problem whereby patients exhibit problematic behaviors, leading to worsening caregiver stress, reducing the caregiver's ability to use behavioral strategies, resulting in further disruptive behaviors. It is also possible that cognitively impaired patients can sense caregiver depression or burnout and, therefore, react with symptoms, such as anxiety, depression, or agitation. The toll of caregiving is substantial, with studies showing high rates of

Table 1
Examples of psychological and environmental approaches

Psychological Factor	Relevant Symptoms	Approaches
Unmet needs (eg, sensory deprivation, lack of social contact)	Agitation, anxiety, depression	Sensory stimulation (massage/touch, music) Social contact (real or simulated) Positive activities Exercise therapy
Reduced stress threshold model (eg, overwhelming stimuli)	Agitation, anxiety	Tailor activities appropriate to cognitive level Relaxation (music, aromatherapy) Caregiver education to simplify interactions
Learning and behavioral theory (ie, behavioral problems inadvertently reinforced by caregiver reactions)	Agitation	Caregiver education to identify and change patterns (antecedent, behavior, and consequence)
Psychotherapy	Depression, anxiety	Cognitive behavioral therapy Problem-solving therapy

Social and Environmental Factor	Relevant Symptom	Approaches
Caregiver strain	All symptoms	Caregiver education and support (see **Table 2**)
Environmental triggers	All symptoms	Adjust environment to remove triggers (eg, noise, poor lighting, presence of strangers, or other specific elements in the environment)

depression, anxiety, and sleep disturbance in caregivers as well as higher rates of nursing home placement.[10,11] When caregiver stress is alleviated, it is not uncommon for patients' psychiatric symptoms to also improve.[12]

Any treatment plan should, therefore, include caregiver support; this has been recognized as a central component of dementia care and has been incorporated into the Centers for Medicare and Medicaid Services Physician Quality Reporting System for physician reimbursement. Many of these support approaches involve patient and caregiver education, and they can be done relatively easily during a clinical visit. Others may require referrals to social services or community support organizations, such as the Alzheimer's Association. Examples of caregiver support approaches are listed in **Table 2**.

Management Overview: Pharmacologic Approaches

When nonpharmacologic approaches have been implemented and practiced on a consistent basis with only minimal to moderate efficacy, then medication trials are recommended.[4,6] Pharmacologic approaches are also considered if symptoms are severe or endanger patients or others. Choosing a medication depends on the specific symptom target, the severity of symptoms, and side effect profiles. Because efficacy is usually only modest, it is important to continue using nonpharmacologic measures. Also, the natural course of many symptoms is to eventually remit, so careful

Table 2 Approaches to caregiver support	
Approach	**Examples**
Caregiver education	Nature of disease and disease course
	Acknowledgment of the high risk of depression and burnout; importance of self-care
	Medications: expected benefits vs side effects
	Referral to community outreach organizations with educational programs, such as the Alzheimer's Association
Direct caregiver support	Referrals to support groups
	Encourage caregiver to maintain outside activities or relationships (friendships, social clubs, classes at a senior center, and so forth)
	Assess for caregiver depression and potential need for a referral to counseling or other mental health services
Respite options	Paid companion or caregiver services
	Adult day health
	Respite (typically short-term stays for dementia patients in a skilled nursing or assisted-living facility)

reductions in doses or even discontinuation of medications should be attempted after a period of stability.[13]

Specific medications are described later in each symptom-specific section. However, a common approach for all medications is to "start low and go slow."[4,14] A reasonable rule of thumb is to start medications at half the usual adult dose and increase slowly over weeks (instead of days), until the lowest effective dose is reached. However, some patients may require rapid escalation to doses in the higher range to attain adequate symptom control. It is best to avoid psychotropic polypharmacy. In situations when multiple medications are used or need to be changed, changing only one medication at a time is prudent unless obvious drug toxicity requires rapid de-escalation or discontinuation.

Acetylcholinesterase inhibitors and memantine

Acetylcholinesterase inhibitors (AChEIs) and memantine are included here because, although not recommended for acute symptom management, they can be incorporated in a longer-term strategy for behavioral symptom reduction. These medications can help delay the progression of functional deficits, but secondary analyses have found a benefit over placebo with regard to behavioral symptoms, including a lower likelihood that symptoms will emerge.[15,16] They may be of benefit for a range of behavioral problems, including agitation, psychosis, and depression.

AChEIs include donepezil, rivastigmine, and galantamine. Beneficial effects have been reported for depression, apathy, and aberrant motor behavior as well as global behavioral measures.[1] Additional support for efficacy comes from a randomized withdrawal study; cessation of donepezil was associated with a significant worsening of behavioral symptoms within 6 weeks.[17] These medications are generally well tolerated, with the most common side effects being gastrointestinal (nausea, vomiting, diarrhea). AChEIs are contraindicated in patients with severe asthma or chronic obstructive pulmonary disease, bradycardia, heart conduction abnormalities, or peptic ulcer disease.

In post hoc analyses, memantine has been associated with superiority over placebo for agitation and psychosis as well as for global behavioral measures.[18] The use of memantine may also reduce the need for additional psychotropic medications.[19,20]

This medication is particularly well tolerated; the more common side effects include confusion, dizziness, and headache.

Identifying Symptoms and Measuring Response: Use of Rating Scales

Several rating scales aid in the assessment of behavioral symptoms in dementia and are described in **Table 3**. Such scales can be used as screening tools to identify the presence of symptoms. Subsequent use provides a tangible measure of symptom change, allowing all parties to better gauge an intervention's effectiveness.

In Summary

- Start with a broad clinical evaluation to rule out and address nonpsychiatric causes of behavioral symptoms.
- Nonpharmacologic approaches are always first line.
- Nonpharmacologic approaches work best when individualized to each patient.
- Caregiver support is a key aspect of the treatment plan.
- Medications are recommended when nonpharmacologic approaches have failed or are insufficient alone.
- AChEIs and memantine can be used as part of a longer-term strategy for behavioral symptom reduction.

Table 3
Rating scales

Symptom	Rating Scale	Description
Useful for all symptoms	NPI[101] and NPI-Q[102] (brief form)	It is clinician administered and based on caregiver input. It measures 12 symptom domains. The NPI-Q (brief form) is easily administered in clinic settings.
	Minimum Data Set–Mood and Behavior[103]	Required for all residents of Medicare and Medicaid skilled nursing facilities, the MDS documents the presence, frequency, and other qualities of mood and behavioral symptoms.
Depression	PHQ-9 and PHQ-9 OV	Self-report and observation based versions are available. It is validated in skilled nursing facility settings.[104]
	Cornell Scale for Depression in Dementia	It is a clinician-administered scale that incorporates input from both patients and caregivers.
	Geriatric Depression Scale	It is based on patient input. It avoids symptoms that may overlap with medical disorders or aging, but questions may be challenging for patients with more advanced cognitive impairment.
	Hamilton Depression Rating Scale	It is clinician-administered and based on patient input. Patients with dementia may have trouble reporting symptoms over time.
	Montgomery-Asberg Depression Rating Scale	It is clinician administered and incorporates patient input. Patients with dementia may have trouble reporting symptoms over time.

Abbreviations: MDS, Minimum Data Set; NPI, Neuropsychiatric Inventory; NPI-Q, Neuropsychiatric Inventory Questionnaire; OV, observational version; PHQ-9, Patient Health Questionnaire-9 item interview.

AGITATION AND AGGRESSION
Introduction

Agitation is an umbrella term that refers to disruptive motor or vocal activity and tends to occur with advanced stages of cognitive impairment.[21] Examples include excessive motor activity (eg, pacing, restlessness), verbal aggression (eg, yelling, using profanity), or physical aggression (eg, grabbing, shoving, hitting others). This constellation of symptoms is also referred to in the literature as *agitation and aggression*.[22]

Agitation negatively impacts the quality of life of both the patients and the caregivers, with caregivers identifying agitation and irritability, along with delusions, as the most distressing psychiatric symptoms in patients.[23] Aggressive behaviors and sleep disturbances are the major precipitants leading to institutionalization.[11] Symptoms of agitation are common problems in patients with cognitive disorders. For example, between 40% and 60% of patients with Alzheimer disease in care facilities have agitation and aggression.[24]

Nonpharmacologic Interventions

Nonpharmacologic interventions should be used as the first-line intervention. Because patients with dementia cannot usually explain in words why they are agitated, clinical observations must be anchored by one or more theoretical frameworks that help to interpret the behavior and guide intervention (see **Table 1**).

One of these approaches is to evaluate for unmet needs.[8] The unmet needs model states that psychiatric symptoms or behaviors can result from an inability to communicate needs. Such needs may include sensory deprivation, boredom, loneliness, pain, and toileting needs. Interventions include appropriate social or sensory stimulation, sensory aids (eyeglasses, hearing aids), safe places to move about, social interaction, pain control, and scheduled toileting. Specific therapies that have been studied include structured activity, exercise therapy, pet therapy, and real or simulated social contact.

Patients with dementia and associated limited cognition may have an impaired ability to process and cope with environmental stimuli, such as sound, light, and human activity around them. This phenomenon has been described in the literature as the reduced (or progressively lowered) stress threshold model.[8,25] Patients may misperceive stimuli or have a lower threshold at which these stimuli become overwhelming. Treatment focuses, therefore, on reducing stimuli and producing a calmer environment. Approaches consistent with this model include relaxation therapies, caregiver education to simplify interactions, and appropriately tailoring activities to patients' cognitive level.

It is also important to identify factors that precipitate and exacerbate agitation. Careful observation of the patients' behaviors, precipitants to agitation, and the response to interventions will clarify what is helpful and what is ineffective. Also known as the *A-B-Cs* (antecedents [A], behavior [B], and consequences [C]) and based on learning/behavioral theory, this approach gives caregivers and clinicians the information needed to change the relationships between the A-B-Cs.[8,26] For example, a patient may be alone in his room needing social contact (antecedent), so starts yelling out (behavior). The staff responds (consequence), inadvertently reinforcing the yelling out behaviors. Providing regular social contact regardless of yelling out could change this pattern, which addresses the antecedent and removes the relationship between behavior and consequence.

A diary tracking the symptoms, including timing, potential triggers, and severity, can be useful. Common triggers include changes to routine, environmental stimulation, and the presence of strangers (caregivers they are not familiar with, relatives they do not recognize). When others try to assist with activities of daily living, particularly toileting, bathing, and dressing, patients with dementia may become agitated. Alternate forms of medications, such as pill crushing or using liquid medications, may help avoid agitation around medication administration.

Finally, it is important to provide education to caregivers. For example, it is common for patients to wander, misplace items, and accuse others of stealing. These symptoms are most amenable to education because they are primarily caused by memory deficits and impaired reasoning and not psychiatric problems per se. This education helps caregivers understand these behaviors as part of the illness and not intentional stubbornness or disruptiveness. Education about interactional styles and simple environmental modifications is also helpful (**Box 2**).

Pharmacologic Interventions

The use of psychotropic medications should be reserved for when nonpharmacologic interventions have failed and behaviors have the potential to be harmful to patients and others. Nursing home residents have historically been overprescribed psychotropic medications.[27] No medication has proven efficacy; often a period of trial and error must occur, and side effects often limit use (as discussed later). It can be helpful to have discussions with patients and families about their goals of care; the palliative care goals of quality of life, comfort, and dignity are often appropriate in this setting.[7] For example, some patients and families are willing to accept sedating side effects if such treatment results in greater patient comfort. Others may wish to avoid side effects or mortality risk and, therefore, accept some degree of ongoing agitation. Quantifying specific treatment targets with caregivers also helps clinicians gauge medication effectiveness (eg, aim to reduce the frequency of verbal aggression from daily to <3 days a week). Polypharmacy should be avoided, and the continued use of psychopharmacologic agents should be periodically reviewed.

Box 2
Family and caregiver education about agitation

Independence

- Use clothing and shoes with Velcro (Velcro USA Inc, Manchester, NH) instead of buttons or zippers.
- Use large-handled utensils or cut food into manageable bites to allow patients to continue to feed themselves.

Style of interaction

- Use clear and simple language and visual cues.
- Approach patients from the front to avoid startling them.
- Stay an arm's length away to lessen the potential for injury from hitting or kicking.
- Maintain consistent routines.

Wandering

- Signs, safety alarms, and difficult-to-operate key latches may reduce the risk.
- The Safe Return program with identification bracelets (Alzheimer's Association) or clothing tags can assist in locating lost patients.

Antipsychotics

Antipsychotics are often used for agitation in dementia; this is an off-label use and is not approved by the Food and Drug Administration (FDA) for this purpose. Typical antipsychotics were widely used until recently, when the atypical agents came onto the market. Since that time, atypical agents have gained in popularity because of their improved side effect profile and tolerability.[27] A large number of randomized clinical trials, meta-analyses, and reviews have examined the efficacy and safety of atypical antipsychotics, including risperidone, olanzapine, quetiapine, and aripiprazole (doses in **Table 4**).[28,29] As a whole, early published efficacy studies demonstrated a modest benefit over placebo.[30–33] Studies examining withdrawal versus continuation of chronic antipsychotic treatment provided more mixed results. Most patients do not experience detrimental effects on behavior after drug discontinuation[34]; however, in the Antipsychotic Discontinuation in Alzheimer's Disease trial, 60% of those who discontinued risperidone experienced a significant symptom recurrence within 16 weeks compared with 33% of those maintained on the medication.[35]

An effectiveness trial funded by the National Institute of Mental Health (NIMH), the Clinical Antipsychotic Trials of Intervention Effectiveness–Alzheimer's Disease study, cast doubt over the benefit of treating agitation and psychosis with atypical antipsychotics.[36] In this trial, risperidone, olanzapine, quetiapine, and placebo were compared head to head with the primary outcome measure being time to discontinuation for any reason, such as lack of efficacy or side effects. No difference was found among the treatment groups or placebo, and the researchers concluded that side effects offset advantages in the efficacy for these drugs.

In April 2005, a meta-analysis of 17 placebo-controlled trials of aripiprazole, olanzapine, quetiapine, and risperidone raised the question of mortality risk associated with these medications.[37] In this analysis, the risk of mortality was 1.6 to 1.7 times greater in elderly patients with dementia treated with atypical antipsychotic medications, primarily because of cardiovascular effects or infection. This finding precipitated the black box warning that the use of atypical agents for the treatment of behavioral symptoms in elderly patients with dementia is associated with increased mortality.

Additional risks include cognitive decline as well as cerebrovascular events; randomized clinical trials of risperidone indicate a 3-fold increase in cerebrovascular compared with placebo.[38] Other significant adverse effects include extrapyramidal symptoms (EPS), sedation, tardive dyskinesia, metabolic syndrome, and gait disturbance; furthermore, these side effects increase the risk of falls, fractures, and head injuries. Peripheral anticholinergic effects include dry mouth, constipation, and urinary hesitation or retention. Central anticholinergic effects include further impairments to cognition and memory, delirium, and oversedation.

Given the evidence that atypical antipsychotic medications can reduce agitation symptoms but have an associated mortality risk and burdensome side effects, guidelines and expert statements continue to include these drugs as treatment options, with

Table 4 Antipsychotic doses in older adults		
Drug	**Starting Dose (mg)**	**Range (mg)**
Olanzapine	2.5	5–10
Quetiapine	12.5–25.0	25–200
Risperidone	0.25–0.5	0.5–4.0
Aripiprazole	2.5–5.0	10–15

the caveat that potential benefits must be carefully weighed against risks.[1,4] In patients with severe agitation causing significant distress or potential harm to themselves and others, the risks of undertreatment are substantial, and many patients and caregivers accept an increased mortality risk if a medication improves quality of life. Informed consent should be obtained and documented, and periodic attempts at dose reduction should be made.[1,4]

Patients with dementia with Lewy bodies (DLB) and Parkinson disease dementia (PDD) experience more frequent and severe extrapyramidal side effects from antipsychotics. This sensitivity is actually a feature that supports the diagnosis of DLB. Whenever possible, antipsychotic agents should be avoided. However, if an antipsychotic must be used, quetiapine—with its low affinity for D2 receptors and limited EPS—appears to have a positive effect on psychosis, agitation, and anxiety and may be the preferred agent for this patient population.[39]

In summary: antipsychotics

- Antipsychotics are modest in efficacy, are associated with adverse effects, and carry an increased risk of mortality.
- Use only when there are significant psychotic symptoms that are distressing to the patients or aggressive behaviors that risk harm to the patients or others.
- Treatment providers should collaborate with the patients' families and caregivers and carefully weigh the risks and benefits, including the risk of increased mortality. This conversation should be documented in the record.
- Low-dose atypical antipsychotics are the recommended agents if an antipsychotic is to be used.
- If patients respond favorably, periodic attempts should be made to reduce or discontinue the medication to see if continued treatment of the original target symptoms is warranted.
- In PDD or DLB, quetiapine is a preferred agent because of its lower risk of EPS.

Antidepressants
Lists of antidepressant medications and doses can be found in **Tables 5–7**. Clinical trials of several antidepressants, including sertraline, fluoxetine, citalopram, and trazodone, as treatments for agitation have generally shown mixed results, with the more promising results for the selective serotonin reuptake inhibitor (SSRI) citalopram. Recently, the Citalopram for Agitation in Alzheimer Disease Study demonstrated superiority over placebo for reducing agitation in patients with Alzheimer disease.[40] Notably, 40% of patients in the citalopram arm were rated as moderately to markedly improved compared with 26% in the placebo arm. This degree of improvement is comparable with that seen in antipsychotic trials. However, citalopram was also associated with a slightly greater decline in cognition as measured by the Mini-Mental State

Table 5		
Selective serotonin reuptake inhibitors: doses in older adults		
Drug	**Starting Dose (mg)**	**Range (mg)**
Citalopram	10	10–20
Escitalopram	5	5–20
Fluoxetine	5	5–60
Paroxetine	10	10–40
Sertraline	12.5–25.0	25–200

Table 6
Serotonin norepinephrine reuptake inhibitors and mirtazapine: dosages in older adults

Drug	Starting Dosage	Range
Venlafaxine (SNRI)	18.75–37.5 mg every morning or twice daily	75–150 mg twice daily
Venlafaxine extended release (SNRI)	37.5 mg every morning	75–150 mg daily
Duloxetine (SNRI)	10–20 mg every morning or twice daily	20–60 mg once to twice daily
Mirtazapine	7.5–15.0 mg every evening	15–60 mg every evening

Abbreviation: SNRI, serotonin norepinephrine reuptake inhibitors.

Examination and lengthening of the QT interval. The target dosage in this trial was 30 mg daily, which exceeds the current FDA advisory limit of 20 mg in older adults because of a dose-dependent risk for QTc prolongation. Citalopram is, therefore, a useful approach; but side effects and the issue of QT prolongation may limit use. Common side effects of SSRIs include nausea, diarrhea, and anorexia; these could be problematic in the elderly if they contribute to discomfort and weight loss.

Anticonvulsants
Anticonvulsants, effective for irritability, aggression, and impulsivity in bipolar disorder, have been used in elderly patients with agitation (**Table 8**). Carbamazepine has demonstrated efficacy in several small studies for treating agitation,[41,42] although its use is limited by drug-drug interactions and side effects. Carbamazepine has a black box warning for hematologic toxicity and can induce hepatic drug metabolizing enzymes. The development of sedation, confusion, and ataxia limits its use in the elderly. For valproate, initial studies suggested efficacy for agitation in patients with dementia, but subsequent randomized trials failed to support this.[43–45] As with carbamazepine, side effects of valproate, including sedation and falls, limit its use in elderly patients. There is insufficient evidence for gabapentin.[46] These agents may be of use in individual cases when other agents have failed, with a low-dose approach.

Antiadrenergic medications
Enhanced behavior responses to norepinephrine may contribute to agitation in dementia. In a randomized placebo-controlled study, propranolol was shown to be

Table 7
Atypical antidepressants: dosages in older adults

Drug	Starting Dosage	Range
Bupropion (immediate release)	75 mg every morning or twice daily	150–450 mg total daily dose, divided 2–3 times per day
Bupropion (sustained release 12 h)	100–150 mg daily	150–400 mg total daily dose, divided twice daily
Bupropion (extended release 24 h)	150 mg daily	150–450 mg total daily dose, once daily
Trazodone[a]	12.5–25.0 mg every evening	50–200 mg

[a] Trazodone is often used for sleep, although it is FDA approved for depression only.

Table 8		
Anticonvulsant dosages in older adults		
Drug	**Starting Dosage**	**Range**
Divalproex sodium[45]	125 mg twice daily	250–1000 mg total daily dose
Carbamazepine[41]	50–100 mg/d	Blood level: 5–8 ug/mL[a]

[a] Although blood levels are provided, patients may respond at lower levels. Dosing toward treatment response and side effect tolerability, rather than blood level, is recommended.

superior to placebo and generally well tolerated; but behavioral effects decreased over time, limiting its clinical effectiveness.[47] A pilot double-blind placebo-controlled trial of prazosin demonstrated efficacy over placebo and good tolerability, suggesting prazosin may be a promising pharmacologic alternative to atypical antipsychotics.[48]

Benzodiazepines

All benzodiazepines can decrease cognitive function, precipitate delirium, and increase the risk of falls and subsequent injury. Their use should be limited to emergent use only, when severe agitation places patients or others at risk of injury and patients have been unresponsive to trials of other agents. A limited trial of a short-acting benzodiazepine (lorazepam, oxazepam, temazepam) in these cases is preferred. These agents do not accumulate, and their metabolism is not affected by age or liver dysfunction. Long-acting agents may have a long half-life and accumulate.

In summary: nonantipsychotic medications for agitation

- There is evidence supporting citalopram's efficacy for treating agitation in dementia. Citalopram is associated with an increased risk for QTc prolongation.
- Carbamazepine can be beneficial for agitation; but its use is limited by potential side effects, such as ataxia, sedation, hematologic effects, and drug-drug interactions.
- Prazosin has preliminary evidence of benefit.
- For dangerous aggression, the brief use of a benzodiazepine may be warranted; but the emergence of adverse effects should be monitored.

PSYCHOSIS

Psychotic symptoms are common in cognitive disorders, with one study estimating a 4-year cumulative incidence of 51% in patients with Alzheimer disease.[49] The criteria for psychosis of Alzheimer disease have been proposed, which require the presence of either or both hallucinations and delusions.[50] Hallucinations may be auditory or visual. Delusions, particularly in Alzheimer disease, tend to be simple, nonbizarre, and of a paranoid nature. Examples include the belief that one's current living situation is not really their home, caregivers are stealing from them, or they misidentify their caregivers. It can be questionable whether delusions reflect a true psychotic process or are patients' misinterpretations of their surroundings caused by cognitive impairment.

In DLB, visual hallucinations are a diagnostic criterion; they also occur commonly in PDD.[51] In both of these syndromes, visual hallucinations usually start as benign, such as images of small children or animals. Patients often understand that these images are hallucinations and, therefore, find them nondistressing. However, as dementia progresses in severity, patients' hallucinations can become threatening and patients can lose insight. Delusions similar to those experienced by patients with AD can also occur in patients with DLB and PDD as their cognitive impairment reaches more severe stages.

If hallucinations or delusions are not distressing, it is preferred to not treat with medications. These symptoms are often more distressing to caregivers than patients themselves, so careful education and finding nonpharmacologic adaptation strategies provide more benefit. For patients with PDD, decreasing or changing dopaminergic medications is often a good first step because these drugs can produce psychotic symptoms. In cases whereby delusions are in fact a reflection of cognitive impairment, a cholinesterase inhibitor or memantine may be helpful.

If psychotic symptoms are distressing to patients and impair their quality of life, an atypical antipsychotic medication is recommended (see **Table 4**). However, as described in the earlier section on agitation, antipsychotic treatment has limited efficacy, significant side effects, and an increased risk of mortality in patients with dementia. For patients with DLB and PDD, antipsychotic use is especially complicated by the high likelihood of worsening their already present parkinsonian symptoms. The 2 medications least likely to worsen parkinsonism are clozapine and quetiapine.[52] Clozapine carries a risk for agranulocytosis and, therefore, requires prescribers to have specific training and access to appropriate monitoring with weekly blood tests. Quetiapine is, therefore, more commonly used.

In Summary: Hallucinations and Delusions

- There is uncertainty as to whether some delusions are more accurately characterized as misinterpretation caused by cognitive impairment. For example, delusions of theft may reflect patients' inability to recall the location of their possessions.
- If psychotic symptoms are nondistressing, caregiver education is the best treatment strategy.
- If psychotic symptoms are distressing and problematic, antipsychotic medications are the agents of choice.
- Psychotic symptoms are common in DLB and PDD. Particular care must be taken when prescribing antipsychotic medications in these individuals because of parkinsonian side effects. Quetiapine is a preferred agent in patients with DLB and PDD.

DEPRESSION
Introduction

A significant percentage of patients living with cognitive impairment suffer from depression. Prevalence estimates range from 26% to 50%.[53–55] Major depression in Alzheimer disease persists over time,[53,56] and depression is more common in Alzheimer disease than mild cognitive impairment (25% compared with 16%).[57] Depression leads to worsening functioning and greater caregiver burden while increasing the risk of sleep disturbances, anxiety, aggressiveness, and suicide.[57–61]

The diagnosis of depression in dementia is complicated by the overlap with other symptoms common in cognitive disorders, such as apathy, decreased ability to think and function, insomnia, and psychomotor abnormalities. Further, depression in dementia may differ from major depressive disorder symptoms in cognitively normal individuals; severity of depressive signs and symptoms may be less and may co-occur with social isolation, withdrawal, irritability, decline in motivation, and delusions.[62] Patients may have difficulty conveying their distress because of aphasia, and many do not complain of sad mood.[63] Apathy must be differentiated from depression because the cause and treatment of these conditions are significantly different.

Although patients with apathy may seem to lack interest and have difficulty enjoying activities, they do not exhibit the emotional pain, despair, and negativism of thought seen in depression.

To aid in diagnosis, in 2002, the NIMH proposed diagnostic criteria for depression in Alzheimer disease.[62] Key differences from the *Diagnostic and Statistical Manual of Mental Disorders (DSM)* criteria for major depressive disorder include fewer symptoms required and changes in several criteria to better accommodate cognitive impairment. Specifically, the symptom of "poor concentration" is not found in the diagnostic criteria for depression in Alzheimer disease, and "loss of interest or pleasure in most or all activities" was replaced by "decreased positive affect or pleasure." The criteria for irritability and social isolation were added. The NIMH's criteria demonstrated 94% sensitivity and 85% specificity when compared with the criteria of the *DSM* (Fourth Edition) for a major depressive episode.[55] Nonetheless, controversy remains regarding whether the NIMH's criteria or the *DSM*'s criteria are most appropriate for use in the diagnosis of depression in dementia.[64]

The diagnosis of depression in dementia is made most effectively through thorough history taking, clinical examination, and interview of patients and their caregivers. Several rating scales may aid the assessment and diagnosis of depression in dementia and are described in **Table 3**.

In Summary: Introduction to Depression

- Depression is a common and persistent comorbidity in dementia, complicating the outcomes for patients and their caregivers.
- To make the diagnosis of depression in dementia, it is important to distinguish it in presentation from apathy and dementia itself.
- Sad mood may not be the chief complaint of depressed patients with dementia.
- Social withdrawal, decreased positive affect, loss of pleasure, and negativism may be useful markers distinguishing depression from other conditions.

Nonpharmacologic Approaches

Good evidence exists for physical activity and exercise for improving depression in dementia. Just as elderly exercisers have less depressed mood,[65] patients with Alzheimer disease with higher levels of activity have lower levels of depression.[66] A randomized-controlled trial of patients with Alzheimer disease in the community, extending over several years, showed that patients assigned to a combined exercise and caregiver program were less depressed and showed a trend for lower rates of institutionalization because of behavioral disturbance (19% vs 50%).[67]

In addition to exercise, increasing pleasurable activities in general is effective in reducing depression in dementia. Behavioral activation, based on cognitive behavioral theory, emphasizes regularly scheduling activities associated with positive mood.[68] In studies adapting behavioral activation in patients with dementia with depression, significant improvements for both patients and their caregivers were seen, with gains maintained at 6 months' follow-up.[69] Resources in the community that promote behavioral activation include activities provided through senior centers and adult day health programs. Occupational therapy, in which cognitive and behavioral interventions are used to train patients with dementia in adaptation strategies, has also been shown to have long-lasting beneficial effects on the mood and quality of life for patients and caregivers.[70]

Psychotherapy options for patients with early dementia include modified cognitive behavioral therapy and problem-solving therapy.[71] Such approaches are adaptable and make allowances for the patients' cognitive losses. Problem-solving therapy teaches patients with executive dysfunction a structured approach to selecting a problem to solve and a method for reviewing and selecting potential solutions, as described in **Box 3**.[72]

Pharmacologic Approaches

Controversy exists over the efficacy of antidepressants for the treatment of depression in dementia (dosages described in **Tables 5–7**). Several smaller studies and a recent meta-analysis provide evidence suggestive of efficacy and good tolerability.[73–75] A study that observed patients whose antidepressant was discontinued found an increase in depressive symptoms compared with those who remained on drug treatment.[76]

However, 2 large randomized clinical trials cast doubt over efficacy and highlighted the side effect burden associated with these drugs. Depression in Alzheimer's Disease-2, a multicenter, randomized, placebo-controlled trial of sertraline, which also provided structured psychosocial treatment of caregivers of all patients, found no difference in response between placebo and sertraline.[77] Higher numbers of gastrointestinal and respiratory side effects were seen in patients on sertraline. The extension of the trial to 24 weeks did not demonstrate a significant difference among those treated with sertraline or placebo.[78] The Health Technology Assessment Study of the Use of Antidepressants for Depression in Dementia trial compared sertraline, mirtazapine, and placebo.[79] No difference in response to all interventions was found, whereas more adverse reactions were seen in the sertraline and mirtazapine groups.

In spite of these mixed results, antidepressant medications remain the mainstay for pharmacologic treatment of depression in cognitively impaired patients. There exists greater supportive evidence for this class than other pharmacologic agents, and side effects are well tolerated by most patients. It is also important to note that studies do not specifically examine efficacy in patients with the most severe illness. In these situations, the potential benefit of a medication trial can outweigh the risks of undertreatment.

Other Treatment Considerations

One should always keep in mind the potential for electroconvulsive therapy (ECT) for the treatment of depression in dementia. A safe and effective treatment of major depressive disorder, it has also been found to be effective for depression in dementia,

---

Box 3
Steps of problem-solving therapy

Educate patients and caregivers about the importance of learning how to problem solve

Create a list of problems

1. Problem orientation
2. Problem definition
3. Goal setting
4. Solution generation
5. Decision making
6. Implementation
7. Solution verification

although the number of studies describing such intervention is limited.[80] Because one of the most bothersome side effects of ECT is short-term memory loss, these studies do in fact report worsening cognitive difficulties in the patients undergoing ECT. It was found that patients with dementia who received antidementia treatment during ECT experienced fewer cognitive losses.[81]

Red flags that should prompt clinicians to consider aggressive treatment, such as hospitalization or ECT, are listed in **Box 4**.

In Summary: Treatment Recommendations for Depression in Dementia

- Stress the importance of exercise and behavioral activation.
- Provide psychological support to patients and caregivers.
- Use available resources in the community; adult day health or senior centers may provide the structure and pleasant activities that will assist with behavioral activation.
- In those with milder dementia, problem-solving therapy may prove useful.
- In patients who show no signs of improvement despite the interventions listed earlier, consider using a carefully chosen antidepressant.
- In patients who show red flag signs (see **Box 4**), consider hospitalization and ECT.

ANXIETY
Introduction

Estimates of prevalence of anxiety in dementia vary. Depending on the population and measure of anxiety used, the results of studies are as high as 70%.[54,82,83] When the criteria for specific disorders are used, estimates are far lower; a study of a consecutive series of patients with Alzheimer disease found an overall prevalence of anxiety disorders of 7%, 5% of which were generalized anxiety disorder and 2% panic disorder.[56] Anxiety in dementia is associated with a higher rate of behavioral disturbance,[83,84] decreased independence,[85] activities of daily living impairment,[83] higher caregiver distress,[86] and earlier nursing home placement.[87]

Anxiety and depression in dementia are closely related, with anxiety a frequent comorbid condition of major depression.[88,89] Some experts suggest that anxiety should be considered a component of depression in Alzheimer disease.[64] Further, there is evidence that generalized anxiety disorder in Alzheimer disease occurs more frequently in those patients who suffered from depression in their adult life.[56]

Diagnosis is challenging, as there is significant variability in the literature as to how anxiety is best measured and defined. Most rating scales used in cognitively normal patients, such as the Beck Anxiety Inventory and the Geriatric Anxiety Inventory, have not been robustly validated in dementia populations. One rating scale specific

Box 4
Red flags for depression requiring aggressive interventions
Severe functional impairment
Inability to care for self not related to cognitive impairment
Rapid weight loss related to depression
Psychotic symptoms
Suicidal ideation with intent or plan

to anxiety in dementia is the Structured Interview Guide for the Rating for Anxiety in Dementia (RAID-SI).[90] The RAID-SI attempts to differentiate medical symptoms commonly experienced by older adults from the symptoms of anxiety. However, the time needed to administer this scale may limit its usefulness in busy clinic settings. The Geriatric Anxiety Inventory-Short Form has been studied in a memory clinic setting and may be a useful screening tool.[91] The *DSM*'s criteria for generalized anxiety disorder is also appropriate for use in this population, as research suggests patients who meet the criteria warrant clinical attention. Patients with dementia who meet the *DSM*'s criteria are more likely to exhibit other problematic behaviors, such as irritability, overt aggression, and pathologic crying.[56]

Nonpharmacologic Approaches

One study that described the views of patients with dementia and their caregivers on anxiety listed the following interventions perceived as helpful: socialization; attendance of day centers and day hospitals; being with other people experiencing similar problems; person-centered care; memory aids, such as keeping a diary; medication boxes to help take medications correctly; engaging in meaningful enjoyable activities; and managing physical and environmental problems. Notably, resorting to medications was seen as the last option for most patients and their caregivers, though the patients who had experiences with medications described potential benefit from using them.[92]

Further, there has been an upsurge in trials of Cognitive Behavioral Therapy (CBT) for anxiety in dementia. A form of CBT for anxiety in persons with dementia is Peaceful Mind, described in detail by Paukert and colleagues.[93] Peaceful Mind is provided over the course of 6 months, with 12 sessions delivered in the participant's home for the first 3 months and with booster phone sessions occurring during the second half of the treatment. Collaterals are extensively involved in this treatment modality, attending each session and acting as a coach for patients. The clinician manual includes modules teaching self-awareness, breathing, calming statements, increasing activity, and sleep skills, although not all skills could be taught to all participants. Several modifications to traditional CBT distinguish Peaceful Mind: emphasis on skills rather than cognitive interventions, focusing on one skill at a time with fewer skills being taught, and spending a significant amount of time in each session on repetition and practice. In a randomized controlled trial of Peaceful Mind compared with usual care, although improvements were seen at 3 months' time, there was no difference between Peaceful Mind and usual care at 6 months' time.[94] The lack of difference between CBT-based intervention and usual care at 6 months' time may be related to the fact that all patients' anxiety and caregiver distress improved over that period of time or to the small size of the trial.

Similarly modifying CBT for cognitive impairment, another group of clinicians described using this approach for 2 patients with Alzheimer disease and anxiety, both of them experiencing significant benefits through treatment.[95] The researchers hypothesized that transmission of hope and improving communication between patients and caregivers may have played an important role in the patients' improvement. Further trials of CBT modified for cognitively impaired individuals are planned.[96]

Music therapy has been widely studied and is commonly used in various care settings. As defined by the American Music Therapy Association's Web site, "music therapists structure the use of both instrumental and vocal music strategies to improve functioning or facilitate changes that contribute to life quality. They may improvise or compose music with clients, accompany and conduct group music experiences, provide instrument instruction, direct music and movement activities, or structure music listening opportunities." (http://www.musictherapy.org/assets/1/7/MT_Alzheimers_2006.pdf). The results of this intervention were summarized in a meta-analysis that included all available studies, including cohort, controlled, and randomized clinical trials, including studies from Japan. The largest effect of music therapy was found for anxiety symptoms in dementia, both as a short-term and a long-term intervention.[97]

Pharmacologic Approaches

There are very few systematic studies of medications used to treat the symptoms of anxiety in dementia. A retrospective chart review of patients residing in nursing facilities showed that patients older than 65 years with major depressive disorder or another depression diagnosis, who were prescribed mirtazapine, received fewer prescriptions for the anxiolytic lorazepam.[98] Although this study was not conducted on the patients with anxiety and dementia, it leads to the consideration of using mirtazapine in hopes that a prescription for benzodiazepine may not become necessary. There is also a positive case report of buspirone for use in anxiety and agitation in dementia.[99]

An open-label study investigated the effects of quetiapine compared with haloperidol on behavioral disturbances in patients with Alzheimer disease, focusing on anxiety as one of the outcome measures. Quetiapine was found to be beneficial on anxiety and depression measures compared with haloperidol, with better tolerability; though in the quetiapine group, there were also notable medical problems, namely, reversible syncope and gastroenteritis.[100]

Given the lack of guidance in the literature regarding what medications to use for the treatment of anxiety in dementia, SSRIs are recommended first, as one would for patients without dementia (doses found in **Table 5**). The choice of the antidepressant should be selected based on the lack of drug-drug interactions for those patients on many other medications and on minimizing side effects. Benzodiazepines, although effective for treatment of anxiety, should be used sparingly and briefly, given the potential of these medications to cause falls, confusion, and potentially promote tolerance and dependence to these substances.

In Summary: Treatment Recommendations for Anxiety in Dementia

- Recommend socialization and memory aids.
- Minimize changes in the caregivers and environment.
- Consider using music therapy, particularly in settings such as adult family homes and nursing homes.
- Use medications sparingly, aiming to minimize drug-drug interactions and side effects. Consider using SSRIs, mirtazapine, and buspirone.
- Reserve benzodiazepines for acute crises, and only use them sparingly and briefly.

SUMMARY

This review aims to provide clinicians an overview on how to conceptualize psychiatric problems in patients with cognitive disorders and to construct treatment plans that include both nonpharmacologic and pharmacologic approaches. It begins with a general approach to treatment, followed by specific discussions on agitation, psychosis, depression, and anxiety, for which evidence-based treatment options are presented. There are validated treatment options discussed as well as therapies limited by mixed results or even lack of studies available in the literature.

Limitations aside, there are several well-supported and guideline-recommended key elements to successful management and treatment. First, it is important to understand that all types of behavioral symptoms in cognitively impaired patients stem from a combination of physiologic, psychological, and environmental factors. Therefore, successful treatment depends on a combination of treatment modalities; limiting treatment to just a medication is often not sufficient. Nonpharmacologic approaches are recommended as the first-line treatment because medication efficacy is uncertain and the risk of side effects can be substantial, particularly in the case of atypical antipsychotics for agitation and psychosis. Some nonpharmacologic measures can be performed in the office (eg, caregiver education), others require referrals (eg, adult day health), and others involve specialists (eg, cognitive behavioral therapy). When considering a medication, informed consent with the patients or their surrogate decision maker is important, as side effects can be significant. Finally, because symptoms may change over time, ongoing reassessments and gradual dose reductions of medications improve chances of successful treatment and minimization of side effects.

In conclusion, common psychiatric problems in cognitively impaired patients are treatable, particularly when care is given to understanding the roles of the nonpharmacologic and pharmacologic options available. While research continues to develop and validate new tools, clinicians can still, with the tools on hand and the concepts described earlier, improve the quality of life for patients and their families.

REFERENCES

1. Gauthier S, Cummings J, Ballard C, et al. Management of behavioral problems in Alzheimer's disease. Int Psychogeriatr 2010;22(3):346–72.
2. Okura T, Plassman BL, Steffens DC, et al. Neuropsychiatric symptoms and the risk of institutionalization and death: the aging, demographics, and memory study. J Am Geriatr Soc 2011;59(3):473–81.
3. Stern Y, Tang MX, Albert MS, et al. Predicting time to nursing home care and death in individuals with Alzheimer disease. JAMA 1997;277(10):806–12.
4. APA Work Group on Alzheimer's Disease other Dementias, Rabins PV, Blacker D, et al. American Psychiatric Association practice guideline for the treatment of patients with Alzheimer's disease and other dementias. Second edition. Am J Psychiatry 2007;164(Suppl 12):5–56.
5. Azermai M, Petrovic M, Elseviers MM, et al. Systematic appraisal of dementia guidelines for the management of behavioural and psychological symptoms. Ageing Res Rev 2012;11(1):78–86.
6. Lyketsos CG, Colenda CC, Beck C, et al. Position statement of the American Association for Geriatric Psychiatry regarding principles of care for patients with dementia resulting from Alzheimer disease. Am J Geriatr Psychiatry 2006; 14(7):561–72.
7. Passmore MJ, Ho A, Gallagher R. Behavioral and psychological symptoms in moderate to severe Alzheimer's disease: a palliative care approach emphasizing recognition of personhood and preservation of dignity. J Alzheimers Dis 2012;29(1):1–13.
8. Cohen-Mansfield J. Nonpharmacologic interventions for inappropriate behaviors in dementia: a review, summary, and critique. Am J Geriatr Psychiatry 2001;9(4):361–81.
9. Passmore MJ, Gardner DM, Polak Y, et al. Alternatives to atypical antipsychotics for the management of dementia-related agitation. Drugs Aging 2008;25(5):381–98.

10. Schneider J, Murray J, Banerjee S, et al. EUROCARE: a cross-national study of co-resident spouse carers for people with Alzheimer's disease: I–Factors associated with carer burden. Int J Geriatr Psychiatry 1999;14(8):651–61.

11. Yaffe K, Fox P, Newcomer R, et al. Patient and caregiver characteristics and nursing home placement in patients with dementia. JAMA 2002;287(16):2090–7.

12. Selwood A, Johnston K, Katona C, et al. Systematic review of the effect of psychological interventions on family caregivers of people with dementia. J Affect Disord 2007;101(1–3):75–89.

13. Ballard CG, Margallo-Lana M, Fossey J, et al. A 1-year follow-up study of behavioral and psychological symptoms in dementia among people in care environments. J Clin Psychiatry 2001;62(8):631–6.

14. Shi S, Klotz U. Age-related changes in pharmacokinetics. Curr Drug Metab 2011;12(7):601–10.

15. Gauthier S, Wirth Y, Mobius HJ. Effects of memantine on behavioural symptoms in Alzheimer's disease patients: an analysis of the Neuropsychiatric Inventory (NPI) data of two randomised, controlled studies. Int J Geriatr Psychiatry 2005;20(5):459–64.

16. Rodda J, Morgan S, Walker Z. Are cholinesterase inhibitors effective in the management of the behavioral and psychological symptoms of dementia in Alzheimer's disease? A systematic review of randomized, placebo-controlled trials of donepezil, rivastigmine and galantamine. Int Psychogeriatr 2009; 21(5):813–24.

17. Holmes C, Wilkinson D, Dean C, et al. The efficacy of donepezil in the treatment of neuropsychiatric symptoms in Alzheimer disease. Neurology 2004;63(2): 214–9.

18. Grossberg GT, Pejovic V, Miller ML, et al. Memantine therapy of behavioral symptoms in community-dwelling patients with moderate to severe Alzheimer's disease. Dement Geriatr Cogn Disord 2009;27(2):164–72.

19. Lachaine J, Beauchemin C, Crochard A, et al. The impact of memantine and cholinesterase inhibitor initiation for Alzheimer disease on the use of antipsychotic agents: analysis using the Regie de l'Assurance Maladie du Quebec database. Can J Psychiatry 2013;58(4):195–200.

20. Vidal JS, Lacombe JM, Dartigues JF, et al. Evaluation of the impact of memantine treatment initiation on psychotropics use: a study from the French national health care database. Neuroepidemiology 2008;31(3):193–200.

21. American Psychiatric Association. Diagnostic and statistical manual of mental disorders. Fifth edition. Arlington, VA: American Psychiatric Association; 2013.

22. Salzman C, Jeste DV, Meyer RE, et al. Elderly patients with dementia-related symptoms of severe agitation and aggression: consensus statement on treatment options, clinical trials methodology, and policy. J Clin Psychiatry 2008; 69(6):889–98.

23. Fauth EB, Gibbons A. Which behavioral and psychological symptoms of dementia are the most problematic? Variability by prevalence, intensity, distress ratings, and associations with caregiver depressive symptoms. Int J Geriatr Psychiatry 2014;29(3):263–71.

24. Margallo-Lana M, Swann A, O'Brien J, et al. Prevalence and pharmacological management of behavioural and psychological symptoms amongst dementia sufferers living in care environments. Int J Geriatr Psychiatry 2001;16(1):39–44.

25. Hall GR, Buckwalter KC. Progressively lowered stress threshold: a conceptual model for care of adults with Alzheimer's disease. Arch Psychiatr Nurs 1987; 1(6):399–406.

26. Moniz Cook ED, Swift K, James I, et al. Functional analysis-based interventions for challenging behaviour in dementia. Cochrane Database Syst Rev 2012;(2): CD006929.

27. Kamble P, Chen H, Sherer JT, et al. Use of antipsychotics among elderly nursing home residents with dementia in the US: an analysis of National Survey Data. Drugs Aging 2009;26(6):483–92.

28. Ballard C, Waite J. The effectiveness of atypical antipsychotics for the treatment of aggression and psychosis in Alzheimer's disease. Cochrane Database Syst Rev 2006;(1):CD003476.

29. Maher AR, Maglione M, Bagley S, et al. Efficacy and comparative effectiveness of atypical antipsychotic medications for off-label uses in adults: a systematic review and meta-analysis. JAMA 2011;306(12):1359–69.

30. Katz IR, Jeste DV, Mintzer JE, et al. Comparison of risperidone and placebo for psychosis and behavioral disturbances associated with dementia: a randomized, double-blind trial. Risperidone Study Group. J Clin Psychiatry 1999;60(2): 107–15.

31. Street JS, Clark WS, Gannon KS, et al. Olanzapine treatment of psychotic and behavioral symptoms in patients with Alzheimer disease in nursing care facilities: a double-blind, randomized, placebo-controlled trial. The HGEU Study Group. Arch Gen Psychiatry 2000;57(10):968–76.

32. Streim JE, Porsteinsson AP, Breder CD, et al. A randomized, double-blind, placebo-controlled study of aripiprazole for the treatment of psychosis in nursing home patients with Alzheimer disease. Am J Geriatr Psychiatry 2008;16(7): 537–50.

33. Zhong KX, Tariot PN, Mintzer J, et al. Quetiapine to treat agitation in dementia: a randomized, double-blind, placebo-controlled study. Curr Alzheimer Res 2007; 4(1):81–93.

34. Declercq T, Petrovic M, Azermai M, et al. Withdrawal versus continuation of chronic antipsychotic drugs for behavioural and psychological symptoms in older people with dementia. Cochrane Database Syst Rev 2013;(3):CD007726.

35. Devanand DP, Mintzer J, Schultz SK, et al. Relapse risk after discontinuation of risperidone in Alzheimer's disease. N Engl J Med 2012;367(16):1497–507.

36. Schneider LS, Tariot PN, Dagerman KS, et al. Effectiveness of atypical antipsychotic drugs in patients with Alzheimer's disease. N Engl J Med 2006;355(15): 1525–38.

37. Schneider LS, Dagerman KS, Insel P. Risk of death with atypical antipsychotic drug treatment for dementia: meta-analysis of randomized placebo-controlled trials. JAMA 2005;294(15):1934–43.

38. Herrmann N, Lanctot KL. Do atypical antipsychotics cause stroke? CNS Drugs 2005;19(2):91–103.

39. Aupperle P. Management of aggression, agitation, and psychosis in dementia: focus on atypical antipsychotics. Am J Alzheimers Dis Other Demen 2006;21(2): 101–8.

40. Porsteinsson AP, Drye LT, Pollock BG, et al. Effect of citalopram on agitation in Alzheimer disease: The CitAD randomized clinical trial. JAMA 2014;311(7): 682–91.

41. Tariot PN, Erb R, Leibovici A, et al. Carbamazepine treatment of agitation in nursing home patients with dementia: a preliminary study. J Am Geriatr Soc 1994;42(11):1160–6.

42. Tariot PN, Erb R, Podgorski CA, et al. Efficacy and tolerability of carbamazepine for agitation and aggression in dementia. Am J Psychiatry 1998;155(1):54–61.

43. Herrmann N, Lanctot KL, Rothenburg LS, et al. A placebo-controlled trial of valproate for agitation and aggression in Alzheimer's disease. Dement Geriatr Cogn Disord 2007;23(2):116–9.

44. Porsteinsson AP, Tariot PN, Erb R, et al. Placebo-controlled study of divalproex sodium for agitation in dementia. Am J Geriatr Psychiatry 2001;9(1):58–66.

45. Tariot PN, Raman R, Jakimovich L, et al. Divalproex sodium in nursing home residents with possible or probable Alzheimer disease complicated by agitation: a randomized, controlled trial. Am J Geriatr Psychiatry 2005;13(11):942–9.

46. Kim Y, Wilkins KM, Tampi RR. Use of gabapentin in the treatment of behavioural and psychological symptoms of dementia: a review of the evidence. Drugs Aging 2008;25(3):187–96.

47. Peskind ER, Tsuang DW, Bonner LT, et al. Propranolol for disruptive behaviors in nursing home residents with probable or possible Alzheimer disease: a placebo-controlled study. Alzheimer Dis Assoc Disord 2005;19(1):23–8.

48. Wang LY, Shofer JB, Rohde K, et al. Prazosin for the treatment of behavioral symptoms in patients with Alzheimer disease with agitation and aggression. Am J Geriatr Psychiatry 2009;17(9):744–51.

49. Paulsen JS, Salmon DP, Thal LJ, et al. Incidence of and risk factors for hallucinations and delusions in patients with probable AD. Neurology 2000;54(10):1965–71.

50. Jeste DV, Finkel SI. Psychosis of Alzheimer's disease and related dementias. Diagnostic criteria for a distinct syndrome. Am J Geriatr Psychiatry 2000;8(1):29–34.

51. McKeith IG, Dickson DW, Lowe J, et al. Diagnosis and management of dementia with Lewy bodies: third report of the DLB Consortium. Neurology 2005;65(12):1863–72.

52. Miyasaki JM, Shannon K, Voon V, et al. Practice parameter: evaluation and treatment of depression, psychosis, and dementia in Parkinson disease (an evidence-based review): report of the Quality Standards Subcommittee of the American Academy of Neurology. Neurology 2006;66(7):996–1002.

53. Starkstein SE, Chemerinski E, Sabe L, et al. Prospective longitudinal study of depression and anosognosia in Alzheimer's disease. Br J Psychiatry 1997;171:47–52.

54. Steinberg M, Shao H, Zandi P, et al. Point and 5-year period prevalence of neuropsychiatric symptoms in dementia: the Cache County Study. Int J Geriatr Psychiatry 2008;23(2):170–7.

55. Teng E, Ringman JM, Ross LK, et al. Diagnosing depression in Alzheimer disease with the national institute of mental health provisional criteria. Am J Geriatr Psychiatry 2008;16(6):469–77.

56. Chemerinski E, Petracca G, Manes F, et al. Prevalence and correlates of anxiety in Alzheimer's disease. Depress Anxiety 1998;7(4):166–70.

57. Van der Mussele S, Bekelaar K, Le Bastard N, et al. Prevalence and associated behavioral symptoms of depression in mild cognitive impairment and dementia due to Alzheimer's disease. Int J Geriatr Psychiatry 2013;28(9):947–58.

58. Dunkin JJ, Anderson-Hanley C. Dementia caregiver burden: a review of the literature and guidelines for assessment and intervention. Neurology 1998;51(1 Suppl 1):S53–60 [discussion: S5–7].

59. Garcia-Alberca JM, Lara JP, Cruz B, et al. Sleep disturbances in Alzheimer's disease are associated with neuropsychiatric symptoms and antidementia treatment. J Nerv Ment Dis 2013;201(3):251–7.

60. Porta-Etessam J, Tobaruela-Gonzalez JL, Rabes-Berendes C. Depression in patients with moderate Alzheimer disease: a prospective observational cohort study. Alzheimer Dis Assoc Disord 2011;25(4):317–25.

61. Seyfried LS, Kales HC, Ignacio RV, et al. Predictors of suicide in patients with dementia. Alzheimers Dement 2011;7(6):567–73.

62. Olin JT, Schneider LS, Katz IR, et al. Provisional diagnostic criteria for depression of Alzheimer disease. Am J Geriatr Psychiatry 2002;10(2):125–8.

63. Lee HB, Lyketsos CG. Depression in Alzheimer's disease: heterogeneity and related issues. Biol Psychiatry 2003;54(3):353–62.

64. Starkstein SE, Dragovic M, Jorge R, et al. Diagnostic criteria for depression in Alzheimer disease: a study of symptom patterns using latent class analysis. Am J Geriatr Psychiatry 2011;19(6):551–8.

65. Kritz-Silverstein D, Barrett-Connor E, Corbeau C. Cross-sectional and prospective study of exercise and depressed mood in the elderly: the Rancho Bernardo study. Am J Epidemiol 2001;153(6):596–603.

66. Vital TM, Hernandez SS, Stein AM, et al. Depressive symptoms and level of physical activity in patients with Alzheimer's disease. Geriatr Gerontol Int 2012;12(4):637–42.

67. Teri L, Gibbons LE, McCurry SM, et al. Exercise plus behavioral management in patients with Alzheimer disease: a randomized controlled trial. JAMA 2003; 290(15):2015–22.

68. Sturmey P. Behavioral activation is an evidence-based treatment for depression. Behav Modif 2009;33(6):818–29.

69. Teri L, Logsdon RG, Peskind E, et al. Treatment of agitation in AD: a randomized, placebo-controlled clinical trial. Neurology 2000;55(9):1271–8.

70. Graff MJ, Vernooij-Dassen MJ, Thijssen M, et al. Effects of community occupational therapy on quality of life, mood, and health status in dementia patients and their caregivers: a randomized controlled trial. J Gerontol A Biol Sci Med Sci 2007;62(9):1002–9.

71. Regan B, Varanelli L. Adjustment, depression, and anxiety in mild cognitive impairment and early dementia: a systematic review of psychological intervention studies. Int Psychogeriatr 2013;25(12):1963–84.

72. Alexopoulos GS, Raue PJ, Kanellopoulos D, et al. Problem solving therapy for the depression-executive dysfunction syndrome of late life. Int J Geriatr Psychiatry 2008;23(8):782–8.

73. Fischer CE, Schweizer TA, Joy J, et al. Determining the impact of dementia on antidepressant treatment response in older adults. J Neuropsychiatry Clin Neurosci 2011;23(3):358–61.

74. Lyketsos CG, DelCampo L, Steinberg M, et al. Treating depression in Alzheimer disease: efficacy and safety of sertraline therapy, and the benefits of depression reduction: the DIADS. Arch Gen Psychiatry 2003;60(7):737–46.

75. Nelson JC, Devanand DP. A systematic review and meta-analysis of placebo-controlled antidepressant studies in people with depression and dementia. J Am Geriatr Soc 2011;59(4):577–85.

76. Bergh S, Selbaek G, Engedal K. Discontinuation of antidepressants in people with dementia and neuropsychiatric symptoms (DESEP study): double blind, randomised, parallel group, placebo controlled trial. BMJ 2012;344: e1566.

77. Rosenberg PB, Drye LT, Martin BK, et al. Sertraline for the treatment of depression in Alzheimer disease. Am J Geriatr Psychiatry 2010;18(2):136–45.

78. Weintraub D, Rosenberg PB, Drye LT, et al. Sertraline for the treatment of depression in Alzheimer disease: week-24 outcomes. Am J Geriatr Psychiatry 2010;18(4):332–40.
79. Banerjee S, Hellier J, Dewey M, et al. Sertraline or mirtazapine for depression in dementia (HTA-SADD): a randomised, multicentre, double-blind, placebo-controlled trial. Lancet 2011;378(9789):403–11.
80. Oudman E. Is electroconvulsive therapy (ECT) effective and safe for treatment of depression in dementia? A short review. J ECT 2012;28(1):34–8.
81. Hausner L, Damian M, Sartorius A, et al. Efficacy and cognitive side effects of electroconvulsive therapy (ECT) in depressed elderly inpatients with coexisting mild cognitive impairment or dementia. J Clin Psychiatry 2011;72(1):91–7.
82. Echavarri C, Burgmans S, Uylings H, et al. Neuropsychiatric symptoms in Alzheimer's disease and vascular dementia. J Alzheimers Dis 2013;33(3):715–21.
83. Teri L, Ferretti LE, Gibbons LE, et al. Anxiety of Alzheimer's disease: prevalence, and comorbidity. J Gerontol A Biol Sci Med Sci 1999;54(7):M348–52.
84. Ferretti L, McCurry SM, Logsdon R, et al. Anxiety and Alzheimer's disease. J Geriatr Psychiatry Neurol 2001;14(1):52–8.
85. Porter VR, Buxton WG, Fairbanks LA, et al. Frequency and characteristics of anxiety among patients with Alzheimer's disease and related dementias. J Neuropsychiatry Clin Neurosci 2003;15(2):180–6.
86. Hynninen MJ, Breitve MH, Rongve A, et al. The frequency and correlates of anxiety in patients with first-time diagnosed mild dementia. Int Psychogeriatr 2012; 24(11):1771–8.
87. Gibbons L, Teri L, Logsdon R, et al. Anxiety symptoms as predictors of nursing home placement in patients with Alzheimer's disease. Journal of Clinical Geropsychology 2002;8(4):335–42.
88. Petracca GM, Chemerinski E, Starkstein SE. A double-blind, placebo-controlled study of fluoxetine in depressed patients with Alzheimer's disease. Int Psychogeriatr 2001;13(2):233–40.
89. Starkstein SE, Jorge R, Petracca G, et al. The construct of generalized anxiety disorder in Alzheimer disease. Am J Geriatr Psychiatry 2007;15(1):42–9.
90. Snow AL, Huddleston C, Robinson C, et al. Psychometric properties of a structured interview guide for the rating for anxiety in dementia. Aging Ment Health 2012;16(5):592–602.
91. Sweeney EB, Greene E, Lawlor BA. Use of the Geriatric Anxiety Inventory–short form as a screening tool for detection of generalised anxiety in a memory clinic population. Int J Geriatr Psychiatry 2013;28(7):767–8.
92. Qazi A, Spector A, Orrell M. User, carer and staff perspectives on anxiety in dementia: a qualitative study. J Affect Disord 2010;125(1–3):295–300.
93. Paukert AL, Calleo J, Kraus-Schuman C, et al. Peaceful mind: an open trial of cognitive-behavioral therapy for anxiety in persons with dementia. Int Psychogeriatr 2010;22(6):1012–21.
94. Stanley MA, Calleo J, Bush AL, et al. The peaceful mind program: a pilot test of a cognitive-behavioral therapy-based intervention for anxious patients with dementia. Am J Geriatr Psychiatry 2013;21(7):696–708.
95. Kraus CA, Seignourel P, Balasubramanyam V, et al. Cognitive-behavioral treatment for anxiety in patients with dementia: two case studies. J Psychiatr Pract 2008;14(3):186–92.
96. Spector A, Orrell M, Lattimer M, et al. Cognitive behavioural therapy (CBT) for anxiety in people with dementia: study protocol for a randomised controlled trial. Trials 2012;13:197.

97. Ueda T, Suzukamo Y, Sato M, et al. Effects of music therapy on behavioral and psychological symptoms of dementia: a systematic review and meta-analysis. Ageing Res Rev 2013;12(2):628–41.
98. Gardner ME, Malone DC, Sey M, et al. Mirtazapine is associated with less anxiolytic use among elderly depressed patients in long-term care facilities. J Am Med Dir Assoc 2004;5(2):101–6.
99. Cooper JP. Buspirone for anxiety and agitation in dementia. J Psychiatry Neurosci 2003;28(6):469.
100. Savaskan E, Schnitzler C, Schroder C, et al. Treatment of behavioural, cognitive and circadian rest-activity cycle disturbances in Alzheimer's disease: haloperidol vs. quetiapine. Int J Neuropsychopharmacol 2006;9(5):507–16.
101. Cummings JL, Mega M, Gray K, et al. The Neuropsychiatric Inventory: comprehensive assessment of psychopathology in dementia. Neurology 1994;44(12):2308–14.
102. Kaufer DI, Cummings JL, Ketchel P, et al. Validation of the NPI-Q, a brief clinical form of the Neuropsychiatric Inventory. J Neuropsychiatry Clin Neurosci 2000;12(2):233–9.
103. Saliba D, Buchanan J. Making the investment count: revision of the Minimum Data Set for nursing homes, MDS 3.0. J Am Med Dir Assoc 2012;13(7):602–10.
104. Saliba D, DiFilippo S, Edelen MO, et al. Testing the PHQ-9 interview and observational versions (PHQ-9 OV) for MDS 3.0. J Am Med Dir Assoc 2012;13(7):618–25.

Palliative Care in Advanced Dementia

 CrossMark

Susan Merel, MD[a],*, Shaune DeMers, MD[b], Elizabeth Vig, MD, MPH[c,d]

KEYWORDS

- Dementia • Palliative care • End-of-life care • Cognitive impairment
- Skilled nursing facilities • Advance directives

KEY POINTS

- Neurodegenerative dementias are progressive and ultimately fatal diseases for which currently there is no cure. A palliative approach focusing on comfort, quality of life, and support of family and caregivers is appropriate.
- Primary care providers for patients with dementia should become proficient in the following: basic discussions of prognosis and goals of care, advance care planning, avoidance of polypharmacy when possible, pain management, and initial management of behavior and mood issues.
- There is no evidence that enteral feeding improves survival or comfort in patients with advanced dementia, and it may increase the risk of pressure ulcers and aspiration pneumonia. Careful hand-feeding is the recommended alternative.
- Infections are common in advanced dementia; antibiotics may very modestly prolong life, but may decrease comfort and contribute to antibiotic resistance and burdensome care transitions at the end of life.
- Patients with advanced dementia and behavioral disturbance should be assessed for delirium and pain, and empiric treatment of pain is often warranted.

Cure sometimes, treat often, comfort always.

— Hippocrates

THE EPIDEMIOLOGY OF ADVANCED DEMENTIA

Approximately 35.6 million people worldwide are thought to be currently living with dementia, approximately 0.5% of the population, and numbers will increase as more

---

The authors have no conflicts of interest to disclose.

[a] Division of General Internal Medicine, Department of Medicine, University of Washington, 1959 Northeast Pacific Street, Box 356429, Seattle, WA 98195-6429, USA; [b] Department of Psychiatry and Behavioral Sciences, University of Washington, 1959 Northeast Pacific Street, Box 359760, Seattle, WA 98195-6429, USA; [c] Geriatrics and Extended Care, VA Puget Sound Health Care System, University of Washington, 1660 South Columbian Way, S 182 GEC, Seattle, WA 98108, USA; [d] Division of Gerontology and Geriatric Medicine, Department of Medicine, University of Washington, Seattle, WA, USA
* Corresponding author.
E-mail address: smerel@uw.edu

Clin Geriatr Med 30 (2014) 469–492
http://dx.doi.org/10.1016/j.cger.2014.04.004

individuals live into advanced age. In the United States, the number of people with dementia is estimated to increase from 4.4 million in 2010 to 11 million in 2050.[1] Alzheimer disease (AD) is the most common type of dementia, representing 50% to 80% of cases (depending on whether "pure" or "mixed" cases are included), followed by vascular dementia (20%–30%), frontotemporal dementia (5%–10%), and dementia with Lewy bodies (<4–7.5%).[2,3] These types of dementia have different neuropathologies and variable symptoms, but all are progressive and incurable. This article focuses on common issues in advanced dementia in elderly patients with AD or vascular or mixed dementia; similar principles apply to younger patients in the final stages of these and other dementing diseases.

THE RATIONALE BEHIND A PALLIATIVE APPROACH IN DEMENTIA

Many clinicians and family members of people with dementia do not consider dementia to be a progressive and ultimately fatal illness.[4] In 2010, however, AD was noted as the sixth leading cause of death in the United States, and the fifth leading cause of death in those 65 years or older.[5] Understanding the trajectory and prognosis of dementia are essential to people with dementia and their family members as they plan for the future. Recent research has attempted to understand the trajectory of dementia, and to identify risk factors for poorer prognosis. In a recent review, Todd and colleagues noted the median survival from dementia to range from approximately 3 to 12 years after onset and approximately 3 to 7 years after diagnosis.[6] Increased age at diagnosis and impaired functional status are associated with greater mortality.

Unfortunately, 2 recent reviews noted that previous studies have not found consistent factors that increase the risk of death in people with dementia.[6,7] Although tools to help estimate prognosis in dementia exist, this lack of clarity on which factors increase the risk of death has prevented these tools from being widely adopted.[7] Without good tools to estimate prognosis in dementia and with dementia progressing at different rates in different individuals, it can be difficult for clinicians to correctly estimate prognosis, and to recognize when a patient may be eligible for hospice. The occurrence of an acute illness in a patient with advanced dementia does suggest a poor prognosis, however, and can be an opportunity to readdress prognosis and goals of care. One study of nursing home residents with dementia found a 6-month mortality rate for residents with pneumonia of 47%, a febrile episode of 45%, and "an eating problem" of 38.6%.[8]

In addition to difficulty estimating prognosis, clinicians face numerous other challenges in providing the best possible care to those living with dementia. First, there are not enough physicians trained in geriatric medicine and geriatric psychiatry to care for every patient with dementia. Palliative medicine faces similar workforce issues, and generalists will need to provide primary care, including palliative care for patients with life-limiting illnesses including dementia.[9] Second, caring for someone with dementia can be economically and psychologically costly to families.[10] Thus, caring for an individual with dementia should involve sensitivity to the needs of that individual's significant others. Third, there is no cure for dementia, and available medications have modest effects at slowing dementia progression. For these reasons, a palliative approach, including identifying the patient's goals, maximizing quality of life, aggressively managing bothersome symptoms, and focusing not only on the needs of the patient, but also the patient's family is an optimal way to care for this population.

The National Consensus Project for Quality Palliative Care's Clinical Practice Guidelines identify that palliative care is appropriate for "patients at all ages living with a persistent or recurring medical condition that adversely affects their daily functioning or will predictably reduce life expectancy," including "people living with progressive chronic conditions."[11] Although palliative care has been a growing field and a palliative approach is now more accepted for many patients with advanced illness, the palliative approach is not uniformly applied near the end of life for patients with dementia, especially those in nursing homes.[4,12] Patients with dementia in nursing homes often have burdensome symptoms and are subjected to nonbeneficial interventions, including artificial nutrition, diagnostic procedures, and hospitalizations. They are referred to hospice much less frequently than patients dying from cancer.

Applying a palliative approach more uniformly to patients with advanced dementia has potential benefit for individual patients, families, and the health system. Hospice and palliative care can improve symptoms and support families while reducing the cost of care by reducing hospitalizations and nonbeneficial interventions, and by allowing patients to die at home rather than in an institution if that is their preference.[13,14] Fortunately, the use of a palliative approach is gaining support, with access to hospice and palliative care for patients with dementia improving in the past 2 decades. A study using the Minimum Data Set (MDS) and Medicare claims showed an increase in hospice use from approximately 15% of those with advanced and 13% of those with mild-moderate dementia in 1999 to approximately 43% and 38%, respectively, in 2006. Mean length of stay in hospice also increased significantly.[15] Guidelines for optimal palliative care in patients with dementia were recently released by the European Association for Palliative Care (see **Box 1** for a list of palliative care domains).[16] In the United States, the National Hospice and Palliative Care Organization provides a set of care guidelines.[17]

What follows is a discussion of the aspects of dementia that may be amenable to a palliative approach. Because of the workforce issues discussed previously, primary care providers caring for elderly patients will need to become comfortable providing primary palliative care for patients with dementia at all stages. See **Fig. 1** for a list of relevant issues for primary care providers to address with patients with dementia and their families.

THE END OF LIFE IN DEMENTIA

Although dementias may present with different symptoms and progress at different rates, the terminal stage of all dementias is similar. People with dementia develop apraxia, dysphagia, decreased mobility, and decreased ability to report early symptoms that lead to infection, malnutrition, and other adverse outcomes.[4] The main causes of death in patients with advanced dementia are pneumonia, other infections, and cardiovascular and cerebrovascular events; the latter are more common in patients with vascular or mixed dementia.[4,18] See **Box 2** for a summary of contributing factors to death from dementia, common causes of death, and common end-of-life symptoms.

Recent studies have described the experience of dying from dementia, including symptom prevalence and the nature and frequency of transitions of care near the end of life. In a study of 323 nursing home residents with advanced dementia in the United States, Mitchell found high symptom prevalence in the last 18 months of life. She also found increased prevalence of pain, dyspnea, agitation, aspiration, and pressure ulcers in the last 3 months of life, with prevalence between 25% and 35% for each symptom.[8] Hospital transfers of nursing home residents with advanced dementia are frequent in the United States, but may not be beneficial. Gozalo and colleagues[19] examined MDS data from nearly 475,000 US nursing home residents with advanced dementia. They found that 19% of the population had at least one transfer in the last 120 days of life. Risk factors for hospital transfer included nonwhite race, male

---

Box 1
Eleven domains of optimal palliative care, with selected recommendations from the European Association for Palliative Care (all domains included; recommendations selected from the full list of 57)

1. Applicability of palliative care

    1.2. Improving quality of life, maintaining function, and maximizing comfort, which also are goals of palliative care, can be considered appropriate in dementia throughout the disease trajectory, with the emphasis on particular goals changing over time.

2. Person-centered care, communication, and shared decision making

3. Setting care goals and advance planning

    3.2. Anticipating progression of the disease, advance care planning is proactive. This implies it should start as soon as the diagnosis is made, when the patient can still be actively involved and patient preferences, values, needs, and beliefs can be elicited.

4. Continuity of care

    4.4. Transfers between settings require communication on care plans between former and new professional caregivers and patients and families.

5. Prognostication and timely recognition of dying

    5.2. Prognostication in dementia is challenging and mortality cannot be predicted accurately. However, combining clinical judgment and tools for mortality predictions can provide an indication that may facilitate discussion of prognosis.

6. Avoiding overly aggressive, burdensome, or futile treatment

    6.4. Hydration, preferably subcutaneous, may be provided if appropriate, such as in the case of infection; it is inappropriate in the dying phase (*only moderate consensus*).

    6.6. Antibiotics may be appropriate in treating infections with the goal of increasing comfort by alleviating the symptoms of infection. Life-prolonging effects need to be considered, especially in the case of treatment decisions around pneumonia.

7. Optimal treatment of symptoms and providing comfort

    7.3. Tools to assess pain, discomfort, and behavior should be used for screening and monitoring of patients with moderate and severe dementia, evaluating effectiveness of interventions.

8. Psychosocial and spiritual support

    8.3. Religious activities, such as rituals, songs, and services, may help the patient because these may be recognized even in severe dementia.

9. Family care and involvement

10. Education of the health care team

11. Societal and ethical issues

    11.6. Economic and systemic incentives should encourage excellent end-of-life care for patients with dementia.

From Van der Steen JT, Radbruch L, Hertogh CM, et al. White paper defining optimal palliative care in older people with dementia: a Delphi study and recommendations from the European Association for Palliative Care. Palliat Med 2014;28(3):197–209.

---

sex, lack of an advance directive, lack of a do not resuscitate order, and lack of a do not hospitalize order. Givens and colleagues[20] examined emergency room and hospital transfers of 323 nursing home residents with advanced dementia. In this population, 16% were hospitalized and 10% visited an emergency room over an 18-month

Element	Stage of dementia

Communicating the diagnosis
Communicating prognosis
Helping patient and family with anticipatory grief
Assessing decisional capacity
Helping patient assign a surrogate decision maker
Discussing goals of care
Discussing the role of artificial nutrition
Discussing the role of antibiotics
Helping patient and surrogate complete advance directives
Planning for transitions in living situation if necessary
Assessing medication appropriateness
Assessing for comorbid depression
Assessing and treating pain
Assessing and treating delirium
Reassessing goals of care and appropriateness of hospital transfer
Making hospice referral when appropriate
Managing terminal pain and delirium
Responding to family's grief after patient death
Expressing condolences
Referring to community resources for grief counseling

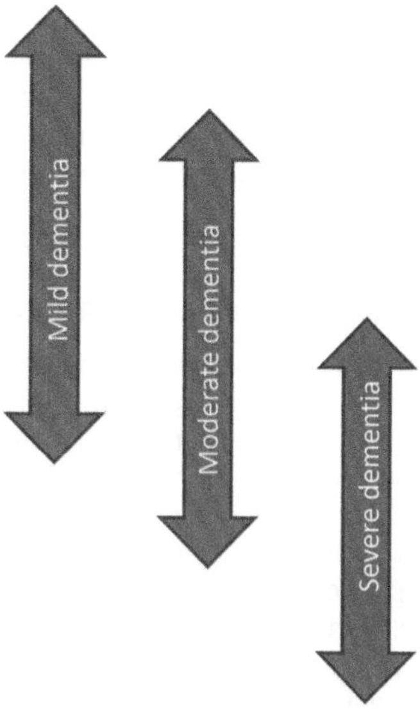

Mild dementia

Moderate dementia

Severe dementia

Fig. 1. Essential elements of primary palliative care in patients with dementia.

Box 2
Contributing factors, causes of death, and common symptoms at the end of life

Contributing factors

  Apraxia

  Dysphagia

  Malnutrition

  Decreased mobility

  Decreased ability to report symptoms

Common symptoms

  Pain

  Agitation

  Shortness of breath

  Aspiration

  Pressure ulcers

Causes of death

  Pneumonia

  Cardiac events

  Cerebrovascular events

  Other infections

Data from Refs.[4,18,116]

period. The most frequent reason for hospitalization was suspected infection and the most frequent reason for emergency room transfer was feeding tube problems. Clinicians, patients, and caregivers should consider discussing likely future causes of death, common end-of-life symptoms, and the possibility of end-of-life transfers between facilities. As will be discussed in subsequent sections, burdensome end-of-life transitions can often be avoided with clear advance directives and thoughtful management of symptoms and acute events.

MANAGEMENT DECISIONS RELATED TO CARE OF PATIENTS WITH ADVANCED DEMENTIA
The Role of Artificial Nutrition at the End of Life

Up to one-third of nursing home residents with advanced dementia had feeding tubes, based on 1999 MDS data. There is wide geographic and socioeconomic variation in the prevalence of this practice.[21] Placement of percutaneous endoscopic gastrostomy (PEG) tubes in elderly hospitalized patients increased between 1993 and 2003, and placement in hospitalized patients with Alzheimer dementia doubled from 5% to 10%.[22] The intention of PEG placement is to improve nutritional status, reduce aspiration, and improve patient comfort and longevity. Financial incentives to both skilled nursing facilities and hospitals favor placement of PEG tubes. Placement of a new feeding tube qualifies a patient for skilled nursing services under Medicare, and patients with advanced dementia who are hand-fed require more staff time than those with feeding tubes. Although weight loss is part of dementia progression, this may be mistaken for negligence or mistreatment by nursing homes.[23]

There is no evidence that enteral feeding improves patient outcomes, and there is significant evidence that feeding tubes may be harmful.[24] A 2009 Cochrane review found no evidence that enteral feeding prolongs survival, improves quality of life, improves nutrition, or decreases the risk of pressure sores. Some evidence suggests that enteral feeding increases the risk of aspiration pneumonia in patients with dementia.[25] A prospective cohort study of more than 30,000 nursing home residents with advanced dementia and eating problems found no survival benefit with feeding tubes.[26] A second cohort study of nursing home residents with advanced dementia and eating difficulties found that residents with a PEG tube were 2.27 times more likely to develop a new pressure ulcer (95% confidence interval 1.95–2.65), and less likely to have an existing ulcer heal. Decreased mobility and increased diarrhea with artificial nutrition are the likely mechanisms for this association.[27] Both the American Geriatrics Society and the American Academy of Hospice and Palliative Medicine recommend against placement of percutaneous feeding tubes in patients with advanced dementia. The practice was recently included on both organizations' lists of "Five Things Physicians and Patients Should Question" as part of the national Choosing Wisely campaign.[24,28] Please see **Box 3** for more information.

The recommended approach in patients with advanced dementia and dysphagia is careful hand-feeding for comfort. A paradigm of "Comfort Feeding Only" has been suggested for discussions with families and nursing home staff, emphasizing the importance of focusing on the patient's comfort in all interactions around nutrition.[29] Optimal hand-feeding in patients with advanced dementia includes upright positioning, use of preferred foods and foods with strong flavors, offering smaller boluses, and frequent reminders to swallow.[24] A systematic review of oral feeding options in patients with dementia concluded that high-calorie supplements help people with dementia and feeding problems gain weight; one study found better pressure ulcer healing with supplementation, but no study showed improvements in function, cognition, or mortality with high-calorie supplements.[30]

Box 3
The case against artificial nutrition in advanced dementia

Feeding tubes in patients with advanced dementia:

Are risky and associated with morbidity, mortality, and frequent hospitalization.

- Periprocedural mortality of patients with dementia is estimated at 6% to 28%[113]
- 64% mortality in the year after placement with a median survival of 56 days[114]
- Approximately 20% require replacement or repositioning, within a median of 145 days after placement[114]
- Nursing home residents with dementia and feeding tubes have an average of 9 hospitalized days per patient in the year after placement[114]

Do not improve survival, nutrition, quality of life, or the risk of aspiration pneumonia.

- Meaningful improvement in nutritional parameters has not been proven[113]
- Tube feeding does not improve survival or the risk of aspiration pneumonia[25]
- No evidence that tube feeding improves quality of life[25,31]

Cause harm and suffering.

- Increase social isolation by removing the necessity for patients to participate in mealtime
- Are associated with increased use of physical and chemical restraints[115]
- Are associated with an increased risk of developing a new pressure ulcer[27]
- Respondents whose loved ones died with a feeding tube were less likely to report excellent end-of-life care than those whose loved ones did not have a feeding tube[31]

There is room for improvement in shared decision making with families about PEG tube placement in patients with advanced dementia. In a mortality follow-back survey of 486 family members whose loved one died of dementia, approximately one-third of those whose loved one died with a feeding tube did not recall discussing risks associated with feeding tube insertion, and approximately half felt the health care provider was strongly in favor of feeding tube insertion.[31] A written or audio decision aid was tested in a randomized controlled trial of nursing home residents with advanced dementia and feeding problems and their surrogate decision makers. Surrogates who used the decision aid reported less decisional conflict, more certainty in their preference for oral feeding, decreased expectations of benefits from tube feeding, and more discussion of feeding options with a health care provider.[32]

Infections and the Role of Antibiotics in Advanced Dementia

Infections are a common cause of death in patients with advanced dementia, and unexplained febrile episodes are also common. Antimicrobials are given often in this setting, but evidence suggests that although antimicrobials in patients with advanced dementia may modestly prolong life, even oral antibiotics are associated with decreased comfort. One prospective cohort study of 214 nursing home residents with advanced dementia found that 66% received at least one course of antibiotics, with a mean number of 4 courses per resident during an average of 322 days of follow-up. Quinolones and third-generation cephalosporins were the most commonly prescribed antimicrobials in this study. Among the 99 patients who died during the study period, approximately 42% received antimicrobials during the 2 weeks preceding death, and nearly 42% were parenteral.[33] Another study found that severity of dementia was the most important predictor of mortality from pneumonia, rather than type of treatment of pneumonia.[34] A study of fever in institutionalized patients with AD showed no difference in survival between patients with the most advanced dementia given antibiotics and those treated with comfort measures.[35] A retrospective cohort study of patients with severe dementia and gram-negative bacteremia showed that patients with decubitus ulcers and bacteremia who received appropriate antibiotics did not survive longer than those given inappropriate antimicrobials.[36]

Studies of patients with advanced dementia and pneumonia have suggested a survival benefit from antibiotics, but no improvement in comfort. In a prospective study of nursing home residents with advanced dementia, 56% to 64% of those treated with oral, intramuscular, or intravenous antibiotics were alive 90 days after the episode of pneumonia, as compared with 33% not treated with antimicrobials. Notably, intravenous antibiotics did not confer a survival benefit over oral antibiotics in this cohort. Comfort levels, as measured by a standardized scale completed by a nurse, were inversely associated with aggressiveness of treatment. Those not receiving antibiotics had the highest comfort levels, and those receiving intravenous antibiotics had the lowest.[37] A similar study of nursing home residents with advanced dementia and pneumonia found an association between antibiotics and decreased 10-day mortality, but no association between antibiotic use and 6-month mortality.[38] Frequent antibiotic use in the nursing home setting adds to the burden of antimicrobial resistance, with E coli susceptibility to ciprofloxacin as low as 59% in some sites in a study of antimicrobial susceptibilities in long-term care facilities.[39] In the setting of unclear mortality benefit, no clear improvement in comfort with antibiotics, and possible harm to the population, antibiotic use should be considered carefully in patients with advanced dementia. In patients whose surrogates think they have an unacceptable quality of life, antibiotics should generally be avoided.[40]

Polypharmacy and Medication Appropriateness

Most patients with dementia have multiple comorbidities and are on multiple medications, and medications may be added for symptom management as dementia progresses. In one study of nursing home residents with advanced dementia, patients were prescribed a mean of approximately 15 medications during the 6 months before study enrollment. In patients who died, the total number of medications did not decrease as illness progressed. Some medications were stopped as others were added for symptom management.[41] Adding medications increases the likelihood of adverse drug reactions, drug-drug reactions, and drug-disease interactions. In a small study of patients with advanced dementia enrolled in a palliative care program who underwent medication review by 12 geriatricians using a modified Delphi process, patients were taking an average of 6.5 medications. Ten (29%) of the 34 patients were taking a medication considered inappropriate in patients with advanced dementia.[42] Clinicians caring for patients with dementia should be familiar with the Beers Criteria for potentially inappropriate medication use in older adults, the shorter list of medications frequently associated with adverse drug events requiring hospitalization, and lists of medications that may be inappropriate in patients with advanced dementia.[42–45] In addition, beneficial medications in patients with longer life expectancy should be readdressed as patients enter the more advanced stages of dementia. See **Box 4** for a list of medications that are potentially inappropriate in patients with advanced dementia.

Management of Pain in Advanced Dementia

Patients with advanced dementia may have painful comorbid conditions, such as osteoarthritis, and some common infectious complications of advanced dementia, such as decubitus ulcers, pneumonia, or urinary tract infections, can be painful. Assessment and management of pain in patients with dementia can be challenging. Patients often

---

Box 4
Medications that may be inappropriate in patients with advanced dementia

Lipid-lowering medications

Cytotoxic chemotherapy

Antiplatelet agents, excluding aspirin

Immunomodulators

Sex hormones

Hydralazine

Sulfonylureas

Bisphosphonates

Insulin

Warfarin

Appetite stimulants

Digoxin

Clonidine

Alpha-blockers

Data from Refs.[42–45]

---

cannot report pain, and often manifest pain as nonspecific symptoms such as agitation or decreased oral intake.[4] Pharmacologic management of pain in patients with dementia also can be challenging because patients cannot report side effects and are susceptible to adverse effects from medications. Pain is often undertreated in patients with dementia, which can lead to functional disturbance and decreased quality of life.[46,47]

Patients with advanced dementia may not manifest typical pain behaviors, such as guarding or moaning, but instead may appear fearful, combative, agitated, or withdrawn.[46] Careful assessment of the patient's behavior and facial expressions is essential in assessing pain. A study comparing patients with and without dementia receiving dressing changes for decubitus ulcers concluded that clinician observation of facial expressions and vocalizations are accurate in assessing the presence but not the intensity of pain in patients with dementia.[48] Common pain behaviors in cognitively impaired older patients include changes in sleep patterns or gait, decreased social interactions or withdrawal, rapid blinking or distorted expression, or increased crying.[49] A number of structured tools for pain assessment in nonverbal patients are available, including the Pain Assessment in Advanced Dementia; these tools can be helpful but should be used as only one element of a complete history and physical examination.[49] The Assessment of Discomfort in Dementia (ADD) protocol, a structured protocol for nursing assessment of discomfort and treatment with nonpharmacologic interventions with escalation to nonopioid and then opioid analgesics, has been shown to decrease discomfort and behavioral disturbances without an increase in the use of antipsychotic medications. Nonpharmacologic interventions suggested in the ADD protocol include distraction with pleasant activities or interaction; cold and heat applied to painful areas; supervised ambulation or other physical activity, including use of a glide rocker; sensory stimulation, such as pet or music therapy; and conversation, storytelling, or life review for patients who are still verbal.[50] A similar protocol for empiric treatment of pain with acetaminophen, morphine, or other agents in nursing home residents with moderate to severe dementia showed reduced agitation in the intervention group compared with the control group.[51] Empiric treatment for pain should always be considered in patients with dementia and new behavioral disturbance.

Guidelines for pain management in the frail elderly population are applicable to patients with dementia; acetaminophen is first line and nonsteroidal anti-inflammatory drugs should be avoided in this group because of significant toxicities.[52] Opioids should be considered in all patients with pain or behavioral disturbance not responsive to acetaminophen. Patients with dementia should be monitored closely on initiation of opioids because of side effects, including nausea, constipation, and sedation; opioids can cause impaired sleep architecture but can improve sleep if they reduce pain.[46]

Role of Specific Pharmacologic Agents for Dementia

There are 4 medications approved by the Food and Drug Administration (FDA) for the treatment of symptoms of dementia; 3 acetylcholinesterase inhibitors (AChEIs: donepezil, rivastigmine, galantamine) and 1 N-methyl-D-aspartate receptor antagonist (memantine). Although no treatment has been found to be disease-modifying, modest improvements in cognitive function, activities of daily living (ADLs), and behavior have been observed in some patients treated with AChEIs, memantine, or both in combination.[53–55] The decision to prescribe these medications is based on identification of appropriate target symptoms in individual patients, keeping in mind possible side effects (primarily gastrointestinal, sleep-related, and bradycardia in the case of AChEIs).

Although beneficial effects of these medications appear to be independent of dementia severity, experts have questioned their use in the later stages of neurodegenerative diseases, a time when polypharmacy is both common and associated with greater mortality.[45,56–58] Despite this, approximately 20% of persons with dementia are taking either an AChEI or memantine at the time of transition to hospice care.[56] Stopping these medications may precipitate swifter decline in some patients or increase behavioral problems.[59–61] The decision to stop AChEIs or memantine, like the decision to start them, should be done thoughtfully with involvement of family and care staff monitoring for alterations in levels of alertness, confusion, and changes in behavior.[62]

Management of Terminal Delirium in Patients with Advanced Dementia

Delirium at the end of life (terminal delirium) is common, affecting up to 88% of patients during their final week of life, and is challenging to treat.[63] There are several essential questions in determining the approach to terminal delirium in patients with advanced dementia. First, is the patient actively dying? Although delirium in the last months of life may be reversible with treatment of underlying causes, such as infection, reversal is unlikely within days to weeks of death. Brain function inevitably unravels as part of the dying process, and attempts to reverse this may not be fruitful. Second, what is the family caregiver's perception of the patient's quality of life before the delirium, and does the caregiver think the delirium is causing the patient to suffer? In patients who seemed comfortable and content before an acute episode of presumed terminal delirium, a judicious, spare medical workup may sometimes be appropriate. This might include a thorough physical examination, basic screening laboratory tests, and perhaps a urinalysis or chest radiograph as directed by the physical examination. Third, if family members, caregivers, or nursing staff express distress regarding a patient's terminal delirium, does this reflect the patient's suffering or the observers' anticipatory grief? Dying patients' delirium can cause their loved ones to suffer. In several studies, hallucinations and motor agitation were the features most associated with caregiver and family distress.[64–66] Family caregivers may sometimes ask for aggressive interventions at the end of life as a part of their grieving process, and supportive listening and grief counseling are as important as attention to the patient's symptoms.

In most cases of true terminal delirium in advanced dementia, an aggressive search for an underlying cause is not appropriate. Before embarking on any search for a cause, it is important to readdress goals of care with the family decision maker and assess whether the decision maker perceives the patient's quality of life to be acceptable based on his or her prior discussions and knowledge. Families often need permission to abandon the usual medical approach to new problems and to focus solely on symptom management.

Although most dying patients will experience delirium, there are few studies examining treatment strategies. A 2012 Cochrane Collaboration review of pharmacologic treatment of terminal delirium found only one trial that met their inclusion criteria.[67] This study, by Breitbart and colleagues in 1996, randomized 30 hospitalized patients with AIDS and delirium to receive an antipsychotic (chlorpromazine or haloperidol) or the benzodiazepine lorazepam.[68] Both antipsychotics were equally effective at improving symptoms of delirium, but all patients who received lorazepam developed either oversedation and/or increased confusion. Nonpharmacological strategies, resolution of underlying medical problems, and avoidance of deliriogenic medications are the foundations of management for all types of delirium. If medications are necessary, low-dose haloperidol is the treatment of choice, followed by atypical antipsychotics (quetiapine, risperidone, olanzapine) as second-line agents.[69] Many clinicians will be more liberal with the dose and frequency of antipsychotics in terminal delirium than in other forms of delirium, giving low doses as often as every one or two hours.[70] Opioids are also a mainstay of treatment of patients with dementia at the very end of life, as with patients dying of any disease, and should generally be added empirically, as pain can always be a contributor to delirium. Although opioids can contribute to delirium, a patient with true terminal delirium should generally have a trial of opioids in the hopes of improving comfort.

Management of Mood and Behavior

The neuropsychiatric complications of AD have been well-characterized in several studies, and affect up to 60% of community-dwelling and 80% of institutionalized patients with dementia.[71–74] Patients with advanced dementia may experience apathy, fearfulness, agitation, and psychotic symptoms that can be difficult to diagnose and manage.[75] Caregivers and medical providers should be vigilant for signs of an acute medical problem as the cause for any new behavioral or mental status change, as it is often difficult to distinguish between delirium and depression, for example, in patients with advanced dementia; see **Table 1** for more details.

Diagnosing depression in persons with advanced dementia is frequently complicated by the presence of vegetative symptoms (poor sleep, low energy, anorexia) due to comorbid medical disorders or medication effects.[76] Therefore, some experts advocate for a focus on emotional symptoms of depression, such as sadness and hopelessness, but this is challenging to assess in patients with limited communication. Persons with advanced dementia may express their depression behaviorally, by refusing to eat or engage with caregivers, or by becoming agitated and irritable.[77]

There is insufficient evidence to recommend the routine use of antidepressants for depression in patients with advanced dementia. A small placebo-controlled study of sertraline in patients with dementia with a minimum Mini-Mental State Examination (MMSE) score of 10 and a mean MMSE of approximately 17 suggested improvement in scores on a standardized scale for depression in dementia, behavioral disturbance,

Table 1
Distinguishing depression from delirium in patients with advanced dementia

Features	Depression	Delirium
Onset	Gradual (weeks to months)	Abrupt (hours to days)
Mood	Sad, hopeless	Labile; frequent mood shifts
Affect	Withdrawn, irritable	Confused
Course	Mostly stable, with some good and bad days	Variable depending on underlying disorder
Level of awareness	Generally alert, does not fluctuate	Prominent fluctuations throughout the day, may be somnolent or agitated
Level of attention	Minor impairment	Major impairment, easily distracted
Psychotic symptoms	Uncommon	Delusions, hallucinations common

ADLs, and caregiver distress, but a Cochrane meta-analysis of trials in patients with a mean MMSE score of 19 (mild to moderate stage) concluded that there is only weak evidence for the efficacy of antidepressants in dementia.[78,79] Small studies suggest that psychostimulants may be effective in treating symptoms of depression in the terminally ill, with a response seen quickly, but these have not been studied extensively in advanced dementia and we do not use these routinely in practice.[80] The management of depression in advanced dementia requires both a high index of suspicion and a creative care plan that involves caregiver support; there is no evidence to support the initiation of antidepressants in patients with severe dementia (eg, MMSE <10) but a trial may be warranted in select patients with severe symptoms, such as anxiety, fearfulness, or dysphoria.

Difficult behaviors that may manifest in advanced dementia include agitation, aggression, combativeness, and resistance to care, sometimes driven by hallucinations and delusions. Potentially effective strategies to manage difficult behaviors include skills training and education for caregivers, pleasant activity planning, environmental redesign, music therapy, and exercise. Involving caregivers is critical.[81,82] Because some of these behaviors seem driven by psychotic symptoms, antipsychotics are frequently prescribed, despite no FDA approval for this indication.[83] A meta-analysis of 16 randomized controlled trials concluded that risperidone and olanzapine are associated with both a significant improvement in aggression and psychosis and a significantly higher incidence of serious adverse cerebrovascular events and extrapyramidal side effects; most subjects included in the meta-analysis had severe dementia with a mean MMSE between 5 and 8.[84] The evidence for negative outcomes led the FDA to add a warning to atypical antipsychotics about the risk of cerebrovascular events and death in patients with dementia. There are some limitations to these studies (designed and powered to study efficacy of antipsychotic, not causal relationship between drug and cerebrovascular accident or death; cerebrovascular events not validated in all studies; limited information on causes of death, comorbidity, concurrent medications), however, and although mechanisms for the adverse outcomes have been suggested, none have been proven.[74] Although caution is warranted with antipsychotics in patients with mild to moderate dementia and behavioral disturbances that do not significantly impair the patient's quality of life, clinicians and families may opt to use them more liberally in patients with more advanced dementia and significant behavioral disturbance if the benefits to the patient's quality of life outweigh potential risks. A careful risk-benefit discussion should be had with the family, weighing the risk of adverse events against the potential to improve the patient's quality of life if behavioral symptoms are causing severe distress.

The only other class of psychotropics that has some proven efficacy in management of behavioral disturbances in persons with dementia is the acetylcholinesterase inhibitors, although like antidepressants these have not been studied for this indication in patients with severe dementia. A Cochrane review showed modest but significant benefit in neuropsychiatric symptom scores in patients with an MMSE between 10 and 26.[85] There is no evidence for efficacy of antidepressants, mood stabilizers, benzodiazepines, or trazodone. See **Box 5** for a basic approach to the treatment of problematic behaviors in patients with advanced dementia.

Role of Hospice and Barriers to Eligibility

Hospice care is likely beneficial to patients with dementia and their families. Two studies identified that bereaved families of people dying with advanced dementia reported fewer unmet needs, a higher rating of the quality of care, and a better quality of dying if the person with dementia received hospice before death.[86,87] People with advanced dementia who receive hospice services are less likely to die in the hospital than others with dementia who do not receive hospice.[13,14] One small study found lower rates of depression and anxiety in bereaved spouses of people with AD when the person with dementia received hospice before death.[88] However, studies have not found a clear improvement in pain assessment and management in patients enrolled in hospice, although one study showed that nursing home residents with advanced dementia enrolled in hospice were more likely to receive scheduled opioids for pain and treatment for dyspnea than those not receiving hospice services.[13,14,89]

Although the use of hospice by people with advanced dementia has been increasing, this may change in the future. One reason is that "debility," a hospice diagnosis used until 2013 to qualify people with less advanced dementia plus other chronic

---

Box 5
Approach to the treatment of behavioral disturbances in patients with advanced dementia

- Evaluate for occult medical problems and pain; treat if present.

- Simplify the patient's medication list if possible, reducing or stopping medications that may be deliriogenic.

- Look for environmental triggers and teach caregivers ways to manage behavior. Consider medications if these fail.

- Consider a trial of antidepressants if the patient shows signs of dysphoria or anxiety.

- Consider a trial of antipsychotics if the patient seems to be experiencing considerable distress from delusions and agitation.

  - Although a very cautious approach is warranted in moderate dementia with behavioral disturbance, a more liberal approach may be warranted in patients with advanced dementia.

  - Have a risk-benefit discussion with the patient's surrogate discussing the possible increased risk of stroke or death before starting antipsychotics.

    - Consider checking a baseline electrocardiogram for prolonged QT interval depending on the risk-benefit discussion with the surrogate and their tolerance for risk.

    - Reevaluate periodically for efficacy and side effects.

Data from Sink K, Holden K, Yaffe K. Pharmacological treatment of neuropsychiatric symptoms of dementia: a review of the evidence. JAMA 2005;293(5):596–608.

conditions and evidence of decline, is no longer an acceptable hospice diagnosis. In late 2014, providers will be required to designate the type of dementia when certifying a patient for hospice.[90] Although Medicare has hospice eligibility criteria for AD, it does not have specific criteria for other dementias. If a patient with advanced non-AD has comfort-focused goals, to certify that individual for hospice care it will be important to make a clear case that the patient has declined, and has had complications of end-stage dementia, such as infections and/or weight loss. The hospice organization will work with the provider to determine if the patient is hospice eligible. If a patient is not deemed to be hospice eligible, providers should be aware of additional resources in their communities, such as home care and palliative care programs. In addition to regulatory barriers to hospice enrollment by people with advanced dementia, additional barriers include dementia not being recognized as a terminal illness, difficulty in estimating prognosis in advanced dementia, and challenges reimbursing for hospice services in nursing facilities. The current hospice eligibility criteria for dementia are noted in **Box 6**.

ADVANCE CARE PLANNING IN PATIENTS WITH DEMENTIA

Advance care planning is an essential part of care in persons with dementia and should start soon after diagnosis. Dementia management quality measures call for

---

Box 6
Medicare hospice eligibility criteria for dementia

This section is specific for Alzheimer dementia and related disorders, and may not be appropriate for other types of dementia, such as vascular dementia.

Patients with dementia should show all the following characteristics:

1. Stage 7 or beyond according to the Functional Assessment Staging Tool (FAST)
2. Unable to ambulate without assistance
3. Unable to dress without assistance
4. Unable to bathe without assistance
5. Urinary and fecal incontinence, intermittent or constant
6. No consistently meaningful verbal communication: stereotypical phrases only or the ability to speak is limited to 6 or fewer intelligible words

Patients should have 1 of the following within the past 12 months:

1. Aspiration pneumonia
2. Pyelonephritis or other upper urinary tract infection
3. Septicemia
4. Decubitus ulcers, multiple, stage 3 or 4
5. Fever, recurrent after antibiotics
6. Inability to maintain sufficient fluid and calorie intake with 10% weight loss during the previous 6 months or serum albumin less than 2.5 g/dL

Note that these criteria may exclude some patients with dementia who have a life expectancy of less than 6 months, and may include others who will live longer than 6 months, and may be discharged from hospice. When patients have significant comorbidities, these should be considered when making a hospice referral.

Adapted from Centers for Medicare and Medicaid Services. Local Coverage Determination (LCD): Hospice Determining Terminal Status (L32015).

comprehensive counseling regarding end-of-life decision making, the assignment of a surrogate decision maker, and plans for symptom management at the end of life within 2 years of diagnosis.[91] In the United States, aggressive life-sustaining care, including cardiopulmonary resuscitation (CPR), is the default, despite its futility in patients with a terminal illness, such as advanced dementia. Studies suggest that most elderly patients would not want CPR or other life-prolonging measures if they were to develop dementia; however, many patients with dementia continue to receive CPR and other life-sustaining treatments.[92] Advance directives are imperfect, and some have suggested a paradigm shift in which aggressive care would not be the default for patients with dementia; barring such a dramatic change in policy, advance directives and continued thoughtful conversations about goals of care are necessary.[93,94] Early discussions with the patient and family should focus on detailed information about prognosis and the natural course of dementia. This allows the patient and family to come to terms with the diagnosis and understand what they may face in the future. Early completion of a power of attorney for health care, finances, and other legal decisions is also important, to ensure that the patient's affairs will be managed appropriately when they lose the ability to do so.

Traditional health care advance directives are inadequate for patients with dementia and many other chronic debilitating illnesses because they often address the person's wishes in the case of a persistent vegetative state or immediately terminal condition, but do not recognize the many end-of-life circumstances that can occur. The Five Wishes Advance Directive, which is a legal advance directive in most states, is more comprehensive and may be helpful for people with dementia and their families. It does not require legal assistance or a notary in many states, although there is a small charge for its use.[95] Video decision support tools for advance directives are now used by some health systems and have been used to assist in decisions regarding future care if an individual were to develop dementia. Studies suggest that the use of these videos may result in patients with dementia being less likely to choose aggressive care at the end of life, having more stable preferences over time, and being more likely to concur with their surrogate about their end-of-life choices.[96,97] Advance care planning conversations with patients with dementia and their surrogates should include discussions about sites of future care, preferences regarding nutrition and antibiotics, and reassurances that every effort to ensure comfort will be taken, regardless of their other care choices. A discussion of whether the patient should be hospitalized near the end of life is an important element of advance care planning with patients with dementia in nursing facilities. End-of-life hospitalizations can be burdensome to frail elders with dementia, but are common. "Do Not Hospitalize" orders are reasonable for many patients with advanced dementia, and can be enacted but are relatively rare nationally.[98] Although advance care planning is helpful, it is not universal among patients with dementia and their families.[99] Barriers include lack of knowledge or avoidance on the part of providers, failure to discuss the prognosis of dementia in detail, and the burdens of illness and caregiving.[99] Important elements in advance care planning for people with dementia are listed in **Box 7**.

The POLST program, although not specific to patients with dementia, has been an important recent development, and is especially relevant to patients with advanced dementia living in nursing facilities. The National POLST Paradigm Program started in Oregon in 1991 as an effort to increase the ability to honor patient preferences for end-of-life care. The POLST system identifies patients' wishes regarding medical treatment and creates portable medical orders, including wishes regarding resuscitation status, hospitalization, artificial nutrition, and antibiotics. Mature, endorsed, or developing POLST programs are available in 43 states.[100] The POLST program has

---

Box 7
Important elements of advance care planning for patients with dementia

- Determination of the patient's decisional capacity to appoint a surrogate decision maker and make decisions about care
- Selection of a surrogate decision maker for health care decisions as well as a financial power of attorney
- Discussion of current and future sites of care and their safety
  - Discussion of the role of nursing facility care and/or home hospice care at the end of life
- Completion of detailed advanced directives covering the following issues
  - Resuscitation status
  - Hospitalization status
  - Decision about artificial nutrition
  - Decision about the role of hydration
  - Decision about when antibiotics might be used or avoided
- Completion of Physician Orders for Life-Sustaining Treatment[100] form or similar if available in your state
  - If not available, consider "Do Not Hospitalize" order if in a facility

---

been proven to increase the number of patients in nursing facilities who have documented treatment preferences that are honored by the facility and their providers.[101]

Clinicians caring for patients with advanced dementia must become comfortable with helping surrogates make decisions for their loved ones. A study of surrogate decision makers who had recently made decisions for elderly hospitalized patients identified communication needs of surrogates as frequent communication, information, and emotional support, and found that the surrogates formed strong relationships with medical teams rather than individuals in the inpatient setting.[102] Although surrogates should be making decisions using the principle of substituted judgment, they need education to ensure that this occurs. One study of surrogate decision makers in Germany using experimental vignettes suggested that family surrogates of patients with dementia tend to refer to their own preferences and decide intuitively, as compared to professional guardians. The family decision makers were less likely to consent to aggressive measures including a feeding tube.[103]

Physician-assisted suicide is legal in 4 states in the United States, but the related laws specify that those requesting physician-assisted suicide must have decisional capacity. Those with advanced dementia, however, are no longer able to make their own medical decisions; thus, they are currently not eligible for physician-assisted suicide. Advance directives for euthanasia are legally recognized in the Netherlands, but are rarely used.[104] Two US ethicists recently speculated on whether advance directives for physician-assisted suicide could be implemented in the United States, but this seems unlikely to become legal in the current political climate.[105]

THE CAREGIVER IN ADVANCED DEMENTIA

Being the primary caregiver for a person with dementia is an arduous and potentially dangerous occupation. Numerous studies have noted the serious negative effects on physical health, quality of life, and mortality for primary caregivers of people with dementia.[106–108] The dementia caregiving experience often lasts for years, extending the

Table 2
Patient and caregiver experiences and possible interventions

Patient Characteristics	Caregiver Experiences	Possible Interventions
Mild dementia (MMSE ~30–20)		
• Mild forgetfulness and word-finding trouble • Difficulty remembering appointments • Trouble with complex planning or multistep instructions • May have social withdrawal • May develop depression or anxiety related to cognitive decline	• Having to help more with planning, remembering, finances • Fearfulness about diagnosis and the future	• Diagnose and stage dementia in patient • Diagnose and treat any mood problems in patient • Counsel patient and family about legal issues, driving, advance care planning • Refer to memory clinic for diagnostic dilemmas or complex behavioral problems
Moderate dementia (MMSE ~20–10)		
• More language impairment • Difficulty with short-term memory, sequences, chronologies • More trouble with IADLs • Some trouble with ADLs • No longer able to drive or perform complex tasks • Beginnings of paranoia or fearfulness • May wander or get lost, leave stove on, succumb to scams	• Increasing burden of care • Frustration at memory trouble, language • Having to decrease working/activities to provide care • Increased vigilance, as may not be able to leave patient alone • Poor sleep • Depression, anxiety, resentment, anger, grief	• Refer to caregiver support groups • Counsel regarding getting more help in the home • Refer patient for driving evaluation • Monitor caregiver for emergence of depression, fatigue • Involve family and friends to provide material and emotional support • Begin discussion about next steps in care: hiring help in the home, move to supported living situation
Severe dementia (MMSE<10)		
• Physical manifestations begin: weakness, gait impairment, falls, swallowing trouble • Difficulty recognizing familiar people • Unable to perform any IADLs • Marked difficulty with ADLs • Apraxia • May have paranoia, delusions, agitation, aggression	• Fatigue may be severe • Medical complications emerge (eg, hypertension) • May feel guilt for placing patient in supervised care setting	• Refer to palliative medicine for goals of care discussion • Encourage caregiver to have close follow-up with their own PCP • Encourage respite, scheduled time away, exercise, self-care • Encourage support group and/or personal therapy
End-stage		
• May be mute, bed-bound • Requires complete care for ADLs	• Significant burden of daily care • Grief and/or relief at time of death	• Transition to hospice, either at home or in facility • Refer to bereavement support groups

Abbreviations: ADLs, activities of dialing; IADLs, instrumental ADLs; PCP, primary care provider.

grief process.[109] Dementia caregivers experience significant levels of depressive symptoms and more than half describe being "on duty" 24 hours a day at the end of their loved ones' lives.[110] Difficult behaviors are cited as the most stressful part of dementia caregiving, and tend to increase in the later stages of disease.[111] Clinicians should be aware of the psychic toll of caregiving over years, addressing it gently but directly in the course of assisting these surrogate decision makers who are also under considerable stress. For example, a wife who is now a caregiver for her husband and who has cooked for and fed him for 20 years of marriage may be very conflicted over decisions related to artificial nutrition near the end of life. After eliciting her understanding of the situation and her understanding of her husband's prior wishes, the clinician could gently explore the possibility that she is experiencing guilt and anticipatory grief relating her inability to continue to nurture him with food as she always has. Possible interventions to help caregivers are usually stage dependent, and the patient/caregiver dyad often needs additional help when the patient progresses to a new stage (eg, from mild to moderate dementia). Caregivers continue to need support after the death of the person with dementia, as the grief process is often complicated and prolonged by depression and feelings of guilt.[112] Primary care providers for bereaved family members who have lost a loved one with dementia or any illness should be aware of the natural course of grief, and in the case of dementia should be aware that caregiving is often a more prolonged and intense role. Please see **Table 2** for a summary of important issues related to caregiving in dementia.

FUTURE DIRECTIONS

Although end-of-life care in general has improved over time with the growth of palliative care as a specialty and stronger evidence for improved outcomes for patients and families, many people with dementia still receive suboptimal end-of-life care.[4] Barriers to excellent end-of-life care in people with dementia still exist and were discussed in detail in this article.

An ambitious "wish list" for addressing these barriers might include the following:

- More palliative care education at all levels of medical and nursing training, which would include education about end-of-life care in dementia, caregiver support, and grief counseling.
- Reforms in the payment structure, which would provide more resources for nonpharmacologic interventions and caregiver support.
- Targeted educational interventions for specialist and generalist physicians involved in the placement of percutaneous feeding tubes in patients with dementia emphasizing the lack of evidence for this practice.
- Changes in Medicare rules liberalizing access to palliative care and hospice services for patients with dementia who have comfort-oriented goals.

As the population ages, with more individuals being afflicted by dementia, we need to find ways to ensure that these vulnerable adults receive quality end-of-life care.

REFERENCES

1. Abbott A. Dementia: a problem for our age. Nature 2011;475:S2–4.
2. Karantzoulis S, Galvin J. Distinguishing Alzheimer's disease from other major forms of dementia. Expert Rev Neurother 2011;11(11):1579–91.
3. Vann Jones SA, O'Brien JT. The prevalence and incidence of dementia with Lewy bodies: a systematic review of population and clinical studies. Psychological Medicine 2014;44(14):673–83.

4. Sachs GA, Shega JW, Cox-Hayley D. Barriers to excellent end-of-life care for patients with dementia. J Gen Intern Med 2004;19(10):1057–63.
5. Murphy SL, Xu J, Kochanek KD. National vital statistics reports deaths: final data for 2010. Natl Vital Stat Rep 2013;61(4):1–10.
6. Todd S, Barr S, Roberts M, et al. Survival in dementia and predictors of mortality: a review. Int J Geriatr Psychiatry 2013;28(11):1109–24.
7. Brown MA, Sampson EL, Jones L, et al. Prognostic indicators of 6-month mortality in elderly people with advanced dementia: a systematic review. Palliat Med 2013;27(5):389–400.
8. Mitchell S, Teno J, Kiely DK, et al. The clinical course of advanced dementia. N Engl J Med 2009;361(16):1529–38.
9. Quill TE, Abernethy AP. Generalist plus specialist palliative care — creating a more sustainable model. N Engl J Med 2013;368(13):1173–5.
10. Hurd L, Martorell P, Delavande A, et al. Monetary costs of dementia in the United States. N Engl J Med 2013;368(14):1326–34.
11. American Academy of Hospice and Palliative Medicine; Center to Advance Palliative Care; Hospice and Palliative Nurses Association; Last Acts Partnership; National Hospice and Palliative Care Organization. Clinical practice guidelines for quality palliative care. 3rd edition. Pittsburgh (PA): National Consensus Project for Quality Palliative Care; 2013.
12. Torke AM, Holtz LR, Hui S, et al. Palliative care for patients with dementia: a national survey. J Am Geriatr Soc 2010;58(11):2114–21.
13. Shega JW, Hougham GW, Stocking CB, et al. Patients dying with dementia: experience at the end of life and impact of hospice care. J Pain Symptom Manage 2008;35(5):499–507.
14. Miller SC, Lima JC, Mitchell SL. Influence of hospice on nursing home residents with advanced dementia who received Medicare-skilled nursing facility care near the end of life. J Am Geriatr Soc 2012;60(11):2035–41.
15. Miller SC, Lima JC, Mitchell SL. Hospice care for persons with dementia: the growth of access in US nursing homes. Am J Alzheimers Dis Other Demen 2010;25(8):666–73.
16. Van der Steen JT, Radbruch L, Hertogh CM, et al. White paper defining optimal palliative care in older people with dementia: a Delphi study and recommendations from the European Association for Palliative Care. Palliat Med 2014;28(3):197–209.
17. National Hospice and Palliative Care Organization. Caring for persons with Alzheimer's and other dementias. Alexandria (VA): National Hospice and Palliative Care Organization; 2008.
18. Michel JP, Pautex S, Zekry D, et al. End-of-life care of persons with dementia. J Gerontol A Biol Sci Med Sci 2002;57(10):M640–4.
19. Gozalo P, Teno JM, Mitchell SL, et al. End-of-life transitions among nursing home residents with cognitive issues. N Engl J Med 2011;365(13):1212–21.
20. Givens JL, Selby K, Goldfeld KS, et al. Hospital transfers of nursing home residents with advanced dementia. J Am Geriatr Soc 2012;60(5):905–9.
21. Mitchell S. A 93-year-old man with advanced dementia and eating problems. JAMA 2007;298(21):2527–36.
22. Mendiratta P, Tilford JM, Prodhan P, et al. Trends in percutaneous endoscopic gastrostomy placement in the elderly from 1993 to 2003. Am J Alzheimers Dis Other Demen 2012;27(8):609–13.
23. Finucane TE, Christmas C, Leff BA. Tube feeding in dementia: how incentives undermine health care quality and patient safety. J Am Med Dir Assoc 2007;8(4):205–8.

24. AGS Choosing Wisely Workgroup. American Geriatrics Society identifies five things that healthcare providers and patients should question. J Am Geriatr Soc 2013;61(4):622–31.
25. Sampson E, Candy B, Jones L. Enteral tube feeding for older people with advanced dementia. Cochrane Database Syst Rev 2009;(2):CD007209.
26. Teno JM, Gozalo PL, Mitchell SL, et al. Does feeding tube insertion and its timing improve survival? J Am Geriatr Soc 2012;60(10):1918–21.
27. Teno JM, Gozalo P, Mitchell SL, et al. Feeding tubes and the prevention or healing of pressure ulcers. Arch Intern Med 2012;172(9):697–701.
28. Fischberg D, Bull J, Casarett D, et al. Five things physicians and patients should question in hospice and palliative medicine. J Pain Symptom Manage 2013; 45(3):595–605.
29. Palecek EJ, Teno JM, Casarett DJ, et al. Comfort feeding only: a proposal to bring clarity to decision-making regarding difficulty with eating for persons with advanced dementia. J Am Geriatr Soc 2010;58(3):580–4.
30. Hanson LC, Ersek M, Gilliam R, et al. Oral feeding options for people with dementia: a systematic review. J Am Geriatr Soc 2011;59(3):463–72.
31. Teno JM, Mitchell SL, Kuo SK, et al. Decision-making and outcomes of feeding tube insertion: a five-state study. J Am Geriatr Soc 2011;59(5):881–6.
32. Snyder EA, Caprio AJ, Wessell K, et al. Impact of a decision aid on surrogate decision-makers' perceptions of feeding options for patients with dementia. J Am Med Dir Assoc 2013;14(2):114–8.
33. D'Agata E, Mitchell SL. Patterns of antimicrobial use among nursing home residents with advanced dementia. Arch Intern Med 2008;168(4):357–62.
34. Van der Steen JT, Ooms ME, Mehr DR, et al. Severe dementia and adverse outcomes of nursing home-acquired pneumonia: evidence for mediation by functional and pathophysiological decline. J Am Geriatr Soc 2002;50(3): 439–48.
35. Fabiszewski K, Volicer B, Volicer L. Effect of antibiotic treatment on outcome of fevers in institutionalized Alzheimer patients. JAMA 1990;263(23):3168–72.
36. Reisfeld S, Paul M, Gottesman BS, et al. The effect of empiric antibiotic therapy on mortality in debilitated patients with dementia. Eur J Clin Microbiol Infect Dis 2011;30(6):813–8.
37. Givens JL, Jones RN, Shaffer ML, et al. Survival and comfort after treatment of pneumonia in advanced dementia. Arch Intern Med 2010;170(13):1102–7.
38. Van der Steen JT, Lane P, Kowall NW, et al. Antibiotics and mortality in patients with lower respiratory infection and advanced dementia. J Am Med Dir Assoc 2012;13(2):156–61.
39. Viray M, Linkin D, Maslow JN, et al. Longitudinal trends in antimicrobial susceptibilities across long-term-care facilities: emergence of fluoroquinolone resistance. Infect Control Hosp Epidemiol 2005;26(1):56–62.
40. Schwaber M, Carmeli Y. Antibiotic therapy in the demented elderly population: redefining the ethical dilemma. Arch Intern Med 2008;168(4):349–50.
41. Blass D, Black B, Phillips H, et al. Medication use in nursing home residents with advanced dementia. Int J Geriatr Psychiatry 2008;23:490–6.
42. Holmes HM, Sachs GA, Shega JW, et al. Integrating palliative medicine into the care of persons with advanced dementia: identifying appropriate medication use. J Am Geriatr Soc 2008;56(7):1306–11.
43. The American Geriatrics Society 2012 Beers Criteria Update Expert Panel. American Geriatrics Society updated Beers Criteria for potentially inappropriate medication use in older adults. J Am Geriatr Soc 2012;60(4):616–31.

44. Budnitz DS, Lovegrove MC, Shehab N, et al. Emergency hospitalizations for adverse drug events in older Americans. N Engl J Med 2011;365(21):2002–12.

45. Parsons C, Hughes CM, Passmore AP, et al. Withholding, discontinuing and withdrawing medications in dementia patients at the end of life: a neglected problem in the disadvantaged dying? Drugs Aging 2010;27(6):435–49.

46. Shega J, Emanuel L, Vargish L, et al. Pain in persons with dementia: complex, common, and challenging. J Pain 2007;8(5):373–8.

47. Shega JW, Hougham GW, Stocking CB, et al. Management of noncancer pain in community-dwelling persons with dementia. J Am Geriatr Soc 2006;54(12): 1892–7.

48. Manfredi PL, Breuer B, Meier DE, et al. Pain assessment in elderly patients with severe dementia. J Pain Symptom Manage 2003;25(1):48–52.

49. Bruckenthal P, Reid MC, Reisner L. Special issues in the management of chronic pain in older adults. Pain Med 2009;10(Suppl 2):S67–78.

50. Kovach CR, Noonan PE, Griffie J, et al. The assessment of discomfort in dementia protocol. Pain Manag Nurs 2002;3(1):16–27.

51. Husebo BS, Ballard C, Sandvik R, et al. Efficacy of treating pain to reduce behavioural disturbances in residents of nursing homes with dementia: cluster randomised clinical trial. BMJ 2011;343:d4065.

52. American Geriatrics Society Panel on Pharmacological Management of Persistent Pain in Older Persons. Pharmacological management of persistent pain in older persons. J Am Geriatr Soc 2009;57(8):1331–46.

53. Rolinski M, Fox C, Maidment I, et al. Cholinesterase inhibitors for dementia with Lewy bodies, Parkinson's disease dementia and cognitive impairment in Parkinson's disease. Cochrane Database Syst Rev 2012;(3):CD006504.

54. McShane R, Areosa Sastre A, Minakaran N. Memantine for dementia. Cochrane Database Syst Rev 2006;(2):CD003154.

55. Van Dyck CH, Schmitt FA, Olin JT. A responder analysis of memantine treatment in patients with Alzheimer disease maintained on donepezil. Am J Geriatr Psychiatry 2006;14(5):428–37.

56. Weschules DJ, Maxwell TL, Shega JW. Acetylcholinesterase inhibitor and N-methyl-D-aspartic acid receptor antagonist use among hospice enrollees with a primary diagnosis of dementia. J Palliat Med 2008;11:738–45.

57. Onder G, Liperoti R, Foebel A, et al. Polypharmacy and mortality among nursing home residents with advanced cognitive impairment: results from the SHELTER study. J Am Med Dir Assoc 2013;14:450.e7–12.

58. Di Santo SG, Prinelli F, Adorni F, et al. A meta-analysis of the efficacy of donepezil, rivastigmine, galantamine, and memantine in relation to severity of Alzheimer's disease. J Alzheimers Dis 2013;35(2):349–61.

59. Feldman H, Gauthier S, Hecker J, et al. Efficacy and safety of donepezil in patients with more severe Alzheimer's disease: a subgroup analysis from a randomized, placebo-controlled trial. Int J Geriatr Psychiatry 2005;20:559–69.

60. Daiello LA, Ott BR, Lapane KL, et al. Effect of discontinuing cholinesterase inhibitor therapy on behavioral and mood symptoms in nursing home patients with dementia. Am J Geriatr Pharmacother 2009;7:74–83.

61. Singh S, Dudley C. Discontinuation syndrome following donepezil cessation. Int J Geriatr Psychiatry 2003;18:282–4.

62. Morrison LJ, Liao S. Dementia medications in palliative care #174. J Palliat Med 2008;11:634–5.

63. LeGrand SB. Delirium in palliative medicine: a review. J Pain Symptom Manage 2012;44:583–94.

64. Bruera E, Bush SH, Willey J, et al. Impact of delirium and recall on the level of distress in patients with advanced cancer and their family caregivers. Cancer 2009;115:2004–12.

65. Brajtman S. The impact on the family of terminal restlessness and its management. Palliat Med 2003;17:454–60.

66. Breitbart W, Gibson C, Tremblay A. The delirium experience: delirium recall and delirium-related distress in hospitalized patients with cancer, their spouses/caregivers, and their nurses. Psychosomatics 2002;43(3):183–94.

67. Candy B, Jackson KC, Jones L, et al. Drug therapy for delirium in terminally ill adult patients. Cochrane Database Syst Rev 2012 Nov 14;11:CD004770.

68. Breitbart W, Marotta R, Platt MM, et al. A double-blind trial of haloperidol, chlorpromazine, and lorazepam in the treatment of delirium in hospitalized AIDS patients. Am J Psychiatry 1996;153:231–7.

69. Vella-Brincat J, Macleod AD. Haloperidol in palliative care. Palliat Med 2004;18:195–201.

70. Moyer DD. Review article: terminal delirium in geriatric patients with cancer at end of life. Am J Hosp Palliat Care 2011;28(1):44–51.

71. Lyketsos CG, Lopez O, Jones B, et al. Prevalence of neuropsychiatric symptoms in dementia and mild cognitive impairment: results from the Cardiovascular Health Study. JAMA 2002;288(12):1475–83.

72. Mézière A, Blachier M, Thomas S, et al. Neuropsychiatric symptoms in elderly inpatients: a multicenter cross-sectional study. Dement Geriatr Cogn Dis Extra 2013;3(1):123–30.

73. Aalten P, Verhey FR, Boziki M, et al. Consistency of neuropsychiatric syndromes across dementias: results from the European Alzheimer Disease Consortium. Dement Geriatr Cogn Disord 2008;25(1):1–8.

74. Jeste DV, Blazer D, Casey D, et al. ACNP White Paper: update on use of antipsychotic drugs in elderly persons with dementia. Neuropsychopharmacology 2008;33(5):957–70.

75. Kverno KS, Black BS, Blass DM, et al. Neuropsychiatric symptom patterns in hospice-eligible nursing home residents with advanced dementia. J Am Med Dir Assoc 2008;9:509–15.

76. Lyness JM. End-of-life care: issues relevant to the geriatric psychiatrist. Am J Geriatr Psychiatry 2004;12(5):457–72.

77. Verkaik R, Francke AL, van Meijel B, et al. Comorbid depression in dementia on psychogeriatric nursing home wards: which symptoms are prominent? Am J Geriatr Psychiatry 2009;17:565–73.

78. Lyketsos CG, DelCampo L, Steinberg M, et al. Treating depression in Alzheimer disease: efficacy and safety of sertraline therapy, and the benefits of depression reduction: the DIADS. Arch Gen Psychiatry 2003;60:737–46.

79. Bains J, Birks JS, Dening TR. The efficacy of antidepressants in the treatment of depression in dementia. Cochrane Database Syst Rev 2002;(4):CD003944.

80. Kerr CW, Drake J, Milch RA, et al. Effects of methylphenidate on fatigue and depression: a randomized, double-blind, placebo-controlled trial. J Pain Symptom Manage 2012;43:68–77.

81. Brodaty H. Meta-analysis of nonpharmacological interventions for neuropsychiatric symptoms of dementia. Am J Psychiatry 2012;169:946.

82. Ayalon L, Gum AM, Feliciano L, et al. Effectiveness of nonpharmacological interventions for the management of neuropsychiatric symptoms in patients with dementia: a systematic review. Arch Intern Med 2006;166:2182–8.

83. Weiss E, Hummer M, Koller D, et al. Off-label use of antipsychotic drugs. J Clin Psychopharmacol 2000;20:695–8.
84. Ballard C, Waite J. The effectiveness of atypical antipsychotics for the treatment of aggression and psychosis in Alzheimer's disease. Cochrane Database Syst Rev 2006;(1):CD003476.
85. Trinh NH, Hoblyn J, Mohanty S, et al. Efficacy of cholinesterase inhibitors in the treatment of neuropsychiatric symptoms and functional impairment in Alzheimer disease: a meta-analysis. JAMA 2003;289:210–6.
86. Kiely DK, Givens JL, Shaffer ML, et al. Hospice use and outcomes in nursing home residents with advanced dementia. J Am Geriatr Soc 2010;58(12): 2284–91.
87. Teno JM, Gozalo PL, Lee IC, et al. Does hospice improve quality of care for persons dying from dementia? J Am Geriatr Soc 2011;59(8):1531–6.
88. Irwin SA, Mausbach BT, Koo D, et al. Association between hospice care and psychological outcomes in Alzheimer's spousal caregivers. J Palliat Med 2013;16(11):1450–4.
89. Albrecht JS, Gruber-Baldini AL, Fromme EK, et al. Quality of hospice care for individuals with dementia. J Am Geriatr Soc 2013;61(7):1060–5.
90. Department of Health and Human Services. Medicare program; FY 2014 hospice wage index and payment rate update; Hospice quality reporting requirements; and Updates on payment reform. Federal Register 2013;78(152):1–49.
91. Odenheimer G, Borson S, Sanders AE, et al. Quality improvement in neurology: dementia management quality measures. Neurology 2013;81(17):1545–9.
92. Volandes AE, Abbo ED. Flipping the default: a novel approach to cardiopulmonary resuscitation in end-stage dementia. J Clin Ethics 2007;18(2):122–39.
93. Tonelli M. Pulling the plug on living wills: a critical analysis of advance directives. Chest 1996;110:816–22.
94. Tulsky JA. Beyond advance directives: importance of communication skills at the end of life. JAMA 2005;294(3):359–65.
95. Five Wishes Online. Available at: www.agingwithdignity.org/five-wishes.php. Accessed May 15, 2014.
96. Volandes A. Video decision support tool for advance care planning in dementia: randomised controlled trial. BMJ 2009;338:b2159.
97. Volandes AE, Mitchell SL, Gillick MR, et al. Using video images to improve the accuracy of surrogate decision-making: a randomized controlled trial. J Am Med Dir Assoc 2009;10(8):575–80.
98. Mitchell SL, Teno JM, Intrator O, et al. Decisions to forgo hospitalization in advanced dementia: a nationwide study. J Am Geriatr Soc 2007;55(3): 432–8.
99. Dening KH, Jones L, Sampson EL. Advance care planning for people with dementia: a review. Int Psychogeriatr 2011;23(10):1535–51.
100. National Polst Paradigm. POLST: Physician orders for life-sustaining treatment. Available at: www.polst.org. Accessed May 15, 2014.
101. Hickman SE, Nelson CA, Moss AH, et al. The consistency between treatments provided to nursing facility residents and orders on the physician orders for life-sustaining treatment form. J Am Geriatr Soc 2011;59(11):2091–9.
102. Torke A, Petronio S, Purnell C, et al. Communicating with clinicians: the experiences of surrogate decision makers for hospitalized older adults. J Am Geriatr Soc 2012;60(8):1401–7.
103. Jox RJ, Denke E, Hamann J, et al. Surrogate decision making for patients with end-stage dementia. Int J Geriatr Psychiatry 2012;27(10):1045–52.

104. De Boer ME, Dröes RM, Jonker C, et al. Advance directives for euthanasia in dementia: how do they affect resident care in Dutch nursing homes? Experiences of physicians and relatives. J Am Geriatr Soc 2011;59(6):989–96.

105. Menzel P, Steinbock B. Advance directives, dementia, and physician assisted death. J Law Med Ethics 2013;41(2):484–500.

106. Schulz R, Beach SR, Lind B, et al. Caregiving as a risk factor for mortality: the Caregiver Health Effects Study. JAMA 1999;285(24):2215–9.

107. Schulz R, O'Brien AT, Bookwala J. Psychiatric and physical morbidity effects of dementia caregiving: prevalence, correlates, and causes. Gerontologist 1995; 35(6):771–91.

108. Mausbach B, Chattillion E, Roepke S, et al. A comparison of psychosocial outcomes in elderly Alzheimer caregivers and noncaregivers. Am J Geriatr Psychiatry 2013;21(1):5–13.

109. Meuser TM, Marwit SJ. A comprehensive, stage-sensitive model of grief in dementia caregiving. Gerontologist 2001;41(5):658–70.

110. Schulz R, Mendelsohn AB, Haley WE, et al. End-of-life care and the effects of bereavement on family caregivers of persons with dementia. N Engl J Med 2003;349:1936–42.

111. Diwan S, Hougham GW, Sachs GA. Strain experienced by caregivers of dementia patients receiving palliative care: findings from the Palliative Excellence in Alzheimer Care Efforts (PEACE) Program. J Palliat Med 2004;7:797–807.

112. Peacock SC. The experience of providing end-of-life care to a relative with advanced dementia: an integrative literature review. Palliat Support Care 2013;11(2):1–14.

113. Dharmarajan TS, Unnikrishnan D, Pitchumoni CS. Percutaneous endoscopic gastrostomy and outcome in dementia. Am J Gastroenterol 2001;96(9): 2556–63.

114. Kuo S, Rhodes RL, Mitchell SL, et al. Natural history of feeding tube use in nursing home residents with advanced dementia. J Am Med Dir Assoc 2010; 10(4):264–70.

115. Gillick MR. Rethinking the role of tube feeding in patients with advanced dementia. N Engl J Med 2000;342(3):206–10.

116. Hendriks SA, Smalbrugge M, Hertogh CM, et al. Dying with dementia: symptoms, treatment and quality of life in the last week of life. J Pain Symptom Manage 2014;47(4):710–20.

Partnering with Caregivers

Joseph E. Gaugler, BA, MS, PhD[a],*, Teddie Potter, PhD, RN[b],
Lisiane Pruinelli, RN, MSN[b]

KEYWORDS

- Informal long-term care • Long-term care • Burden • Stress • Caregiver intervention
- Chronic disease • Partnership-based care

KEY POINTS

- Family caregivers provide extensive long-term care to older adults in the United States; 85% of older adults in need rely on family members.
- Family caregivers indicate several unmet needs related to care provision, and are often at risk for negative health outcomes when compared to noncaregivers.
- Existing evidence suggests that caregiving interventions have moderate, positive benefits although more intensive, multicomponent models hold the most promise.
- A family-centered, partnership-based framework offers a clinical strategy that can enhance the assessment of or intervention with family caregivers.
- Family caregiving research and clinical practice must continue to evolve toward family-centered and person-centered partnership models to best meet the complex needs of families.

INTRODUCTION

There is no consistent definition of family caregiving. Some organizations such as the Alzheimer's Association define caregiving as "attending to one's health needs."[1(p29)] Many studies rely on family members' self-identification as a caregiver, whereas others tend to use more objective measures to define family caregiving, such as the number of activities of daily living (ADLs) that a family member helps a relative with. If the latter definitional scope is selected, it is important to acknowledge the wide range of tasks that family caregiving often encompasses: family caregiving may include not only basic or instrumental ADL tasks but also management of specific disease symptoms (eg, behavior problems caused by a relative's dementia; nausea that is a result of a relative's cancer therapy), financial help, or care coordination between health care professionals.[2,3]

---

[a] Center on Aging, School of Nursing, University of Minnesota, 6-153 Weaver-Densford Hall, 1331, 308 Harvard Street Southeast, Minneapolis, MN 55455, USA; [b] School of Nursing, University of Minnesota, Minneapolis, MN, USA
* Corresponding author.
E-mail address: gaug0015@umn.edu

Clin Geriatr Med 30 (2014) 493–515
http://dx.doi.org/10.1016/j.cger.2014.04.003
0749-0690/14/$ – see front matter © 2014 Elsevier Inc. All rights reserved.

Other approaches focus on the reasons why family members provide support; for example, Schulz and Quittner[4] defined caregiving as "extraordinary care that exceeds the bounds of what is considered normative for others." Family caregiving is said to occur when the support and help provided by 1 family member to another are not routine and are based on a care recipient's health need. Use of this definition can help health care providers and practitioners better ascertain whether family caregiving is occurring, even in instances in which a family member does not consider that what they are doing is caregiving. The unwillingness of some family members to consider themselves caregivers even when extraordinary assistance is provided has led some organizations to launch public awareness campaigns for community members to become aware that "I am a caregiver" (see http://www.whatisacaregiver.org/).

Describing Family Caregivers

In 2009, the National Alliance of Caregiving (NAC) and the American Association of Retired Persons (AARP)[5] conducted a telephone survey of a representative sample of family caregivers in the United States. The following points summarize statistics from this and other, similar sources that describe family caregiving as it is delivered in the United States:

- 18.9%, or 43.5 million Americans, care for someone 50 years of age or older.[5]
- 65.7 million people in the United States have provided unpaid care to an adult or child in the past 12 months.[5]
- 66% of family caregivers in the United States are women.[5]
- Family caregivers are 61 years old, on average.[5]
- 74% of caregivers live within 20 minutes of the care recipient, and more than 95% of primary family caregivers live within 30 minutes of their care recipients.[5,6]
- The average amount of family care provided on a weekly basis is 20.4 hours.[5]
- 72% of family caregivers in the United States are white, 13% are African American, 2% are Hispanic, and 2% are Asian American. The household prevalence of caregiving across racial and ethnic groups is more evenly distributed: 30% of Hispanic households are engaged in family caregiving, 28% of African American households are caregiving, 25% white households are involved in family caregiving, and 17% of Asian American households are caregiving.[5]
- The typical family caregiver is a 46-year-old woman with some college education who provides more than 20 hours of week of help to her mother.[7]
- 85% of help provided to all older adults in the United States is from family members.[8]
- On average, care recipients are close to 80 years of age and close to 70% are women.[6]
- Close to half of care recipients are widowed, whereas approximately 40% of care recipients live alone.[6]

Much of the research available on family caregiving for older adults tends to focus on the primary family caregiver, or the 1 person who is most responsible for providing assistance to an older relative.[9] It is possible that this focus on primary family caregivers is due to ease of analysis, because including multiple family caregivers, an entire family, or various combinations that include unpaid caregivers who are not members of the family is more complex analytically. This emphasis on primary family caregivers obscures how caregiving actually operates in US families, particularly in ethnically or racially diverse contexts. For example, older care recipients in African American families tend to rely on a more complex array of family members and extended kin supports than white families (the reasons for this range from sociocultural history to lack of health care access).[10–12]

Types of Care Provision

As noted earlier, family caregiving can consist of various types of assistance. As reported in the NAC/AARP 2009 report[5]:

- 58% of family caregivers provide help to an adult care recipient on at least 1 ADL.
- 43% of family caregivers provided assistance getting in and out of beds and chairs; 32% helped the care recipient dress; 26% assisted the care recipient bathe or shower; 25% of caregivers helped the care recipient get to and from the toilet; 19% helped to feed the care recipient; and 19% assisted the care recipient with incontinence issues.
- 100%, or all respondents in the 2009 NAC/AARP survey, provided help to an adult care recipient with at least 1 instrumental ADL.
- 83% helped the care recipient with driving or arranging transportation; 75% helped with housework; 75% assisted with grocery shopping; 65% assisted the care recipient prepare meals; 64% helped the care recipient manage finances; 41% gave medications, pills, or injections to the care recipient; and 34% arranged or supervised paid services for the care recipient.

This substantial assistance shows that families are on the front lines of long-term care provision in the United States. The importance of ADL assistance provided by family caregivers becomes particularly apparent when considering predictors of nursing home admission in older adults; our previous meta-analysis[13] found that older adults with 3 or more ADL dependencies were 3.25 times more likely to enter a nursing home. This extent of family care, coupled with the average amount of time that such care is provided by families in the United States (20.4 hours; see earlier discussion) suggests that the economic value of family care is considerable. For example, family care for Alzheimer disease in 2012 was valued at $216 billion, which was more than 8 times the total sales of McDonalds in 2011 ($27 billion).[1]

Several family caregivers provide care to more than 1 person. Although two-thirds of family caregivers in the United States are providing help to 1 relative, slightly more than 20% care for more than 1 care recipient and approximately 10% provide care to 3 or more persons.[5] Although the existing data are not specific, some of these multiple care recipient arrangements may represent caregivers in the sandwich generation, or family members who are providing care to multiple generations in 1 family (eg, a child and an elderly parent). Alternatively, multiple care arrangements may also reflect the general aging of the population; some adults in the United States may be providing care not only to an aging spouse but also an elderly parent(s), because of the increasing proportion of the oldest-old (ie, those who are 85 years of age and older) in the United States.

How Long Do Families Provide Care?

On average, family members have been providing care for 4.6 years.[5] **Fig. 1** provides additional detail on duration of family care in the United States.

More than 70% of caregivers in the NAC/AARP 2009 survey were currently providing assistance to a relative.[5] With regards to the 30% of past caregivers, because of variations in disease context many family members may enter and exit family care responsibilities based on the needs and disease progression of the care recipient. For example, in acute disease contexts family caregivers may engage in

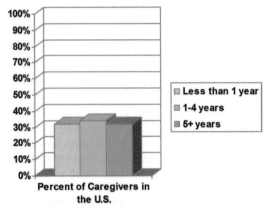

Fig. 1. Duration of family care in the United States, 2009. (*From* Gaugler JE. Informal care supports: the basics. University of Minnesota; 2012. Available at: http://coa.umn.edu/GEM/index.htm. Accessed December 28, 2012; *Data from* National Alliance for Caregiving, American Association of Retired Persons. Caregiving in the U.S. 2009. Washington, DC: National Alliance for Caregiving, American Association of Retired Persons; 2009.)

more extensive care responsibilities and then reduce their care in periods of remission or when a relative's needs decrease.

Some studies have suggested that providing community-based support, such as in-home help, earlier during the course of caregiving can lead to positive outcomes including delayed institutionalization for care recipients.[14] Some studies have examined the onset of family caregiving, because this transition may influence key outcomes on the part of family caregivers and their relatives. We found that caregivers who had provided assistance before a diagnosis of dementia were more likely to delay institutionalization, and they reported lower levels of emotional distress when compared with those whose transition to caregiving was more abrupt (ie, based on a new diagnosis of dementia).[15] Understanding when and how family caregiving begins may allow clinicians to help families identify potentially helpful services and supports earlier and also assist families to prepare for subsequent transitions that may occur during a relative's disease trajectory (eg, when in-home help/community-based support, respite, psychosocial support, residential long-term care, or end-of-life care should begin for the caregiver or care recipient).[16]

SCOPE OF THE PROBLEM

The prevalence and duration of family caregiving in the United States alone emphasize the public health importance of this phenomenon. Moreover, a considerable segment of the gerontologic and geriatric literature has focused on the emotional, psychological, social, economic, and physiologic implications of family caregiver provision.[8,17] In addition to the overall value of family care summarized earlier, the cost implications of providing care for individual families are considerable. About 7 in 10 family caregivers (69%) have to make changes in their work schedule, decrease their hours, or take unpaid leave because of family care demands. A typical family caregiver can also expect to lose $109 per day in wages on average because of family caregiving responsibilities.[18,19] The economic burdens of family care extend to other domains of health; for example, spousal caregivers with a history of chronic illness have a mortality rate that is 63% higher than similar individuals who are noncaregivers, and family caregiving has been linked to several physiologic mechanisms that may make family care providers susceptible to health problems.[17,20–23] The extensive literature on family caregiving has also shown the association between family caregiving and negative mental health symptoms and burden (or feelings of being overwhelmed with the emotional, psychological, social, and financial aspects of care provision).[24,25] With the array of challenges that family caregiving poses, individuals engaged in these responsibilities note several unmet informational needs, as shown in **Fig. 2**.

Twenty-three percent of family caregivers in 2009[5] reported that they needed more information to effectively communicate with doctors or other health care professionals; this suggests that many primary care providers may be unaware of the importance of engaging (or partnering) with family caregivers. Collectively, these unmet needs along with the extensive health risks and other concerns of family caregivers emphasize the need for effective, sustained clinical engagement with families to achieve optimal chronic care management outcomes.[26] The purpose of the remaining sections of this article is to further highlight existing scientific evidence as to the negative health outcomes associated with family caregiving, review clinical strategies that have shown promise in alleviating negative caregiving outcomes, and propose a partnership-based approach that can serve as the basis to enhance engagement with family caregivers.

CLINICAL CORRELATIONS

The preceding sections have already highlighted some of the general findings related to family caregiving for older adults and its consequences. **Table 1** further summarizes the key conclusions derived from synthesized evidence (meta-analyses, literature reviews) related to family caregiving for older adults in general samples as well as disease-specific contexts. The health implications of family caregiving (and correlates of such outcomes) and clinical interventions that have the potential to reduce negative caregiving outcomes are described in **Table 2**.

When the scientific literature is considered broadly, caregiver intervention benefits are moderate at best. Although family caregiving intervention research has

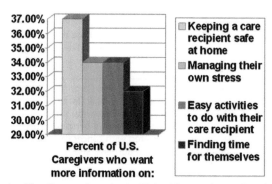

Fig. 2. Unmet needs of family caregivers in the United States. (*From* Gaugler JE. Informal care supports: the basics. University of Minnesota; 2012. Available at: http://coa.umn.edu/GEM/index.htm. Accessed December 28, 2012; *Data from* National Alliance for Caregiving, American Association of Retired Persons. Caregiving in the U.S. 2009. Washington, DC: National Alliance for Caregiving, American Association of Retired Persons; 2009.)

Table 1
Syntheses that describe family caregiving for older adults and its outcomes

Disease Context	Family Caregiving Outcomes and Correlates
General[12,17,25,27–30]	Family caregivers indicate significantly higher rates of depression and stress when compared to noncaregivers
	The amount of care provided and care recipient's physical impairments are associated with caregiver burden and depression
	Uplifts, or perceived positive aspects of caregiving, are possibly associated with the well-being of family caregivers, whereas caregiving stress is linked to depressive symptoms
	Depressive signs and symptoms are associated with negative perceptions of health on the part of family caregivers. Behavior problems on the part of care recipients are also associated with poorer health of family caregivers, as is older age, lower socioeconomic status, and less social support
	When compared to noncaregivers, family caregivers suffer from greater overall and clinical depression and anxiety, less social support, greater physical impairments and disabilities, poorer self-rated health, and acute and chronic conditions than do noncaregivers
	Ethnically and racially diverse family caregivers are more likely to be of lower socioeconomic status, younger, less likely to be a spouse, more likely to receive informal support, have stronger filial obligation beliefs, are more depressed, and experience worse physical health
	There is substantial diversity in caregiving experience and outcomes across various racial and ethnic groups; more attention to acculturation, theory development, and cultural beliefs, values, and norms is needed
Alzheimer disease[1,23,24,31,32]	Family caregivers of persons with Alzheimer disease or a related dementia experience greater emotional, psychological, financial, and physiologic distress when compared to other caregivers or noncaregivers
	Lower current relationship quality is associated with increased depression and strain and decreased self-efficacy; lower previous relationship quality is related to depression, burden, and emotional reactivity
	Personal mastery, self-efficacy, and positive coping strategies can serve to protect dementia caregivers from negative outcomes
	Spouses provide more support but report more depressive symptoms, greater physical and financial burden, and lower levels of psychological well-being than children and children-in-law
	Dementia caregivers show a slightly greater risk for health problems than noncaregivers
Cancer[33–37]	Cancer caregivers who are wives report lower mental health, lower physical health, poorer health-related quality of life, lower life satisfaction, and decreased marital satisfaction; however, they are also more likely to experience personal growth
	The demands associated with cancer care lead to time restraints, employment-related burdens, and financial pressures for family members
	Cancer caregivers are more likely to suffer from negative mental health or other outcomes than noncaregivers
	Care recipient and caregiver emotional distress are highly associated, and correlates of this reciprocal distress varies according to disease stage

(continued on next page)

Table 1 (continued)	
Disease Context	**Family Caregiving Outcomes and Correlates**
Stroke[38–40]	Stroke caregivers indicate increased levels of depression when compared with noncaregivers The longitudinal changes of stroke caregiving distress are not clear; quantitative data suggest little to no change over time, whereas qualitative data imply a more dynamic process Tangible and social companionship is most highly related to psychosocial health in stroke caregivers (less stress, burden, strain, mood, depressive symptoms, and more positive coping)
End-of-life/ palliative care[41–43]	Caregivers experience intense, negative, and conflicting emotions and stress during end-of-life care, such as being unprepared for their role, uncertainty, and anxiety Family caregivers have unmet needs and problems during end-of-life care, but the existing literature also highlights the potential for positive outcomes and gains Caregivers in palliative care situations report difficulty, burden, depression, mental and physical ill health, barriers to accessing services, dissatisfaction with formal services, and lack of informal support
Motor neuron disease[44]	Family caregivers report substantial burden and distress which exacerbate negative health outcomes; caregivers in these contexts experience many challenges within a short period

Table 2 Family caregiving intervention results	
Disease Context	**Results**
General[45–47]	Overall, family caregiver interventions have moderate effects in reducing burden, depression, negative mental health, and improving satisfaction or ability/knowledge of caregivers. Psychoeducational and psychotherapeutic interventions are most consistent in enhancing caregiver outcomes over short-term periods. The positive effects of cognitive-behavioral therapy as an intervention are also apparent Although most high-quality respite evaluations show mixed or no effects, a trend emerges in which long-term term respite use is associated with more positive outcomes on the part of family caregivers
Dementia[48–61]	A synthesis of existing meta-analyses and literature reviews found that multicomponent interventions were the most effective in reducing caregiver stress and negative mental health as well as reducing care recipient institutionalization; psychoeducational and psychotherapeutic interventions were also effective, with supportive interventions less so. Respite was mostly found to be not effective
Cancer[62]	Psychoeducation, skills training, and therapeutic counseling can significantly reduce caregiver burden, improve caregivers' ability to cope, increase self-efficacy, and improve quality of life of cancer caregivers
Palliative care[63]	Psychoeducational interventions appeared to result in the most consistent, positive outcomes for palliative caregivers; interventions that were targeted to caregivers' needs appeared particularly promising
Stroke[64,65]	Supportive and educational interventions for stroke caregivers seem to have moderate effects Vocational educational interventions delivered before a care recipient's discharge from a hospital seem to be the most promising approach to reducing family caregivers' stress and strain

developed considerably over the past 15 years, the quality of evidence available remains mixed; there is not a large surplus of randomized controlled trials that test the efficacy of various clinical approaches. More recent evaluations that yield higher quality evidence do seem to show the potential benefits of clinical interventions for family caregivers. Intervention models that are more intensive (offered more frequently and over longer periods), flexible, and individualized to meet the specific needs of family caregivers seem most effective at alleviating an array of negative outcomes on the part of family caregivers. Given the disease course of many chronic conditions, constructing caregiver support protocols that are individualized to fit the complex schedules of family caregivers but are also sufficiently intensive and long-term seems beneficial.

From a clinical standpoint, implementing evidence-based caregiving interventions requires the appropriate balance between clinical expertise and patient values.[66] Many current interventions are evaluated with fairly select samples, which are not generalizable to other settings or populations. A considerable amount of variation exists in evaluation designs (eg, measures used; length of follow-up), and sample sizes are small. It is also difficult to classify interventions into distinct types; as the literature suggests, there are many ways to intervene on behalf of family caregivers, ranging from psychotherapy to multicomponent approaches.

FAMILY CAREGIVER ASSESSMENT

A key component when collaborating with family caregivers and potentially recommending a clinical treatment approach is assessment. Underlying the caregiving assessment process are 7 principles developed by the Family Caregiver Association, as shown in **Box 1**.[67,68]

Family caregiving assessment is not focused solely on a primary caregiver (see earlier discussion) but instead requires more of a systems perspective, which

---

Box 1
The 7 principles of family caregiver assessment

1. Because family caregivers are a core part of health care and long-term care, it is important to recognize, respect, assess, and address their needs.

2. Caregiver assessment should embrace a family-centered perspective, inclusive of the needs and preferences of both the care recipient and the family caregiver.

3. Caregiver assessment should result in a care plan (developed collaboratively with the caregiver) that indicates the provision of services and intended measurable outcomes.

4. Caregiver assessment should be multidimensional in approach and periodically updated.

5. Caregiver assessment should reflect culturally competent practice.

6. Effective caregiver assessment requires assessors to have specialized knowledge and skills. Practitioners and service providers' education and training should equip them with an understanding of the caregiving process and its effects, as well as the benefits and elements of an effective caregiver assessment.

7. Government and other third-party payers should recognize and pay for caregiver assessment as a part of care for older people and adults with disabilities.

Used with permission of Family Caregiver Alliance. For more information, visit www.caregiver. org or call (800) 445-8106.

considers the person receiving assistance, other family members involved in the care process, the overall environment or context of family care (including history), and services used or available. Health care providers should consider assessing the following individuals: the primary caregiver, other family members, or other individuals involved in the care situation. Whether multiple family members or the care recipient themselves are included in a single assessment depends on several factors, including feasibility and whether multiple family members can feel comfortable sharing their perceptions of their care situation in the presence of one another.[67] The main objectives to achieve in an assessment procedure are to[69]:

- Ascertain the emotional and psychological well-being of the caregiver and care recipient
- Determine what challenges the care recipient's chronic illness, condition, or disability places on both the primary caregiver as well as other family members or care providers
- Identify whether there are precipitating factors, or triggers, which result in either positive or negative outcomes on the part of the caregiver or care recipient

The Family Caregiver Alliance/National Center on Caregiving as well as the American Psychological Association provides substantial guidance as to what clinicians should assess when working with family caregivers.[67,69] Specifically, 7 domains are suggested[69]:

- Background of the caregiver and the caregiving situation
- The caregiver's perception of the health and functional status of the care recipient
- The caregiver's values and preferences
- The health and well-being of the caregiver
- The consequences of caregiving on the caregiver
- Care provision requirements
- Resources to support the caregiver

Although a caregiving assessment may include these 7 domains, content or questions may vary as a result of when the assessment is administered (ie, an initial assessment or a follow-up assessment that determine changes over time); whether the caregiving situation is new or has been ongoing for some time; whether an acute episode, such as a fall or hospital discharge, has led to a change in the caregiving situation; and whether the care recipient is living at home, in a residential setting, or is receiving some other arrangement of services.[67] Although space considerations preclude a detailed overview, please see https://caregiver.org/caregivers-count-too-s3-caregiver-assessment-table for a detailed table that identifies the areas to assess as well as possible questions to consider for each of the 7 caregiving assessment domains described earlier.[67]

Assessments for family caregivers should include measures that have shown reliability and validity (for compendia of family caregiver measures, see Refs.[70–72] and http://www.rosalynncarter.org/caregiver_assessment/), but to maximize usefulness and feasibility, clinical providers are advised to select measures that are short, have been used in care settings that are similar to the clinician's, and are appropriate and practical for family caregivers. Simplicity and directness (eg, reducing response categories on given items),[67,68] identifying measure sections that are most appropriate, and using language that is appropriate to the cultural or socioeconomic contexts of family caregivers are all key issues to consider when developing an assessment protocol. However, the clinical considerations should be balanced with a need to collect information from family caregivers in as systematic way as possible to compare service effectiveness (eg, across families served, across different clinics).[67,68]

An issue that we have observed as it relates to caregiving assessment is the phenomenon of assessment bloat, in which a driving need to assess every possible dimension results in impractical assessment protocols. In some circumstances, the assessment becomes the principal intervention as opposed to using the assessment to allow family caregivers to share their insights and stories and apply the content of the assessment to better inform the design and delivery of services for families. Understanding how to complete given caregiver measures and how to appropriately score and interpret these measures is critical to optimize clinical care provision for family caregivers. Ensuring a family-centric focus and flexible modes of administration is integral (ranging from questionnaires completed by the family caregiver to observational ratings). As recommended by the Family Caregiver Alliance, assessment should take place in a private setting that is comfortable for the family caregiver; although home visits may be ideal to complete such assessments, they likely are not practical for all situations.[67]

Periodic assessment is needed; as summarized earlier, clinical interventions that are delivered over time that mirror the disease trajectory of care recipients are more likely to exert positive benefits for family caregivers in many situations. Similarly, assessments should occur over time to determine whether or how things have changed for the family caregiver. Some clinicians also choose to include an intake or screening process before administering a family caregiver assessment protocol to: (1) determine whether an assessment is required at the time of intake/screening; and (2) inform the content of the family caregiving assessment (for a suggested list of caregiver intake forms and tools see Ref.[71]).

PARTNERING WITH CAREGIVERS

As summarized in the 2013 Dementia Management Quality Measures Report developed by the Dementia Measures Work Group of the American Academy for Neurology,[73] caregivers are integral to the ongoing management of older persons with chronic diseases.[74–79] As noted by the Dementia Measures Work Group,[73] family caregivers' "knowledge, well-being, and sustained engagement with health care providers are critical to the success of both medical and psychosocial components of care" (p. 706). Although some family caregiver intervention approaches have shown important benefits for both family caregivers and their care recipients (see earlier discussion) many of these approaches are not covered by health care insurance or Medicare, and primary care providers are either unaware of caregiver interventions or do not acknowledge their potential benefits.

The following sections summarize partnership-based health care as a possible framework that clinicians can use to better integrate family caregivers into existing health care management regimens. We postulate that partnership-based health care can serve as a strategy within which effective caregiver interventions can be administered.

Partnership-Based Health Care Theory

There is a growing movement in health care toward patient-centered (or person-centered) and family-centered care.[80] Yet, before this model can be fully actualized, it is important that health care providers and consumers share a common foundation or philosophy of what is meant by partnership and collaboration. This section defines partnership-based health care,[81] thereby establishing a framework to support the full partnership of families, patients, and health care providers.

The World Health Organization[82] underscores the confusion that exists around the word collaboration:

> Many health workers believe themselves to be practicing collaboratively, simply because they work together with other health workers. In reality, they may simply be working within a group where each individual has agreed to use their own skills to achieve a common goal. Collaboration, however, is not only about agreement and communication, but about creation and synergy. Collaboration occurs when 2 or more individuals from different backgrounds with complementary skills interact to create a shared understanding that none had previously possessed or could have come to on their own (p. 36).

Just as providers think that they are practicing collaboratively because they are all in the same room, providers can also assume that they are practicing patient-centered and family-centered care because decisions are made in the presence of patients and families. However, full partnership requires an intentional paradigm shift, not just a shift of care team members. Partnership-based health care is grounded in cultural transformation theory.[83] Systems theorist and metahistorian Riane Eisler found that families, organizations, governments, and nations are socially organized on a continuum from domination to partnership. Proximity to one pole rather than the other affects the way that individuals and groups see the world and interact with one another. Cultural transformation theory acknowledges the tendency to operate according to partnership or domination beliefs and values (**Table 3**).

When the domination paradigm guides the interactions of providers, patients (persons), and families, the following characteristics may be present:

- Rigid hierarchies and ranking of individual participants
- Communication that flows only 1 way: top-down or provider to patient and family
- Patients and families do not feel safe to express their personal health care objectives
- Patients and families are afraid to disagree with the treatment and care plans established by providers and nurses

When patient-centered and family-centered care is based on partnership, the characteristics are markedly different:

- Patients, families, and providers welcome and respect each other's input and observations
- Communication flows easily between all members of the team
- Patients and families feel safe to ask questions until they feel fully informed to make the best health care decisions for them
- Patients and families are not afraid to disagree with providers and express their own opinions and their goals for treatment and care

In partnership-based relationships, power and influence still are present but they are used as tools of empowerment rather than oppression. Instead of power over, power is given to or used with patients and families to help them reach their health care goals. Hierarchies may also exist in both domination and partnership systems. For example, parents may make decisions for children who are minors. The difference lies in the use of power. In hierarchies of domination, power is used to maintain compliance, whereas in hierarchies of actualization based on partnership values, power is used to lift others up[84] helping them reach their highest potential.

Table 3
The domination-partnership systems continuum

Component	Domination System	Partnership System
1. Structure	Authoritarian and inequitable social and economic structure of rigid hierarchies of domination in both family and state	Democratic and economically equitable structure of linking and hierarchies of actualization in both family and state
2. Relations	High degree of fear, abuse, and violence from child and wife beating to abuse by superiors in families, workplaces, and society. Children grow up in highly punitive, authoritarian, male-dominated families	Mutual respect and trust with a low degree of fear and violence, because they are not required to maintain rigid rankings of domination. Children grow up in families in which parenting is authoritative rather than authoritarian and adult relations are egalitarian
3. Gender	Ranking of male half of humanity over female half, as well as rigid gender stereotypes with traits and activities viewed as masculine ranked over those viewed as feminine, such as caring and caregiving	Equal valuing of male and female halves of humanity, as well as fluid gender roles with high valuing of empathy, caring, caregiving, and nonviolence in both women and men, as well as in social and economic policy
4. Beliefs	Beliefs and stories justify and idealize domination and violence, which are presented as inevitable, moral, and desirable	Beliefs and stories recognize and give high value to empathic, mutually beneficial, and caring relations, which are considered moral and desirable

Courtesy of the Center for Partnership Studies; with permission. Available at: http://www.partnershipway.org/.

Partnership-based health care exemplar: the Institute for Patient- and Family-Centered Care

The Institute for Patient- and Family-Centered Care (IPFCC) is a primary example of a partnership-based approach to patient-centered and family-centered care. Core concepts of the IPFCC[85] include:

- Dignity and respect
    Health care practitioners listen to and honor patient and family perspectives and choices. Patient and family knowledge, values, beliefs, and cultural backgrounds are incorporated into the planning and delivery of care.
- Information sharing
    Health care practitioners communicate and share complete and unbiased information with patients and families in ways that are affirming and useful. Patients and families receive timely, complete, and accurate information to effectively participate in care and decision making.
- Participation
    Patients and families are encouraged and supported in participating in care and decision making at the level they choose.
- Collaboration
    Patients, families, health care practitioners, and health care leaders collaborate in policy and program development, implementation, and evaluation;

in facility design; and in professional education as well as in the delivery of care (p. 4).

These core concepts include the following partnership themes: mutual respect and trust, 2-way communication, an environment of safety fostered through transparency, and encouragement of patients/families to fully participate in health care decisions and management (**Box 2**).

Management of care implies that the care relationship is based on providers who have the power to manage the care and subordinates (patients and families) who are passive recipients of the care. This type of relationship is based on values and beliefs more closely aligned with the domination end of the cultural transformation continuum. Partnership-based health care on the other hand encourages providers, the patient, and families to come together, each respecting each other's contributions to health care decision making and participation in treatment plans and care. Communication is open, flows both ways, and seeks to fully grasp and affirm each unique individual and family's care objectives. In partnership-based care, power is not used to control those perceived to have lower rank or status. Instead, power is used to encourage patients' families to fully participate in decision making and care to the best of their abilities. Partnership-based care promotes and affirms the full dignity of those giving and receiving care.

In addition to creating a stronger, collaborative partnership between patients, families, and primary care providers, a partnership-based practice would offer an ideal platform from which to deliver or more effectively refer families to appropriate caregiving services. For example, in the scenario in **Box 2**, the primary care provider could do more than simply refer a family member to the appropriate care service but instead: (1) could provide a warm handoff, in which the provider or a representative of the provider works directly with the family to arrange for a consultation or family caregiver assessment; and (2) could develop a partnership with the referral program to ensure that information is shared between the primary care provider and the family caregiver support program to enhance the overall management of the care recipient's cancer.[26] We have found in our community outreach and intervention research that too often family caregivers "fall through the cracks" during the referral process; that is, primary care providers or other health care professionals are passive when attempting to link families to appropriate support services. As partnership-care models suggest, a more engaged, proactive approach to working with families is needed, particularly given the competing life demands as well as the potential stress that family caregivers may experience when helping a relative with a chronic disease.

TRAVERSING THE GAP BETWEEN EVIDENCE AND PRACTICE

The sophistication and quality of evidence supporting clinical interventions for family caregivers have greatly advanced over the past 2 decades. However, the state of the art has not yet progressed to the point where clinical providers have at their disposal the information necessary to guide the selection of interventions that are most appropriate for specific types of caregivers. Evidence-based clinical supports for family caregivers are also not widely available for various disease contexts; for example, although the Administration on Aging has led statewide efforts to translate evidence-based interventions for Alzheimer disease caregivers in various community and health care settings, these initiatives have occurred sporadically in other disease contexts. Here, we present a series of resources and tools that we have used in our various community outreach efforts that may assist clinical providers

Box 2
Scenarios showing the difference between a domination-based approach and partnership-based approach to family caregiving

Domination: a provider is speaking to the family of an 86-year-old patient with end-stage small cell cancer of the lung

> Provider: "You need to take her home as there is nothing more we can do for her."
>
> Family: "But, we have read there may be other treatment options."
>
> Provider: "I would have offered other options if there were any."
>
> Family: "If you discharge her we don't want her told that she is going to die. She does not need to know. Just keep her comfortable." "We are worried however that we may not be able to manage her at home because we both need to work."
>
> Provider: "I'm sure as a family you can figure out a way to rotate so she is never left alone."

Threads of domination:

> The provider directs the family on the action they need to take rather than inviting discussion. The family shows a domination-based relationship with the patient when they ask that the patient be kept from knowing her prognosis. The provider fails to listen and minimizes the family's fears related to external pressures (the need to work).

Partnership: same scenario but from a partnership perspective

> Provider, patient, and family in conference together: "For the last 3 months we have walked a long walk from diagnosis of your cancer to several rounds of treatments, and management of all your symptoms and side effects. We have reached a point that there aren't any more treatments available and your cancer is rapidly growing. I am sorry. I understand this is very difficult news to hear. During the treatment phase I relied heavily on our partnership and that has not changed. Treatments are no longer possible but expert comfort care is. I would like to know what your opinions are about where you would like to receive care and how much your family would like to participate in this care."
>
> Family: "But, we have read there may be other treatment options."
>
> Provider: "You can certainly seek a second-opinion. I am afraid I am not aware of any further treatment options at this late stage of the disease. I may not be able to offer additional treatments but when you feel ready, I am here to make sure she receives excellent management of pain and other symptoms so she can be comfortable."
>
> Family: "We understand, but we are worried that we may not be able to manage her at home because we both need to work."
>
> Provider: "I realize that families are often unable to provide around-the-clock care. If you are open, I'd like to arrange for a hospice consult to see if they can provide supplemental services when your family is away from the home. If they cannot provide care, we can have a further discussion about other respite alternatives or long-term care."

Threads of partnership:

> The key stakeholders are in open and transparent conversation with one another. The provider has respected the patient and family's input throughout their entire relationship. The provider respects the family's need to hold onto hope that another provider may have treatments that have not been tried. The provider is not defensive but rather suggests that the family seek another opinion if that is what they need for peace of mind. The provider does not say, "There is nothing more we can do," but instead offers to stay with the patient and family and provide expert comfort care. The provider hears and validates the family's fears that they will not be able to care for the patient. The provider offers to work in partnership with the patient, family, and other health care workers to find the best delivery of care possible.

who are partnering with family caregivers. Candidate information resources include the following:

- As part of the National Family Caregiver Support program, every Area Agency on Aging (AAA) in the United States includes staff who specialize in providing caregiver support. Family caregiver support specialists can provide consultation directly to families or refer caregivers to local support groups or other resources. To find a local AAA, see http://n4a.org/about-n4a/?fa=aaa-title-VI.
- Disease-specific advocacy organizations often offer up-to-date resources and information for family caregivers. Some examples include the Alzheimer's Association (http://www.alz.org); the American Cancer Society (http://www.cancer.org); the American Heart Association (http://www.heart.org); and the American Stroke Association (http://www.strokeassociation.org).
- Other important informational resources include consumer-oriented National Institutes of Health sites that provide evidence-based information for patients and families. For example, the National Institute on Aging hosts the Alzheimer's Disease Education and Referral site (http://www.nia.nih.gov/alzheimers), which provides several free publications that are available online or can be ordered and placed in a health care provider's office (we have used several of these information resources with considerable success in our outreach efforts). The National Cancer Institute (http://www.cancer.gov) has successfully integrated scientific information alongside several resources for patients and families. The National Institutes of Health sites also provide extensive links to online communities and organizations that offer information and support.
- The Alzheimer's Disease Support Services Program of the Administration on Aging has assembled a resource compendium that provides details on various types of interventions for persons with Alzheimer disease as well as their family caregivers, and translation details (http://www.aoa.gov/AoARoot/AoA_Programs/HPW/Alz_Grants/compendium.aspx#evidence).
- The comprehensive Family Caregiver Alliance Web site includes several general family caregiving resources, information, and services, including a summary section of evidence-based interventions as an annotated bibliography (http://caregiver.org/caregiver/jsp/content_node.jsp?nodeid=2324&chcategory=17).
- The American Psychological Association has assembled a superb online resource for clinical providers who are working with family caregivers: the Caregivers' Briefcase (http://www.apa.org/pi/about/publications/caregivers/practice-settings/intervention/intervention-models.aspx). Included are overviews of various types of intervention models in addition to practice guides that a clinician could follow when partnering with family caregivers.
- The Rosalynn Carter Institute for Caregiving has assembled a comprehensive and up-to-date Web site that includes helpful resources for family caregivers, a directory of family caregiving interventions, and guidance for clinicians as to how to implement these services (http://www.rosalynncarter.org/caregiver_intervention_database/).
- The Caregiving Resource Center of the American Association of Retired Persons (AARP) provides a number of person-centered information, referral, and local resource tools for family caregivers (http://www.aarp.org/home-family/caregiving/).
- There are several decision-making tools that guide family caregivers during the course of a relative's disease. These tools offer a structured format for families to weigh the pros and cons related to critical decisions associated with family caregiving. A library of decision-making tools for various chronic conditions is

available at the Ottawa Hospital Research Institute Web site (http://decisionaid. ohri.ca). For example, Healthwise developed 2 tools for Alzheimer family caregivers: *When should I make the decision to place a relative with Alzheimer's disease or dementia in a nursing home?* (http://decisionaid.ohri.ca/AZsumm.php? ID=1044) and *Should I take medications for Alzheimer's disease?* (http:// decisionaid.ohri.ca/AZsumm.php?ID=1131). The Mayo Clinic offers another decision-making tool related to long-term care in Alzheimer disease (http:// decisionaid.ohri.ca/AZsumm.php?ID=1362).

- The Medicare and Caregivers site (http://nihseniorhealth.gov/medicareandcaregivers/managingmedicalconditions/01.html) provides informational resources not only related to Medicare and its benefits but also various long-term care resources and information (such as an overview of the Center for Medicare and Medicaid Services' Nursing Home Compare tool; http://www.medicare.gov/ nursinghomecompare/search.html).
- Medline Plus provides an extensive resource list of information and videos for patients and families about selected diseases (http://www.nlm.nih.gov/ medlineplus/healthtopics.html).
- Several states and organizations have developed long-term care decision-making aids that can help older persons and their families generate individualized care plans based on their relative's care needs, particularly related to long-term care services. **Table 4** provides a list of these long-term care decision-making tools.

Table 4 Long-term care (LTC) decision-making tools		
Financing long-term care	Department of Family and Social Science, The University of Minnesota	http://www.cehd.umn.edu/ fsos/projects/ccfltc.asp
CalQualityCare.org	California HealthCare Foundation	http://www.calqualitycare.org/
Own Your Future: LTC Planning	Texas LTC Partnership	http://ownyourfuturetexas. org/files/LtcPlanKitEng.pdf
National Clearinghouse LTC Info	Department of Health and Human Services	http://www.longtermcare.gov/ LTC/Main_Site/index.aspx
SeniorLivingGuide.com	SeniorLivingGuide.com	http://www.seniorlivingguide. com/
Aplaceformom.com	A Place for Mom	http://www.aplaceformom. com/
LTC Guide	Clemson University	http://www.clemson.edu/ centers-institutes/aging/ documents/decision-guide. pdf
LTC Information	South Carolina Aging Disability and Resource Center	https://scaccess.agis.com/site/ 401/long_term_care.aspx
Guide to LTC: Explore Your Options	Veterans Administration	http://www.va.gov/geriatrics/ guide/longtermcare/Shared_ Decision_Making.asp
Long-Term Care Choices Navigator	Minnesota Department of Human Services	http://longtermcarechoices. minnesotahelp.info/

Courtesy of Tetyana Shippee, PhD, School of Public Health, University of Minnesota.

Several online resources and now applications (apps) for mobile devices are available, but their quality varies considerably.[86] Specifically, although these online resources and apps seem to hold promise and tend to have user-friendly, convenient features, whether these advances have shown efficacy in helping family caregivers remains largely unknown. **Table 5** presents several online family caregiving resources and apps that we have found helpful for families as part of our community outreach initiatives via the Families and Long-Term Care Research Projects at the University of Minnesota. The Web sites provided may change, but these resources may find a receptive audience among some family caregivers (particularly those seeking easy-to-use apps that can be integrated into day-to-day care responsibilities).

Table 5 is by no means a comprehensive list of smartphone applications; this is a market that is advancing and growing rapidly. As of December, 2013, there were several organizations that had compiled lists of best family caregiving applications; primary care providers and others are encouraged to review these sites to identify additional family caregiving support resources. Simply entering "best apps for family caregivers" in Google.com or another search engine yields several lists for the clinician or caregiver to review. It is important to note that: (1) the links and apps provided here and elsewhere may become quickly outdated given the rapid development of the smartphone application market; (2) some of the apps listed may be promoted based on industry ties and not because of their helpfulness for family caregivers; and (3) the availability and cost of these apps vary depending on the mobile device that the caregiver has available.

KNOWLEDGE NEEDS FOR HEALTH CARE IN THE FUTURE

Family caregiving research remains a mainstay in the disciplines of gerontology and geriatrics, and the ongoing work documenting the emotional, psychological, social, financial, and physiologic burdens of family caregiving has led to the development, evaluation, and to a lesser extent translation of clinical interventions to assist these

Table 5 Online resources for family caregivers	
Resource	**Web Link**
Elder 911 and Elder 411: smartphone application that provides expert advice in emergency situations	http://www.elder411.net/
Caregiver's Touch: smartphone application that stores and shares care-related information in 1 place	http://www.caregiverstouch.com/
Medicine Cabinet: smartphone application that stores medication-related information	http://www.limbua.com/medicineCabinet/index.html
RxMindMe: smartphone application that provides management and reminder alerts for medications	https://itunes.apple.com/us/app/rxmindme-prescription-medicine/id379864173?mt=8
Personal Caregiver: smartphone application that also provides medication management support	http://www.personalcaregiver.com/
iBioMed: smartphone application that provides extensive care management tools	http://www.biomedprofile.com/

families. Many resources are available that are likely to benefit particular family members, ranging from traditional, peer-led support groups to smartphone applications. However, does the current health care system, with its ongoing emphasis on the treatment of acute diseases,[26,87] sufficiently acknowledge the importance of family caregivers (much less partner with them)? The answer is mixed. In some disease contexts (such as Alzheimer disease), exciting and novel efforts have taken place to integrate extensive dementia care management approaches into primary care settings; these initiatives have led to increased use of community-based long-term care services, reduced medication use, reduced family caregiver stress, and enhanced clinical outcomes for the person with dementia.[88–91] Although such systems change efforts are state of the art, it does not seem that these models are gaining traction outside specialty settings.[73] Perhaps with the advent of patient-centered medical homes, health care systems will begin to better incorporate and partner with families to ensure proper chronic disease management and support families. However, this is a development that bears watching.

In keeping with the patient-centered goals of health care change efforts such as medical homes, how person-centered are current family caregiver support services? Although intensive multicomponent intervention models can exert positive benefits for family caregivers, it is not clear that these types of approaches (with their need for sufficient provider training and time commitment on the part of caregivers) work for all families in every type of situation. Online tools, applications, or emerging intervention models should determine, based on family caregivers' preferences and the characteristics of the caregiver or care recipient, the most appropriate support option for family caregivers. A consistent unmet need on the part of family caregivers is a lack of quality information about support strategies or services that can help ease the challenges of their particular caregiving situation. Although evidence-based, comprehensive psychosocial interventions are in various stages of translation across several US states (see http://www.rosalynncarter.org/caregiver_intervention_database/), such services are often presented as "one size fits all" solutions. Whether all caregivers are likely to benefit from or even prefer such comprehensive support protocols is often not considered. Even with the advent of online resources and apps, there remains a lack of individualized information that can directly meet the diverse needs of family caregivers that is concurrently based on scientific evidence. Partnering with family caregivers to establish a relationship that results in improved assessment and more effective referral to individualized support services would help to address an important gap in family caregiving practice and science.

REFERENCES

1. Thies W, Bleiler L, Alzheimer's Association. 2013 Alzheimer's disease facts and figures. Alzheimers Dement 2013;9(2):208–45.
2. Gaugler JE, Kane RL, Kane RA. Family care for older adults with disabilities: toward more targeted and interpretable research. Int J Aging Hum Dev 2002; 54(3):205–31.
3. Gaugler JE. Informal care supports: the basics. 2012. Available at: http://coa. umn.edu/GEM/index.htm. Accessed December 28, 2012.
4. Schulz R, Quittner AL. Caregiving for children and adults with chronic conditions: introduction to the special issue. Health Psychol 1998;17(2):107–11.
5. National Alliance for Caregiving, American Association of Retired Persons. Caregiving in the U.S. 2009. Washington, DC: National Alliance for Caregiving, American Association of Retired Persons; 2009.

6. Wolff JL, Kasper JD. Caregivers of frail elders: updating a national profile. Gerontologist 2006;46(3):344–56.
7. National Alliance for Caregiving, American Association for Retired Persons. Caregiving in the U.S. 2004. Washington, DC: National Alliance for Caregiving, American Association of Retired Persons; 2004.
8. Gitlin LN, Schulz R. Family caregiving of older adults. In: Prohaska TR, Anderson LA, Binsotck RH, editors. Public health for an aging society. Baltimore (MD): Johns Hopkins University Press; 2012. p. 181–204.
9. Fisher GG, Franks MM, Plassman BL, et al. Caring for individuals with dementia and cognitive impairment, not dementia: findings from the aging, demographics, and memory study. J Am Geriatr Soc 2011;59(3):488–94.
10. Dilworth-Anderson P, Williams SW, Copper T. Family caregiving to elderly African-Americans: caregiver types and structures. J Gerontol B Psychol Sci Soc Sci 1999;54B:S237–41.
11. Dilworth-Anderson P. Family issues and the care of persons with Alzheimer's disease. Aging Ment Health 2001;5:S49–51.
12. Dilworth-Anderson P, Williams IC, Gibson BE. Issues of race, ethnicity, and culture in caregiving research: a 20-year review (1980-2000). Gerontologist 2002; 42(2):237–72.
13. Gaugler JE, Duval S, Anderson KA, et al. Predicting nursing home admission in the U.S: a meta-analysis. BMC Geriatr 2007;7:13.
14. Gaugler JE, Kane RL, Kane RA, et al. Early community-based service utilization and its effects on institutionalization in dementia caregiving. Gerontologist 2005; 45:177–85.
15. Gaugler JE, Zarit SH, Pearlin LI. The onset of dementia caregiving and its longitudinal implications. Psychol Aging 2003;18:171–80.
16. Montgomery RJV, Kosloski KD. Family caregiving: change, continuity, and diversity. In: Lawton MP, Rubenstein RL, editors. Interventions in dementia care: toward improving quality of life. New York: Springer; 2000. p. 143–71.
17. Fortinsky RH, Tennen H, Frank N, et al. Health and psychological consequences of caregiving. In: Aldwin C, Park C, Spiro R, editors. Handbook of health psychology and aging. New York: Guilford; 2007. p. 227–49.
18. Feinberg L, Reinhard SC, Houser A, et al. Valuing the invaluable: 2011 update–the growing contributions and costs of family caregiving. Washington, DC: AARP Public Policy Institute; 2011.
19. The Family Caregiver Alliance. Selected long-term care statistics. Available at: http://caregiver.org/selected-long-term-care-statistics. Accessed April 9, 2014.
20. Kiecolt-Glaser JK, Preacher KJ, MacCallum RC, et al. Chronic stress and age-related increases in the proinflammatory cytokine IL-6. Proc Natl Acad Sci U S A 2003;100(15):9090–5. http://dx.doi.org/10.1073/pnas.1531903100.
21. Schulz R, Beach SR. Caregiving as a risk factor for mortality: the caregiver health effects study. JAMA 1999;282:2215–60.
22. Mausbach BT, Chattillion E, Roepke SK, et al. A longitudinal analysis of the relations among stress, depressive symptoms, leisure satisfaction, and endothelial function in caregivers. Health Psychol 2012;31(4):433–40.
23. Harmell AL, Chattillion EA, Roepke SK, et al. A review of the psychobiology of dementia caregiving: a focus on resilience factors. Curr Psychiatry Rep 2011; 13(3):219–24.
24. Vitaliano PP, Zhang J, Scanlan JM. Is caregiving hazardous to one's physical health? A meta-analysis. Psychol Bull 2003;129:946–72.

25. Pinquart M, Sörensen S. Correlates of physical health of informal caregivers: a meta-analysis. J Gerontol B Psychol Sci Soc Sci 2007;62(2):P126–37.
26. Kane RL, Priester R, Totten A. Meeting the challenge of chronic illness. Baltimore (MD): Johns Hopkins University Press; 2005.
27. Pinquart M, Sörensen S. Associations of caregiver stressors and uplifts with subjective well-being and depressive mood: a meta-analytic comparison. Aging Ment Health 2004;8(5):438–49.
28. Pinquart M, Sörensen S. Associations of stressors and uplifts of caregiving with caregiver burden and depressive mood: a meta-analysis. J Gerontol B Psychol Sci Soc Sci 2003;58(2):P112–28.
29. Pinquart M, Sörensen S. Differences between caregivers and noncaregivers in psychological health and physical health: a meta-analysis. Psychol Aging 2003; 18(2):250–67.
30. Pinquart M, Sorensen S. Ethnic differences in stressors, resources, and psychological outcomes of family caregiving: a meta-analysis. Gerontologist 2005; 45(1):90–106.
31. Ablitt A, Jones GV, Muers J. Living with dementia: a systematic review of the influence of relationship factors. Aging Ment Health 2009;13(4):497–511.
32. Pinquart M, Sörensen S. Spouses, adult children, and children-in-law as caregivers of older adults: a meta-analytic comparison. Psychol Aging 2011;26(1):1–14.
33. Sales E, Schulz R, Biegel D. Predictors of strain in families of cancer patients: a review of the literature. J Psychosoc Oncol 1992;10(2):1–26.
34. Given BA, Given CW, Kozachik S. Family support in advanced cancer. CA Cancer J Clin 2001;51:213–31.
35. Haley WE. Family caregivers of elderly patients with cancer: Understanding and minimizing the burden of care. J Support Oncol 2003;1(4 Suppl 2):25–9.
36. Li QP, Mak YW, Loke AY. Spouses' experience of caregiving for cancer patients: a literature review. Int Nurs Rev 2013;60(2):178–87.
37. Northouse LL, Katapodi MC, Schafenacker AM, et al. The impact of caregiving on the psychological well-being of family caregivers and cancer patients. Semin Oncol Nurs 2012;28(4):236–45.
38. Han B, Haley WE. Family caregiving for patients with stroke review and analysis. Stroke 1999;30(7):1478–85.
39. Gaugler JE. The longitudinal ramifications of stroke caregiving: a systematic review. Rehabil Psychol 2010;55(2):108–25.
40. Saban KL, Sherwood PR, DeVon HA, et al. Measures of psychological stress and physical health in family caregivers of stroke survivors: a literature review. J Neurosci Nurs 2010;42(3):128–38.
41. Funk L, Stajduhar K, Toye C, et al. Part 2: home-based family caregiving at the end of life: a comprehensive review of published qualitative research (1998-2008). Palliat Med 2010;24(6):594–607.
42. Hudson P, Payne S. Family caregivers and palliative care: current status and agenda for the future. J Palliat Med 2011;14(7):864–9.
43. Stajduhar K, Funk L, Toye C, et al. Part 1: home-based family caregiving at the end of life: a comprehensive review of published quantitative research (1998-2008). Palliat Med 2010;24(6):573–93.
44. Aoun SM, Bentley B, Funk L, et al. A 10-year literature review of family caregiving for motor neurone disease: moving from caregiver burden studies to palliative care interventions. Palliat Med 2013;27(5):437–46.
45. Sörensen S, Pinquart M, Duberstein P. How effective are interventions with caregivers? an updated meta-analysis. Gerontologist 2002;42(3):356–72.

46. Zabalegui Yarnoz A, Navarro Diez M, Cabrera Torres E, et al. Efficacy of interventions aimed at the main carers of dependent individuals aged more than 65 years old. A systematic review. Rev Esp Geriatr Gerontol 2008;43(3): 157–66 [in Spanish].

47. Shaw C, McNamara R, Abrams K, et al. Systematic review of respite care in the frail elderly. Health Technol Assess 2009;13(20):1–224, iii.

48. Thompson CA, Spilsbury K, Hall J, et al. Systematic review of information and support interventions for caregivers of people with dementia. BMC Geriatr 2007;7:18.

49. Cooper C, Balamurali TB, Selwood A, et al. A systematic review of intervention studies about anxiety in caregivers of people with dementia. Int J Geriatr Psychiatry 2007;22(3):181–8.

50. Selwood A, Johnston K, Katona C, et al. Systematic review of the effect of psychological interventions on family caregivers of people with dementia. J Affect Disord 2007;101(1–3):75–89.

51. Cooke DD, McNally L, Mulligan KT, et al. Psychosocial interventions for caregivers of people with dementia: a systematic review. Aging Ment Health 2001; 5(2):120–35.

52. Peacock SC, Forbes DA. Interventions for caregivers of persons with dementia: a systematic review. Can J Nurs Res 2003;35(4):88–107.

53. Acton GJ, Kang J. Interventions to reduce the burden of caregiving for an adult with dementia: a meta-analysis. Res Nurs Health 2001;24(5):349–60.

54. Mason A, Weatherly H, Spilsbury K, et al. A systematic review of the effectiveness and cost-effectiveness of different models of community-based respite care for frail older people and their carers. Health Technol Assess 2007; 11(15):1–157, iii.

55. Schoenmakers B, Buntinx F, DeLepeleire J. Supporting the dementia family caregiver: the effect of home care intervention on general well-being. Aging Ment Health 2010;14(1):44–56.

56. McNally S, Ben-Shlomo Y, Newman S. The effects of respite care on informal carers' well-being: a systematic review. Disabil Rehabil 1999;21(1):1–14.

57. Lee H, Cameron M. Respite care for people with dementia and their carers. Cochrane Database Syst Rev 2004;(2):CD004396.

58. Brodaty H, Green A, Koschera A. Meta-analysis of psychosocial interventions for caregivers of people with dementia. J Am Geriatr Soc 2003;51(5):657–64.

59. Smits CH, de Lange J, Droes RM, et al. Effects of combined intervention programmes for people with dementia living at home and their caregivers: a systematic review. Int J Geriatr Psychiatry 2007;22(12):1181–93.

60. Olazarán J, Reisberg B, Clare L, et al. Nonpharmacological therapies in Alzheimer's disease: a systematic review of efficacy. Dement Geriatr Cogn Disord 2010;30(2):161–78.

61. Pinquart M, Sörensen S. Helping caregivers of persons with dementia: which interventions work and how large are their effects? Int Psychogeriatr 2006;18(4): 577–95.

62. Northouse LL, Katapodi MC, Song L, et al. Interventions with family caregivers of cancer patients: meta-analysis of randomized trials. CA Cancer J Clin 2010; 60(5):317–39.

63. Hudson PL, Remedios C, Thomas K. A systematic review of psychosocial interventions for family carers of palliative care patients. BMC Palliat Care 2010;9:17.

64. Lee J, Soeken K, Picot SJ. A meta-analysis of interventions for informal stroke caregivers. West J Nurs Res 2007;29(3):344–56 [discussion: 357–64].

65. Legg Lynn A, Quinn Terry J, Mahmood F, et al. Non-pharmacological interventions for caregivers of stroke survivors. Cochrane Database Syst Rev 2011;(10):CD008179.

66. Sackett DL, Rosenberg WM, Gray JA, et al. Evidence based medicine: what it is and what it isn't. BMJ 1996;312(7023):71–2.

67. Family Caregiver Alliance. Caregiver assessment: principles, guidelines and strategies for change. San Francisco (CA): Family Caregiver Alliance; 2006.

68. Feinberg LF. Caregiver assessment. Am J Nurs 2008;108(Suppl 9):38–9.

69. The American Psychological Association. Assessment strategy. 2013. Available at: http://www.apa.org/pi/about/publications/caregivers/practice-settings/assessment/strategy.aspx. Accessed December 28, 2013.

70. Gaugler JE, Kane RA, Langlois J. Assessment of family caregivers of older adults. In: Kane RL, Kane RA, editors. Assessing the well-being of older people: measures, meaning, and practical applications. New York: Oxford University Press; 2000. p. 320–59.

71. The American Psychological Association. Assessment tools. 2013. Available at: http://www.apa.org/pi/about/publications/caregivers/practice-settings/assessment/tools/. Accessed December 29, 2013.

72. Family Caregiver Alliance and the Benjamin Rose Institute on Aging. Selected caregiver assessment measures: a resource inventory for practitioners. 2nd edition. 2012. Available at: http://caregiver.org/caregiver/jsp/content/pdfs/SelCGAssmtMeas_ResInv_FINAL_12.10.12.pdf. Accessed December 29, 2013.

73. Odenheimer G, Borson S, Sanders AE, et al. Quality improvement in neurology: dementia management quality measures (executive summary). Am J Occup Ther 2013;67(6):704–10.

74. American Geriatrics Society 2012 Beers Criteria Update Expert Panel. American Geriatrics Society updated Beers criteria for potentially inappropriate medication use in older adults. J Am Geriatr Soc 2012;60(4):616–31.

75. Banerjee S, Wittenberg R. Clinical and cost effectiveness of services for early diagnosis and intervention in dementia. Int J Geriatr Psychiatry 2009;24(7):748–54.

76. Gitlin LN, Kales HC, Lyketsos CG. Nonpharmacologic management of behavioral symptoms in dementia. JAMA 2012;308(19):2020–9.

77. Nelson JC, Devanand DP. A systematic review and meta-analysis of placebo-controlled antidepressant studies in people with depression and dementia. J Am Geriatr Soc 2011;59(4):577–85.

78. Vigen CL, Mack WJ, Keefe RS, et al. Cognitive effects of atypical antipsychotic medications in patients with Alzheimer's disease: outcomes from CATIE-AD. Am J Psychiatry 2011;168(8):831–9.

79. Resnick B, Fick DM. 2012 Beers criteria update: how should practicing nurses use the criteria? Geriatr Nurs 2012;33(4):253–5.

80. Agency for Healthcare Research and Quality. Expanding patient-centered care to empower patients and assist providers. Rockville (MD): AHRQ Publication; 2002. Available at: http://www.ahrq.gov/research/findings/factsheets/patient-centered/ria-issue5/index.html.

81. Eisler R, Potter TM. Transforming interprofessional partnerships: a new framework for nursing and partnership-based health care. Indianapolis (IN): Sigma Theta Tau International; 2014.

82. World Health Organization. Framework for action on interprofessional education and collaborative practice. Geneva (Switzerland): WHO Press; 2010.

83. Eisler R. The chalice and the blade: our history, our future. San Francisco (CA): Harper Collins; 1987.
84. Eisler R. The power of partnership. Novato (CA): New World Library; 2002.
85. Institute for Patient- and Family-Centered Care. Advancing the practice of patient- and family-centered care in hospitals. Bethesda (MD): Institute for Patient- and Family-Centered Care; 2011.
86. Anderson KA, Nikzad-Terhune KA, Gaugler JE. A systematic evaluation of online resources for dementia caregivers. J Consum Health Internet 2009;13:1–13.
87. Lubkin IM, Larsen PD, editors. Chronic illness: impact and intervention. 8th edition. Burlington (MA): Jones and Bartlett Learning, LLC; 2013.
88. Borson S, Scanlan JM, Watanabe J, et al. Improving identification of cognitive impairment in primary care. Int J Geriatr Psychiatry 2006;21(4):349–55.
89. Boustani M, Sachs G, Callahan CM. Can primary care meet the biopsychosocial needs of older adults with dementia? J Gen Intern Med 2007;22(11):1625–7.
90. Callahan CM, Boustani MA, Weiner M, et al. Implementing dementia care models in primary care settings: the Aging Brain Care Medical Home. Aging Ment Health 2011;15(1):5–12.
91. Reuben DB, Roth CP, Frank JC, et al. Assessing care of vulnerable elders–Alzheimer's disease: a pilot study of a practice redesign intervention to improve the quality of dementia care. J Am Geriatr Soc 2010;58(2):324–9.

Other Mental Health Problems in Older Adults

A Systematic Approach to Pharmacotherapy for Geriatric Major Depression

Benoit H. Mulsant, MD, MS[a,b,*], Daniel M. Blumberger, MD, MSc[b,c], Zahinoor Ismail, MD[a,d], Kiran Rabheru, MD[e], Mark J. Rapoport, MD[b,f]

KEYWORDS

- Major depressive disorder • Geriatrics • Old age • Antidepressant agents
- Drug therapy • Guidelines • Algorithm • Stepped care

KEY POINTS

- The effectiveness of antidepressants depends in large part on the way they are used. Under usual care conditions, the outcomes of antidepressant pharmacotherapy for geriatric depression have been shown to be mediocre at best.
- Trying to individualize treatment by matching each patient with a specific antidepressant based on the patient's symptoms and an antidepressant putative side-effect profile is ineffective. Instead, the outcomes of antidepressant pharmacotherapy for geriatric depression can be improved markedly when antidepressants are prescribed following an algorithmic ("stepped-care").
- Published guidelines and algorithms for the antidepressant pharmacotherapy for geriatric depression are informed by published evidence but they do not necessarily conform to this evidence. This article presents an updated algorithm for the antidepressant pharmacotherapy for geriatric depression that is based on the authors' interpretation of the available evidence.

Funding: This work was supported in part by grant MH083643 from the US National Institute of Mental Health.
Conflicts of Interest: See last page of the article.
[a] Centre for Addiction and Mental Health, 1001 Queen Street West, Toronto, Ontario M6J 1H4, Canada; [b] Department of Psychiatry, Faculty of Medicine, University of Toronto, 250 College Street, Toronto, ON, M5T 1R8, Canada; [c] Temerty Centre for Therapeutic Brain Intervention, Centre for Addiction and Mental Health, 1001 Queen Street West, Toronto, Ontario M6J 1H4, Canada; [d] Hotchkiss Brain Institute, Foothills Hospital, University of Calgary, 1403 29th Street Northwest, Calgary, Alberta T2N 2T9, Canada; [e] Geriatric Psychiatry & ECT Program, Department of Psychiatry, The Ottawa Hospital, University of Ottawa, 75 Bruyere Street, Suite 137 Y, Ottawa, Ontario K1N 5C7, Canada; [f] Sunnybrook Health Sciences Centre, FG37-2075 Bayview Avenue, Toronto, Ontario M4C 5N6, Canada
* Corresponding author. Centre for Addiction and Mental Health, 1001 Queen Street West, Toronto, Ontario M6J 1H4, Canada.
E-mail address: benoit.mulsant@camh.ca

INTRODUCTION

Approximately 14% of older Americans are now taking an antidepressant.[1–3] However, this broad use has not been associated with a notable decrease in the burden of geriatric depression.[4,5] This article, based on a selective review of the literature, explores several explanations for this paradox. First, the possible explanations that antidepressants are not effective in the treatment of depression or that the results of randomized, controlled clinical trials (RCTs) are not applicable to the treatment of depression in real-world clinical settings, are discussed and rejected. Instead, the authors propose that the efficacy of antidepressants depends in large part on the way they are used. Evidence is presented to support the proposition that the use of antidepressant pharmacotherapy is associated with better outcomes when guided by a treatment algorithm (a stepped-care approach) as opposed to an attempt to individualize treatment. Published guidelines and pharmacotherapy algorithms developed for the treatment of geriatric depression are reviewed. Finally an updated algorithm is proposed, based on the authors' interpretation of the available evidence.

ARE ANTIDEPRESSANTS EFFECTIVE FOR THE TREATMENT OF MAJOR DEPRESSIVE DISORDER?

Some investigators have proposed that antidepressants are either not effective or only minimally effective except in patients with the most severe depression, pointing out the small effect sizes in meta-analyses including both published and unpublished placebo-controlled RCTs of antidepressants (eg, Refs.[6–8]). Several analyses have been published specifically to refute these results (eg, Refs.[9–12]) or show that psychotropic medications (including antidepressants) are as efficacious as drugs used to treat general medical conditions.[13] The debate about the true efficacy of antidepressants (ie, whether there is a meaningful difference in the remission or response rates experienced by patients randomized to an antidepressant or a placebo) continues.[14–16] Regardless of the degree to which antidepressants are more efficacious than placebo, patients treated with active antidepressants should experience at least the improvement associated with the use of a placebo. However, some published data suggest that patients whose depression is treated under usual care (nonstudy) conditions are actually less likely to respond to antidepressant treatment or to experience remission of their depressive symptoms than depressed patients who receive a placebo in an RCT. Poor outcomes for depressed patients treated under usual care conditions have been reported in both those treated by primary care providers (PCPs) and those treated by psychiatrists. For instance, Meyers and colleagues[17] reported that only 30% of adult patients with a major depressive disorder (MDD) who were treated by a psychiatrist experienced remission of their major depressive episode after 3 months, a rate lower than the 30% to 40% rate of remission typically associated with placebo in RCTs of adults with MDD.[12,13]

ARE THE RESULTS OF RANDOMIZED CONTROLLED TRIALS OF ANTIDEPRESSANTS APPLICABLE TO REAL-WORLD GERIATRIC PRACTICE?

Some investigators have proposed that antidepressants are not as effective in clinical practice as in RCTs because patients who participate in RCTs are not representative of patients treated in real-world clinical practice. This argument is supported by some published data showing that, because of the required eligibility criteria they have to meet to participate, depressed subjects included in RCTs differ from the population from which they are drawn.[18,19] However, the gap between the efficacy of antidepressants when used in an RCT and their lower effectiveness when used under usual care conditions persists in studies that randomize depressed participants who meet the same eligibility criteria to either an experimental intervention or usual care. For instance, in 2 large geriatric studies, IMPACT[20,21] and PROSPECT,[22–25] older depressed participants who met the same eligibility criteria were randomized to either an experimental intervention or treatment as usual. In these 2 studies, the response rates associated with usual care (IMPACT: 16% after 12 months; PROSPECT: 19% after 4 months) (**Table 1**) were less than half the response rates associated with placebo (mean ± standard deviation: 40% ± 10%; median: 38%; range: 19%–54%) (**Fig. 1**A) in the 9 published placebo-controlled RCTs that have assessed the efficacy of second-generation antidepressants in older patients with MDD.[26–34]

Table 1
Treatment algorithm and outcomes in 2 randomized studies comparing a stepped-care approach with treatment as usual for the treatment of late-life depression

Study (Authors,[Ref.] Year)	No. of Patients	Treatment Algorithm	Outcomes
IMPACT (Unutzer et al,[20,21] 2001, 2002)	1801	Step 1: AD (typically an SSRI) or PST (8–12 wk) Step 2: Nonresponse: switch to other AD or PST Partial response: combine with other AD or PST Step 3: Combine AD and PST Consider ECT or other specialty services	Rate of response (50% reduction in depression score) after 12 mo: Intervention: 45% Usual care: 19%
PROSPECT (Mulsant et al,[22] 2001; Bruce et al,[23] 2004; Alexopoulos et al,[24,25] 2005, 2009)	599	Step 1: Optimize current AD (if applicable) Nonresponse: Switch to: Step 2: citalopram 30 mg once daily Step 3: bupropion SR 100–200 mg twice daily Step 4: venlafaxine XR 150–300 mg once in AM Step 5: nortriptyline (target 80–120 ng/mL) Step 6: mirtazapine 30–45 mg in the evening Partial response: Add: Step 2: bupropion SR 100–200 mg twice daily Step 3: nortriptyline (target 80–120 ng/mL) Step 4: lithium (target 0.60–0.80 mEq/L) Then steps 2, 4, 6 for nonresponders Also, IPT can be used as an alternative to AD or as an augmentation to AD	Rate of response (HDRS score of ≤10) After 4 mo: Intervention: 33% Usual care: 16% After 12 mo: Intervention: 54% Usual care: 45%

Abbreviations: AD, antidepressant; ECT, electroconvulsive therapy; HDRS, Hamilton Depression Rating Scale; IPT, interpersonal therapy; PST, problem-solving therapy; SSRI, selective serotonin reuptake inhibitor; SR, sustained release; XR, extended release.

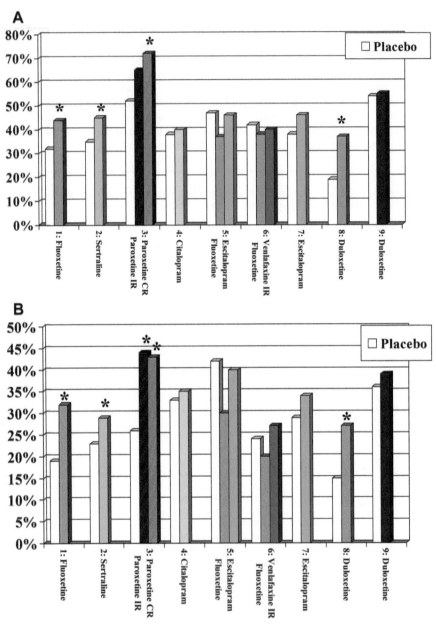

Fig. 1. (*A*) Response rates in 9 published randomized placebo-controlled trials of newer antidepressants. (*B*) Remission rates in 9 published randomized placebo-controlled trials of newer antidepressants. (*C*) Discontinuation rates attributed to adverse effects in 9 published randomized placebo-controlled trials of newer antidepressants. (*D*) Overall discontinuation rates published in 9 published randomized placebo-controlled trials of newer antidepressants. Asterisk indicates significant difference between antidepressant and placebo. CR, controlled release; IR, immediate release. (*Data from* Refs.[26–34])

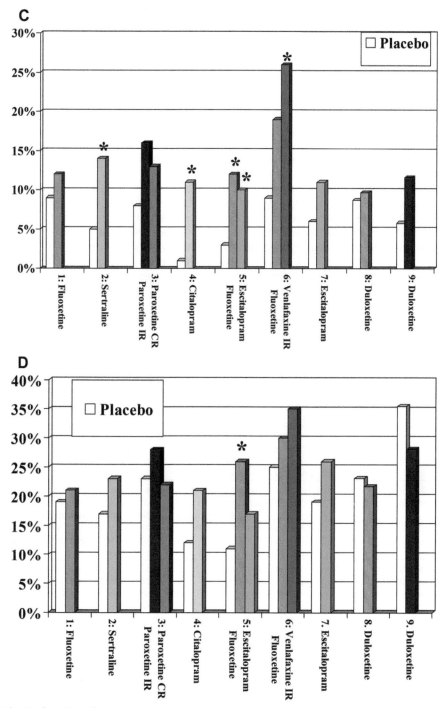

Fig. 1. (*continued*)

The process of care in the experimental intervention group in IMPACT and PROSPECT, or other RCTs, is very different from the process of usual care in primary care or psychiatric practice (**Table 2**). Several lines of evidence suggest that the differences in outcomes are due to these differences in the process of care. For example, a meta-analysis has shown that in placebo-controlled RCTs of antidepressants for adult MDD lasting 6 weeks, 2 additional follow-up visits at weeks 3 and 5 improve outcomes of both placebo and active antidepressants, accounting for 41% of the improvement observed with placebo and 27% for the improvement with an antidepressant.[35] The effect of additional visits was cumulative and proportional (ie, 2 extra visits yielded twice the benefits of 1 additional visit) and was not due to a lower likelihood of dropping out (ie, the dropout rates were similar with 4, 5, or 6 follow-up visits).[35] Similar results have been reported in geriatric trials.[36]

Besides the frequency, duration, and quality of follow-up visits, RCTs and usual care also differ in the quantity and quality of the antidepressant pharmacotherapy offered. In PROSPECT, older patients were systematically screened for the presence of depression, and the PCPs were notified when their patients were found to suffer from a clinically significant depression requiring treatment. However, when assessed after 4, 8, 12, 18, or 24 months, only 50% to 60% of the patients randomized to usual care were found to be receiving any treatment for depression.[25] These low rates of initiation, continuation, and maintenance of treatment in the older participants of PROSPECT are consistent

Table 2
Processes of care when using antidepressants under experimental conditions versus usual care conditions

	Experimental Condition	Usual Care Condition
Schedule of visits	Fixed; 4–6 visits over 6 wk; 6–12 visits over 8–12 wk	Based on physician's and patient's availability; 2–3 visits over 12 wk
Duration of visits	30–60 min	10–20 min
Treatment protocol	Predetermined; minimal adaptations based on patient's characteristics (eg, slower titration for frail patients)	Individualized for each patient based on their characteristics and preferences
Selection of antidepressant	Small number of antidepressants preselected based on best evidence or guidelines and used in a large number of patients	Large number of antidepressants, each used in a small number of patients; matching patient's clinical characteristics with perceived features of specific antidepressants
Dose titration and change in treatment	Predetermined; based on operationalized criteria, protecting clinicians from personal biases or pressures from patients or their families	Negotiated at each visit with each patient based on perceived adverse effects or lack of improvement. Changes often ill-advised or ill-timed
Monitoring of symptoms and adverse effects	Systematic monitoring with use of structured interviews and validated scales	Monitoring based on spontaneous reports and ad hoc clinical interviews
Main focus of clinical interactions	Maximizing treatment adherence with psychoeducation, characterization of changes in patient's symptoms, management of adverse effects	Negotiating whether and how antidepressants should be used, titrated up or down, switched, or augmented; selection of augmenting or alternative agents

with the low rates reported in both older[36] and younger[4,17] adults. By contrast, 80% to 90% of the PROSPECT patients randomized to the intervention were receiving some treatment for depression when assessed after 4, 8, 12, 18, or 24 months.[25]

HOW SHOULD CLINICIANS SELECT ANTIDEPRESSANTS TO TREAT THEIR OLDER PATIENTS?

To make matters worse, barely half of adults who receive depression treatment under usual care receive minimally adequate treatment.[4,17] Again, the low level of the quality of antidepressant pharmacotherapy under usual care is attributable in large part to issues related to the process of care, in particular the way clinicians select antidepressants (see **Table 2**). For instance, despite evidence showing that all antidepressants have comparable efficacy in the acute, continuation, or maintenance treatment of MDD,[37] most physicians try to match each individual patient to a specific antidepressant. The limited empirical data on which strategy physicians use to match patients to antidepressants suggest that they consider 3 main factors: presence of specific target symptoms (particularly insomnia, anxiety, fatigue, or appetite changes); presence of comorbid conditions (particularly panic disorder, generalized anxiety disorder, or posttraumatic disorder); and avoidance of specific side effects (particularly sexual dysfunction, weight gain, fatigue, anticholinergic effects, or agitation).[38]

Avoidance of specific adverse effects makes sense, and is endorsed by the American Psychiatric Association practice guideline for the treatment of patients with MDD.[39] However, there is no convincing evidence that any selective serotonin reuptake inhibitor (SSRI) or serotonin-norepinephrine reuptake inhibitor (SNRI) is superior to other SSRIs or SNRIs in the treatment of anxiety disorders. Similarly, trying to target specific depressive symptoms based on the distinct side-effect profiles of various antidepressants seems to be a futile pursuit, given that response to specific medications is not predicted by specific symptoms or symptom clusters.[40–42] For instance, an analysis assessed whether a "sedating antidepressant" (imipramine) would be better tolerated or more efficacious than an "activating antidepressant" (fluoxetine) in 355 depressed adult patients enrolled in an RCT who presented with insomnia.[43] During 4 weeks of treatment, patients were significantly more likely to discontinue imipramine than fluoxetine, regardless of whether they had a low or high level of insomnia; after 4 weeks, the remission rates for those with a high level of insomnia were 16% with imipramine versus 21% with fluoxetine (and 23% vs 38% for those with a low level of insomnia); there was no significant interaction between level of insomnia and treatment with respect to either discontinuation rates or remission rates.[43]

Minimal empirical data are available to assess other strategies used by physicians to individualize the treatment of depression. In an RCT for chronic depression, initial preference for pharmacotherapy or psychotherapy was a strong predictor of treatment outcome following randomization to pharmacotherapy or psychotherapy (but, surprisingly, not of the likelihood of dropping out).[44] In a retrospective chart review published 20 years ago, 20 of 35 (57%) patients responded to an antidepressant to which they had responded previously, whereas 19 of 24 (79%) were treated with a different antidepressant and responded.[45] To the authors' knowledge, there are no other published data to support or contradict the wisdom of heeding a depressed patient's preference for a specific treatment, or of favoring an antidepressant to which a patient has responded in the past.[40]

Most clinicians are surprised when they hear that individualized interventions under usual care conditions (ie, selection of a specific antidepressant based on a patient's unique characteristics and treatment management based on patient's unique experience) yield significantly worse outcomes than a systematic approach used under experimental conditions (ie, all patients receiving a preselected antidepressant and treatment changes guided by predetermined criteria). However, for the treatment of geriatric depression, the benefits of using a stepped-care approach built around a treatment algorithm are supported not only by the results of IMPACT[20,21] and PROSPECT[22–25] (see **Table 1**) but also by 4 other studies showing that approximately 80% of older patients with MDD seen in psychiatric settings can respond to such an approach.[46–49]

WHAT CAN WE LEARN FROM GUIDELINES ON PHARMACOTHERAPY FOR GERIATRIC DEPRESSION?

Taken together, the data already discussed suggest that clinicians could double the treatment response rates experienced by their older depressed patients if they adopted a more systematic approach to treatment. Treatment guidelines summarizing and interpreting the relevant evidence and expert opinion offer a starting point to clinicians who wish to follow such an approach. To the authors' knowledge, the most recent guidelines on pharmacotherapy for geriatric depression were published in 2006.[50,51] The recommendations from these Canadian guidelines and from earlier United States expert consensus guidelines[52] are summarized in **Table 3**.

Overall, the recommendations from these 2 sets of guidelines are consistent. One could argue that while they are informed by evidence, they reflect more the preference of the experts involved in their creation than the direct results of RCTs. As of April 2014 there are 9 published placebo-controlled trials of the efficacy and tolerability of SSRIs or SNRIs in the acute treatment of older patients with MDD.[26–34] **Fig. 1** displays the response rates, remission rates, dropout rates attributed to adverse effects, and overall dropout rates in these 9 RCTs. Fluoxetine (in 1 of 3 trials), sertraline (in 1 trial), paroxetine (in 1 trial), and duloxetine (in 1 of 2 trials) were more efficacious than placebo; by contrast, the unique placebo-controlled trial that has assessed the efficacy of citalopram and the 2 placebo-controlled trials that have assessed the efficacy of its S-enantiomer, escitalopram, have failed to demonstrate their superiority to placebo (see **Fig. 1**A, B). Nevertheless, in both the United States and Canadian guidelines, citalopram was recommended as a first-line treatment. Experts, including some of the authors of this article,[22] have typically attributed their preference for citalopram to its lack of drug-drug interaction and its good tolerability "in their clinical experience." However, in placebo-controlled trials, all SSRIs except for paroxetine have been associated with significantly higher rates of discontinuation attributed to adverse effects in comparison with placebo (see **Fig. 1**C), and only fluoxetine (in 1 of 3 trials) was associated with a significantly higher likelihood of overall premature discontinuation (ie, discontinuation for any reason) than placebo (see **Fig. 1**D). The Canadian guidelines also recommend the use of bupropion, mirtazapine, or venlafaxine as first-line treatment, and both the United States and Canadian guidelines recommend the use of bupropion or venlafaxine as second-line treatment. Neither bupropion nor mirtazapine has been assessed in a published placebo-controlled trial in older patients with MDD, and the trial that has assessed the efficacy of venlafaxine as a first-line treatment has failed to demonstrate its superiority to placebo.[31] However, in 2 small nonblinded studies, 14 of 27 (52%) older patients responded to a switch to venlafaxine after having failed to respond to 1 to 3 other antidepressants.[47,53]

AN UPDATED ALGORITHM FOR THE PHARMACOLOGIC TREATMENT OF GERIATRIC DEPRESSION

Beyond traditional efficacy trials that address the 2 questions of which antidepressant to use and at what dose, there is a paucity of data in adult depressed patients[54–60] and

Table 3
Recommendations for pharmacotherapy for major depression from the 2001 United States expert consensus guidelines and the 2006 Canadian guidelines

	2001 US Expert Consensus Guidelines	2006 Canadian Guidelines
Preferred treatment	An antidepressant (SSRI or venlafaxine XR preferred) plus psychotherapy	An antidepressant, psychotherapy, or a combination of both if the depression is of mild or moderate severity; a combination of an antidepressant and psychotherapy for severe depressions
Specific antidepressant	Citalopram and sertraline are preferred with paroxetine as another first-line option	Citalopram, sertraline, venlafaxine, bupropion, or mirtazapine
Starting dose	Begin with "somewhat lower doses" than in younger adults	Half of the recommended dose for younger adults
Increases in dose	Wait 2–4 wk before increasing a low dose if there is little or no response and 3–5 wk if there is a partial response	Aim for "an average dose" within 1 mo if the medication is well tolerated. In the absence of improvement after at least 2 wk on "an average dose," increase dose gradually (up to maximum recommended dose) until clinical improvement or limiting side effects are observed
When to change treatment	After 3–6 wk at a "therapeutic" or the maximum tolerated dose if there is little or no response and 4–7 wk if there is a partial response	After at least 4 wk at the maximum tolerated or recommended dose if there is no or minimal response after 4–8 wk if there is some partial response
What to do in case of minimal or no response to initial antidepressant	Preferred option: switch to venlafaxine or bupropion. Alternative option: switch to nortriptyline, mirtazapine, or another SSRI	Consider "all reasonable treatment options" including ECT, combination of antidepressants or mood stabilizers, addition of psychotherapy
What to do in case of partial response to initial antidepressant	Combine or augment initial antidepressant with another agent	Switch to another antidepressant of the same or another class while considering the risk of losing the improvements made with the first treatment
Agents to consider for combination or augmentation	Bupropion, lithium, or nortriptyline	Mirtazapine, bupropion, or lithium

Abbreviations: ECT, electroconvulsive therapy; SSRI, selective serotonin reuptake inhibitor; XR, extended release.
Data from Refs.[50,51,53]

almost none in older patients[47,61–63] that directly address the practical questions faced by clinicians when they treat an actual patient, such as: How long should one wait before making a change in treatment? When is it preferable to substitute another antidepressant or to add a second antidepressant or another psychotropic agent? Which specific antidepressant should one substitute? Which psychotropic agent should one add? Mindful of these limitations in the literature, the 5 authors convened during a workshop held in September 2013 at the annual meeting of the Canadian Academy of Geriatric Psychiatry to discuss what changes, if any, they would consider to the recommendations from the 2001 United States or 2006 Canadian guidelines and to the published algorithms discussed earlier, if they had to propose an updated algorithm for the pharmacotherapy of geriatric depression. Whereas guidelines tend to list several recommended alternatives, treatment algorithms are typically more prescriptive, focusing on a series of well-defined steps (see **Table 1**). Thus the authors tried to arrive at a consensus on what would constitute the preferred steps when treating older patients presenting with nonbipolar, nonpsychotic MDD. However, they did not reach a unanimous endorsement for any steps; **Table 4** presents the preferred choice of the majority with the alternative(s) endorsed by the minority.

Although older depressed patients typically present with comorbid physical conditions and some cognitive impairment, the proposed steps were not tailored for specific comorbid conditions (eg, Parkinson disease, dementia, chronic pain). Given the availability of older published guidelines and algorithms, the authors considered the newer antidepressants available (eg, escitalopram, duloxetine), recent safety data (eg, the data and warnings about the possible cardiovascular effects of citalopram), and newer data and indications for the use of atypical antipsychotics (eg, aripiprazole, quetiapine) in the treatment of MDD. However, the authors reaffirmed their agreement with principles of judicious prescribing, including initiating only 1 medication at a time, avoiding premature changes, and being circumspect about new medications for which rare adverse effects may not yet have been recognized,[64] leading them to favor simpler steps (eg, 1 medication rather than 2) and safer steps (eg, medications less likely to be involved in drug-drug interactions or medications less likely to be associated with serious adverse events). Finally, while acknowledging a role for both psychotherapy (eg, Ref.[65]) and brain stimulation[66,67] in the treatment of geriatric depression, this algorithm focuses on pharmacologic agents. Similarly, while

Table 4	
Updated pharmacotherapy algorithm for the treatment of late-life depression	
	Majority Consensus and Minority Alternative
Step 1	Escitalopram Alternatives: sertraline, duloxetine
Step 2 for minimal or no response	Switch to duloxetine Alternatives: venlafaxine, desvenlafaxine
Step 3 for minimal or no response	Switch to nortriptyline Alternative: bupropion
Step 2–3 for partial response	Augment antidepressant with lithium or an atypical antipsychotic Alternatives: combine SSRI or SNRI with mirtazapine or bupropion
Duration of each step	6 wk Alternatives: 4 wk; 8 wk

Abbreviation: SNRI, serotonin-norepinephrine reuptake inhibitor.

acknowledging the crucial role of long-term continuation and maintenance pharmaco-therapy for the prevention of relapse and recurrence of geriatric depression,[68] the proposed algorithm focuses on the use of antidepressants during the acute phase of treatment.

First-Line Antidepressant

Despite 2 negative geriatric placebo-controlled RCTs (see **Fig. 1**), the authors' updated algorithm recommends escitalopram as the preferred first-line agent (with sertraline and duloxetine as alternatives). The change from citalopram, recommended in the 2001 United States and 2006 Canadian guidelines, reflects the warning from the US Food and Drug Administration that citalopram has now been associated with a dose-dependent QT-interval prolongation (which can cause torsades de pointes, ventricular tachycardia, or sudden death) and the related maximum recommended dose of 20 mg per day for patients older than 60 years.[69] Some may argue that this warning is more a medicolegal concern than a clinical one, given the lack of cardiotoxicity associated with higher doses of citalopram in a pharmacoepidemiology study of more than 600,000 mid-life and late-life patients.[70] However, the significant lengthening of QTc in a recent placebo-controlled trial involving 186 older patients with dementia[71] is a reminder that, when assessing causal relationships, RCTs cannot be replaced by analyses of nonrandomized observational data, even when they attempt to control for a large number of potential confounders.[72]

Second-Step Treatment of Nonresponders

The selection of duloxetine as the preferred second-line agent (with venlafaxine or desvenlafaxine as alternatives) for older patients who fail to improve significantly on escitalopram is congruent with the 2001 United States guidelines recommending to switch to an antidepressant from another class when a patient fails to respond to an SSRI (see **Table 3**). This preference for switching antidepressant classes is not supported by STAR*D, in which adult patients whose treatment was switched from citalopram to bupropion, sertraline, or venlafaxine did not differ significantly with respect to outcomes, tolerability, or adverse events.[56,59] Although there is no geriatric study similar to STAR*D, as discussed earlier the efficacy of venlafaxine in older patients who failed to respond to an SSRI is supported by 2 small studies.[47,53] The authors are not aware of similar geriatric data for duloxetine, although its efficacy is supported by 1 of 2 published placebo-controlled RCTs[33]; also, in these 2 placebo-controlled trials[33,34] duloxetine and placebo had similar discontinuation rates attributed to adverse effects. By contrast, in a single placebo-controlled RCT,[31] the efficacy of immediate-release venlafaxine was not different from placebo, and its discontinuation rate attributed to adverse effects was higher than with placebo (see **Fig. 1**).

Duloxetine was also favored over venlafaxine because of its indication not only for MDD and generalized anxiety disorder but also for the management of several pain syndromes that are common in older depressed patients: neuropathic pain associated with diabetes, fibromyalgia, and chronic musculoskeletal pain.[73] However, these potential advantages of duloxetine are not supported by the much larger number of RCTs conducted in younger patients with MDD: in 2 recent meta-analyses that compared the results of RCTs of duloxetine and other antidepressants in adult patients with MDD, duloxetine was not more efficacious than SSRIs or venlafaxine but was associated with a higher dropout rate than escitalopram or venlafaxine.[74,75] Similarly, in a pooled analysis of 4 head-to-head RCTs in adult patients with MDD, the effect of duloxetine or paroxetine on pain did not differ significantly.[42]

Third-Step Treatment of Nonresponders

When older patients have failed an SSRI and an SNRI, the algorithm recommends the use of nortriptyline (with bupropion as an alternative). Again, preference is given to a switch to an antidepressant of a different class as opposed to augmenting or combining the failed antidepressant. The evidence that 2 psychotropic agents are more efficacious than 1 is relatively strong in younger patients[76] but much less so in older adults,[61] in whom polypharmacy causes more adverse events than monotherapy.[47] The choice of a tricyclic antidepressant (TCA) is supported by several geriatric RCTs that established their efficacy and safety in the 1980s and 1990s.[77] Similarly, the choice of nortriptyline among the TCAs is justified both by available RCTs and by data showing that it is less likely than tertiary amine TCAs (ie, amitriptyline, clomipramine, doxepin, and imipramine) to cause orthostatic hypotension, falls, or anticholinergic side effects.[78,79] However, contrary to the widespread belief of many experienced psychiatrists, there is no convincing evidence that TCAs are more efficacious than SSRIs, but there is strong evidence than SSRIs are better tolerated, particularly by older patients.[80–83]

Second-Step or Third-Step Treatment of Partial Responders

For patients who have experienced a partial response to a first-line or second-line antidepressant (typically an SSRI or an SNRI), the updated algorithm recommends augmenting the antidepressant with lithium or an atypical antipsychotic (or, alternatively, combining it with mirtazapine or bupropion). The preference for an augmentation (or combination) strategy over switching to another agent is consistent with the 2001 United States guidelines and with the caution in the 2006 Canadian guidelines that a partial improvement may be lost during a switch of medications. Although the use of lithium as an augmenting agent is supported by a larger number of geriatric studies than is the use of an atypical antipsychotic,[61,84–86] drug titration and ongoing monitoring of an atypical antipsychotic are easier to implement. In terms of selecting a specific atypical antipsychotic, the use of aripiprazole as an augmenting agent in older patients with MDD who had failed to respond to an antidepressant is supported by a small open study in 24 older patients (remission rate: 50%)[84] and a secondary analysis of 409 subjects aged 50 to 67 years who had participated in 3 different placebo-controlled RCTs (remission rates: 33% vs 17% with placebo).[85] The use of quetiapine is supported by a placebo-controlled RCT in which 338 older patients with MDD had higher remission and response rates with quetiapine monotherapy (50–300 mg/d) than with placebo (remission rates: 56% vs 23%; response rates: 64% vs 30%).[86] In these trials, aripiprazole and quetiapine were well tolerated (the most common adverse effects were akathisia with aripiprazole and somnolence with quetiapine), but clinicians need to remain mindful of the incontrovertible increased risk of mortality associated with atypical antipsychotics in late life.[72]

SUMMARY

More than 60 years after their introduction into clinical practice, antidepressants remain the mainstay of the treatment of depression in older adults. Their continuing use is supported by solid evidence. However, the typical outcomes of antidepressant treatment under usual care conditions are mediocre at best. Following a systematic approach to their use can improve these outcomes. At its core, such a systematic approach requires a treatment algorithm. However, most published RCTs of pharmacotherapy for geriatric depression assess only one treatment step, typically the first one or, more rarely, the second one. Thus, given the current state of knowledge, treatment algorithms on pharmacotherapy for geriatric depression can be informed by evidence, but are not yet truly evidence based.

CONFLICTS OF INTEREST

Dr B.H. Mulsant currently receives research support from the Canadian Institutes of Health Research, the US National Institutes of Health (NIH), Bristol-Myers Squibb (medications for an NIH-funded clinical trial), and Pfizer (medications for an NIH-funded clinical trial). Within the past 3 years he has received research support from Eli-Lilly (medications for an NIH-funded clinical trial). He directly owns stocks of General Electric (less than $5000). Dr D.M. Blumberger currently receives research support from the Canadian Institutes of Health Research and the US NIH. He receives research support and in-kind equipment support from Brainsway Ltd for an investigator-initiated clinical trial and a sponsor-initiated clinical trial. He receives in-kind equipment support from Tonika-Magventure for an investigator-initiated study. Dr Z. Ismail has served as a consultant to Astra-Zeneca, Bristol-Myers Squibb, Eli-Lilly, Janssen, Lundbeck, Merck, Pfizer, and Sunovion. Dr K. Rabheru receives compensation from the Ottawa Hospital, Ottawa, Ontario. He receives research support from the Canadian Institutes of Health Research. Dr M.J. Rapoport receives research funding from the Canadian Institute for Health Research and from the Ontario Ministry of Transportation.

REFERENCES

1. Olfson M, Marcus SC. National patterns in antidepressant medication treatment. Arch Gen Psychiatry 2009;66(8):848–56.
2. Pratt LA, Brody DJ, Gu Q. Antidepressant use in persons aged 12 and over: United States, 2005–2008. NCHS Data Brief; No. 76; 2011. Available at: http://www.cdc.gov/nchs/data/databriefs/db76.pdf. Accessed April 12, 2014
3. Mojtabai R, Olfson M. National trends in long-term use of antidepressant medications: results from the US National Health and Nutrition Examination Survey. J Clin Psychiatry 2014;75(2):169–77.
4. Kessler RC, Berglund P, Demler O, et al, National Comorbidity Survey Replication. The epidemiology of major depressive disorder: results from the National Comorbidity Survey Replication (NCS-R). JAMA 2003;289(23):3095–105.
5. Kessler RC, Birnbaum H, Bromet E, et al. Age differences in major depression: results from the National Comorbidity Survey Replication (NCS-R). Psychol Med 2010;40(2):225–37.
6. Kirsch I, Deacon BJ, Huedo-Medina TB, et al. Initial severity and antidepressant benefits: a meta-analysis of data submitted to the Food and Drug Administration. PLoS Med 2008;5:e45.
7. Kirsch I. The emperor's new drugs: exploding the antidepressant myth. London: The Bodley Head; 2009.
8. Fournier JC, DeRubeis RJ, Hollon SD, et al. Antidepressant drug effects and depression severity: a patient-level meta-analysis. JAMA 2010;12(1):47–53.
9. Fountoulakis KN, Moller HJ. Efficacy of antidepressants: a re-analysis and re-interpretation of the Kirsch data. Int J Neuropsychopharmacol 2011;12(3):405–12.
10. Vöhringer PA, Ghaemi SN. Solving the antidepressant efficacy question: effect sizes in major depressive disorder. Clin Ther 2011;12:B49–61.
11. Thase ME, Larsen KG, Kennedy SH. Assessing the 'true' effect of active antidepressant therapy v. placebo in major depressive disorder: use of a mixture model. Br J Psychiatry 2011;12:501–7.

12. Gibbons RD, Hur K, Brown CH, et al. Benefits from antidepressants: synthesis of 6-week patient-level outcomes from double-blind placebo-controlled randomized trials of fluoxetine and venlafaxine. Arch Gen Psychiatry 2012;69(6): 572–9.

13. Leucht S, Hierl S, Kissling W, et al. Putting the efficacy of psychiatric and general medicine medication into perspective: review of meta-analyses. Br J Psychiatry 2012;200:97–106.

14. Undurraga J, Baldessarini RJ. Randomized, placebo-controlled trials of antidepressants for acute major depression: thirty-year meta-analytic review. Neuropsychopharmacology 2012;12(4):851–64.

15. Huedo-Medina T, Johnson B, Kirsch I, et al. Kirsch et al.'s (2008) calculations are correct: reconsidering Fountoulakis & Moller's re-analysis of the Kirsch data. Int J Neuropsychopharmacol 2012;12:1193–8.

16. Fountoulakis KN, Veroniki AA, Siamouli M, et al. No role for initial severity on the efficacy of antidepressants: results of a multi-meta-analysis. Ann Gen Psychiatry 2013;12(1):26.

17. Meyers BS, Sirey JA, Bruce M, et al. Predictors from early recovery from major depression among people admitted to community-based clinics. Arch Gen Psychiatry 2002;59:729–35.

18. Zimmerman M, Mattia JI, Posternak MA. Are subjects in pharmacological treatment trials of depression representative of patients in routine clinical practice? Am J Psychiatry 2002;159(3):469–73.

19. Zimmerman M, Chelminski I, Posternak MA. Generalizability of antidepressant efficacy trials: differences between depressed psychiatric outpatients who would or would not qualify for an efficacy trial. Am J Psychiatry 2005;162(7): 1370–2.

20. Unutzer J, Katon W, Williams JW Jr, et al. Improving primary care for depression in late life: the design of a multicenter randomized trial. Med Care 2001;39(8): 785–99.

21. Unutzer J, Katon W, Callahan CM, et al. Collaborative care management of late-life depression in the primary care setting. JAMA 2002;288:2836–45.

22. Mulsant BH, Alexopoulos GS, Reynolds CF 3rd, et al. Pharmacological treatment of depression in older primary care patients: the PROSPECT algorithm. Int J Geriatr Psychiatry 2001;16(6):585–92.

23. Bruce ML, Ten Have TR, Reynolds CF 3rd, et al. Reducing suicidal ideation and depressive symptoms in depressed older primary care patients. JAMA 2004; 291(9):1081–91.

24. Alexopoulos GS, Katz IR, Bruce ML, et al. Remission in depressed geriatric primary care patients: a report from the PROSPECT study. Am J Psychiatry 2005; 162:718–24.

25. Alexopoulos G, Reynolds C, Bruce M, et al, the PROSPECT Group. Reducing suicidal ideation and depression in older primary care patients: 24-month outcomes of the PROSPECT Study. Am J Psychiatry 2009;166(8):882–90.

26. Tollefson GD, Bosomworth JC, Heiligenstein JH, et al. A double-blind, placebo-controlled clinical trial of fluoxetine in geriatric patients with major depression. The Fluoxetine Collaborative Study Group. Int Psychogeriatr 1995;7(1):89–104.

27. Schneider LS, Nelson JC, Clary CM, et al, Sertraline Elderly Depression Study Group. An 8-week multicenter, parallel-group, double-blind, placebo-controlled study of sertraline in elderly outpatients with major depression. Am J Psychiatry 2003;160(7):1277–85.

28. Rapaport MH, Schneider LS, Dunner DL, et al. Efficacy of controlled-release paroxetine in the treatment of late-life depression. J Clin Psychiatry 2003; 64(9):1065–74.
29. Roose SP, Sackeim HA, Krishnan KR, et al, Old-Old Depression Study Group. Antidepressant pharmacotherapy in the treatment of depression in the very old: a randomized, placebo-controlled trial. Am J Psychiatry 2004;161(11): 2050–9.
30. Kasper S, de Swart H, Friis Andersen H. Escitalopram in the treatment of depressed elderly patients. Am J Geriatr Psychiatry 2005;13(10):884–91.
31. Schatzberg A, Roose S. A double-blind, placebo-controlled study of venlafaxine and fluoxetine in geriatric outpatients with major depression. Am J Geriatr Psychiatry 2006;14(4):361–70.
32. Bose A, Li D, Gandhi C. Escitalopram in the acute treatment of depressed patients aged 60 years or older. Am J Geriatr Psychiatry 2008;16(1):14–20.
33. Raskin J, Wiltse CG, Siegal A, et al. Efficacy of duloxetine on cognition, depression, and pain in elderly patients with major depressive disorder: an 8-week, double-blind, placebo-controlled trial. Am J Psychiatry 2007;164(6):900–9.
34. Robinson M, Oakes TM, Raskin J, et al. Acute and long-term treatment of late-life major depressive disorder: duloxetine versus placebo. Am J Geriatr Psychiatry 2014;22(1):34–45.
35. Posternak MA, Zimmerman M. Therapeutic effect of follow-up assessments on antidepressant and placebo response rates in antidepressant efficacy trials: meta-analysis. Br J Psychiatry 2007;190:287–92.
36. Rutherford BR, Tandler J, Brown PJ, et al. Clinic visits in late-life depression trials: effects on signal detection and therapeutic outcome. Am J Geriatr Psychiatry, in press. [Epub ahead of print].
37. Gartlehner G, Hansen RA, Morgan LC, et al. Comparative benefits and harms of second-generation antidepressants for treating major depressive disorder: an updated meta-analysis. Ann Intern Med 2011;155:772–85.
38. Zimmerman M, Posternak M, Friedman M, et al. Which factors influence psychiatrists' selection of antidepressants? Am J Psychiatry 2004;161(7):1285–9.
39. American Psychiatric Association. Practice guideline for the treatment of patients with major depressive disorder (2010 revision). Available at: http:// psychiatryonline.org/content.aspx?bookID=28&sectionID=1667485#654274. Accessed April 13, 2014.
40. Simon GE, Perlis RH. Personalized medicine for depression: can we match patients with treatments? Am J Psychiatry 2010;167(12):1445–55.
41. Gartlehner G, Thaler K, Hill S, et al. How should primary care doctors select which antidepressants to administer? Curr Psychiatry Rep 2012;14(4): 360–9.
42. Thaler KJ, Morgan LC, Van Noord M, et al. Comparative effectiveness of second-generation antidepressants for accompanying anxiety, insomnia, and pain in depressed patients: a systematic review. Depress Anxiety 2012;29(6): 495–505.
43. Simon GE, Heiligenstein JH, Grothaus L, et al. Should anxiety and insomnia influence antidepressant selection: a randomized comparison of fluoxetine and imipramine. J Clin Psychiatry 1998;59(2):49–55.
44. Kocsis JH, Leon AC, Markowitz JC, et al. Patient preference as a moderator of outcome for chronic forms of major depressive disorder treated with nefazodone, cognitive behavioral analysis system of psychotherapy, or their combination. J Clin Psychiatry 2009;70(3):354–61.

45. Remillard A, Blackshaw S, Dangor A. Differential responses to a single antidepressant in recurrent episodes of major depression. Hosp Community Psychiatry 1994;45:359–61.

46. Steffens DC, McQuoid DR, Krishnan KR. The Duke Somatic Treatment Algorithm for Geriatric Depression (STAGED) approach. Psychopharmacol Bull 2002; 36(2):58–68.

47. Whyte EM, Basinski J, Farhi P, et al. Geriatric depression treatment in nonresponders to selective serotonin reuptake inhibitors. J Clin Psychiatry 2004; 65(12):1634–41.

48. Kok RM, Nolen WA, Heeren TJ. Outcome of late-life depression after 3 years of sequential treatment. Acta Psychiatr Scand 2009;119(4):274–81.

49. Ribeiz S, Avila R, Martins CB, et al. Validation of a treatment algorithm for major depression in older Brazilian sample. Int J Geriatr Psychiatry 2013;28(6): 647–53.

50. Buchanan D, Tourigny-Rivard MF, Cappeliez P, et al. National guidelines for seniors' mental health: the assessment and treatment of depression. Can J Psychiatry 2006;9(Suppl 2):S52–8.

51. Canadian Coalition for Senior's Mental Health. National guidelines for seniors' mental health – the assessment and treatment of depression. 2006. Available at: http://www.ccsmh.ca/en/projects/depression.cfm. Accessed April 5, 2014.

52. Alexopoulos GS, Katz IR, Reynolds CF 3rd, et al. Pharmacotherapy of depression in older patients: a summary of the expert consensus guidelines. J Psychiatr Pract 2001;7(6):361–76.

53. Mazeh D, Shahal B, Aviv A, et al. A randomized single-blind comparison of venlafaxine with paroxetine in elderly patients suffering from resistant depression. Int Clin Psychopharmacol 2007;22:371–5.

54. Fava M, Alpert J, Nierenberg A, et al. Double-blind study of high-dose fluoxetine versus lithium or desipramine augmentation of fluoxetine in partial responders and nonresponders to fluoxetine. J Clin Psychopharmacol 2002;22(4):379–87.

55. Quitkin FM, Petkova E, McGrath PJ, et al. When should a trial of fluoxetine for major depression be declared failed? Am J Psychiatry 2003;160(4):734–40.

56. Rush A, Trivedi M, Wisniewski S, et al, STAR*D Study Team. Bupropion-SR, sertraline, or venlafaxine-XR after failure of SSRIs for depression. N Engl J Med 2006;354:1231–42.

57. Trivedi M, Fava M, Wisniewski S, et al, STAR*D Study Team. Medication augmentation after the failure of SSRIs for depression. N Engl J Med 2006; 354:1243–52.

58. Thase M, Friedman E, Biggs M, et al. Cognitive therapy versus medication in augmentation and switch strategies as second-step treatments: a STAR*D report. Am J Psychiatry 2007;164:739–52.

59. Rush A, Wisniewski S, Warden D, et al. Selecting among second-step antidepressant medication monotherapies: are clinical, demographic, or first-step treatment results informative? Arch Gen Psychiatry 2008;65:870–80.

60. Posternak MA, Baer L, Nierenberg AA, et al. Response rates to fluoxetine in subjects who initially show no improvement. J Clin Psychiatry 2011;72(7): 949–54.

61. Cooper C, Katona C, Lyketsos K, et al. A systematic review of treatments for refractory depression in older people. Am J Psychiatry 2011;168(7):681–8.

62. Mulsant BH, Houck PR, Gildengers AG, et al. What is the optimal duration of a short-term antidepressant trial when treating geriatric depression? J Clin Psychopharmacol 2006;26(2):113–20.

63. Sackeim HA, Roose SP, Lavori PW. Determining the duration of antidepressant treatment: application of signal detection methodology and the need for duration adaptive designs (DAD). Biol Psychiatry 2006;59(6):483–92.
64. Schiff GD, Galanter WL, Duhig J, et al. Principles of conservative prescribing. Arch Intern Med 2011;171(16):1433–40.
65. Reynolds CF III, Dew MA, Martire LM, et al. Treating depression to remission in older adults: a controlled evaluation of combined escitalopram with interpersonal psychotherapy versus escitalopram with depression care management. Int J Geriatr Psychiatry 2010;25(11):1134–41.
66. Dombrovski AY, Mulsant BH. ECT: the preferred treatment for severe depression in late life. Int Psychogeriatr 2007;19(1):10–4.
67. Blumberger DM, Mulsant BH, Fitzgerald PB, et al. A randomized double-blind sham controlled comparison of unilateral and bilateral repetitive transcranial magnetic stimulation for treatment-resistant major depression. World J Biol Psychiatry 2012;13(6):423–35.
68. Reynolds CF III, Dew MA, Pollock BG, et al. Maintenance treatment of major depression in old age. N Engl J Med 2006;354(11):1130–8.
69. US Food and Drug Administration. FDA Drug Safety Communication: revised recommendations for Celexa (citalopram hydrobromide) related to a potential risk of abnormal heart rhythms with high doses. Available at: http://www.fda.gov/Drugs/DrugSafety/ucm297391.htm. Accessed April 12, 2014.
70. Zivin K, Pfeiffer PN, Bohnert AS, et al. Evaluation of the FDA warning against prescribing citalopram at doses exceeding 40 mg. Am J Psychiatry 2013;170(6):642–50.
71. Porsteinsson AP, Drye LT, Pollock BG, et al, CitAD Research Group. Effect of citalopram on agitation in Alzheimer disease: the CitAD randomized clinical trial. JAMA 2014;311(7):682–91.
72. Mulsant BH. Challenges of the treatment of neuropsychiatric symptoms associated with dementia. Am J Geriatr Psychiatry 2014;22(4):317–20.
73. Physician Drug Reference. Drug Summary - Cymbalta (duloxetine hydrochloride). 2014. Available at: http://www.pdr.net/drug-summary/cymbalta?druglabelid=288&id=2223. Accessed April 14, 2014.
74. Schueler YB, Koesters M, Wieseler B, et al. A systematic review of duloxetine and venlafaxine in major depression, including unpublished data. Acta Psychiatr Scand 2011;123(4):247–65.
75. Cipriani A, Koesters M, Furukawa TA, et al. Duloxetine versus other anti-depressive agents for depression. Cochrane Database Syst Rev 2012;(10):CD006533.
76. Rocha FL, Fuzikawa C, Riera R, et al. Combination of antidepressants in the treatment of major depressive disorder: a systematic review and meta-analysis. J Clin Psychopharmacol 2012;32(2):278–81.
77. Rajji TK, Mulsant BH, Lotrich FE, et al. Use of antidepressants in late-life depression. Drugs Aging 2008;25(10):841–53.
78. Chew ML, Mulsant BH, Pollock BG, et al. Anticholinergic activity of 107 medications commonly used by older adults. J Am Geriatr Soc 2008;56(7):1333–41.
79. American Geriatrics Society 2012 Beers Criteria Update Expert Panel. American Geriatrics Society updated Beers Criteria for potentially inappropriate medication use in older adults. J Am Geriatr Soc 2012;60(4):616–31.
80. Anderson IM. Selective serotonin reuptake inhibitors versus tricyclic antidepressants: a meta-analysis of efficacy and tolerability. J Affect Disord 2000;58(1):19–36.

81. Wilson K, Mottram P. A comparison of side effects of selective serotonin reuptake inhibitors and tricyclic antidepressants in older depressed patients: a meta-analysis. Int J Geriatr Psychiatry 2004;19(8):754–62.

82. Machado M, Iskedjian M, Ruiz I, et al. Remission, dropouts, and adverse drug reaction rates in major depressive disorder: a meta-analysis of head-to-head trials. Curr Med Res Opin 2006;22(9):1825–37.

83. von Wolff A, Hölzel LP, Westphal A, et al. Selective serotonin reuptake inhibitors and tricyclic antidepressants in the acute treatment of chronic depression and dysthymia: a systematic review and meta-analysis. J Affect Disord 2013; 144(1–2):7–15.

84. Sheffrin M, Driscoll HC, Lenze EJ, et al. Pilot study of augmentation with aripiprazole for incomplete response in late-life depression: getting to remission. J Clin Psychiatry 2009;70(2):208–13.

85. Steffens DC, Nelson JC, Eudicone JM, et al. Efficacy and safety of adjunctive aripiprazole in major depressive disorder in older patients: a pooled subpopulation analysis. Int J Geriatr Psychiatry 2011;26(6):564–72.

86. Katila H, Mezhebovsky I, Mulroy A, et al. Randomized, double-blind study of the efficacy and tolerability of extended release quetiapine fumarate (quetiapine XR) monotherapy in elderly patients with major depressive disorder. Am J Geriatr Psychiatry 2013;21(8):769–84.

Choosing Treatment for Depression in Older Adults and Evaluating Response

Patricia A. Arean, PhD*, Grace Niu, PhD

KEYWORDS

- Late life depression • Psychotherapy • Targeted treatment • Mood disorders
- Geriatrics

KEY POINTS

- Late life depression (LLD) has devastating social, clinical, and economic consequences.
- On average, pharmacologic and behavioral interventions are effective for LLD, but many patients have suboptimal response.
- The choice of treatment of LLD should be informed by patient preferences and suspected underlying causes of the presenting symptoms.
- Patients with LLD and comorbid executive dysfunction exhibit a brittle response to serotonin-specific reuptake inhibitor medication, but respond very well to targeted behavioral treatment (ie, problem-solving therapy).
- Future research should continue to investigate subtypes of LLD and develop efficient assessment and treatment tools to target them.

INTRODUCTION
Late Life Depression Defined

Late life depression (LLD) is one of the most common psychiatric problems among older adults,[1,2] and, overall, it is very similar in presentation to major depression in younger populations. The clinical characteristics of this illness include the following:

- Depressed mood nearly every day for at least 2 weeks, OR
- Difficulty fully enjoying pleasant activities (anhedonia) nearly every day for at least 2 weeks.

Funding Sources: National Institute of Mental Health, National Institute of Diabetes and Diseases of the Kidney, and National Institute on Aging (P.A. Arean). National Institute of Mental Health (G. Niu).
Funding: National Institute of Health K24 2MH074717; T32 MH01826.
Conflict of Interest: None to report.
Department of Psychiatry, University of California, San Francisco, 401 Parnassus Avenue, San Francisco, CA 94143, USA
* Corresponding author.
E-mail address: pata@lppi.ucsf.edu

Clin Geriatr Med 30 (2014) 535–551
http://dx.doi.org/10.1016/j.cger.2014.04.005
0749-0690/14/$ – see front matter © 2014 Elsevier Inc. All rights reserved.

To meet criteria for LLD, patients must have at least 1 of the 2 symptoms above and 3 to 4 of the symptoms listed below:

- Marked difficulty with sleep, either too little or too much
- Poor appetite, either too little or too much
- Trouble concentrating or making decisions
- Low energy
- Thoughts of guilt or worthlessness
- Feeling keyed up and tense or moving more slowly than usual
- Thoughts of death or suicide.

Contrary to popular wisdom, LLD is less common than major depression in younger cohorts, despite the increased exposure of older persons to adverse life events.[2] LLD is associated with several negative consequences, however, making it a very important public health problem to address. LLD has been implicated in the following:

- Increased health care costs[3]
- Increased morbidity and mortality[4]
- Greater risk for hospitalization[5]
- Greater risk of death, compared with nondepressed older adults[6]
- High risk for suicide, as older adults are more likely to complete a suicide than any other age group[7]
- More disability leading to greater perceived burden on family members and loved ones (**Table 1**).[8,9]

Effects and Effectiveness of Treatment

Effective treatment of LLD results in very positive outcomes. Treatment of depression leads to improved functioning and quality of life[10–12] and reduces all-health care costs[13–15] and all-cause mortality.[6] Although several existing treatments for LLD can have a positive impact on its sequelae, recent field trials have demonstrated that existing interventions may not be as effective in the general population as they are in clinical trials. For example, in the Improving Mood: Access to Collaborative Treatment (IMPACT) trial, less than 50% of older people accessing depression treatment had clinically significant improvement despite having increased access to depression treatment.[16,17]

Given the significant costs and disability associated with LLD, the treatments must be offered that the physician knows have maximum benefit and the fewest side effects to the general population. The authors suggest that the poorer-than-expected benefits in field trials are largely due to selecting treatments without a full understanding of the determinants involved in their outcomes. This treatment includes heterogeneity in LLD itself that requires suitably tailored treatment choices.

Table 1
Costs of depression and benefits of treatment

Costs	Benefits
Increased health care costs	Decreased all-cause health care costs
Greater rate of hospitalization	Greater productivity
Disability	Reduced all-cause mortality
Increased risk of suicide	Improved quality of life
Caregiver disability	
Caregiver depression risk	

Research is just beginning to explore how to target treatment of depression based on treatment moderators. Moderators are pretreatment patient characteristics that influence how patients respond to different types of treatments. Thus far, research suggests that clinicians could maximize the potential for good treatment outcome by considering several easily identified clinical characteristics (see Selecting Treatment, below). Furthermore, improvements can be maximized through careful monitoring of treatment outcome and proactive corrective action when treatments fail to be effective (see Data-Driven Decision-Making section). Finally, it is also important to be aware of what treatments are evidence-based and what the limitations are to the evidence base (discussed in next section).

EVIDENCE-BASED TREATMENTS REVIEWED

Several effective treatments for LLD exist and include behavioral interventions (eg, psychotherapy), medications, and electroconvulsive therapy (ECT).[17–22] The treatments are only slightly modified for older adults, with modifications addressing illness and disease burden, physical disability, and cognitive impairments.[23] Recent studies have demonstrated that treating late life mood disorders can offset the impact of the disorder. Older adults who responded to depression treatment lived longer,[24] resulting in lower all-cause health costs[25] 5 years after positive treatment response, compared with older adults who did not respond to treatment. Treatments that are considered to be evidence-based, first-line interventions are most antidepressant medications, specifically serotonin-specific reuptake inhibitor (SSRI) antidepressants (see Mulsant review in this issue), cognitive behavioral therapy (CBT[26–28]), problem-solving therapy (PST[29–36]), and interpersonal therapy (IPT[37]). ECT is generally reserved for patients who fail to respond to antidepressant medication and psychotherapy.[38,39]

Recent meta-analyses of treatment impact on LLD have revealed interesting insights. One study found that antidepressant medication and psychotherapy had very similar positive effects on LLD.[40] Another found that among psychotherapies, IPT seemed to have a slightly larger effect size compared with CBT and PST, but patients given PST are less likely to drop out of treatment.[41] Although all interventions have been found to be effective in primary care medicine, only PST has been used successfully in patients with mild dementia,[42,43] and as telephone-/Internet-based treatment of LLD.[34–36] Despite clinical wisdom that the combination of psychotherapy and medication is the best option, particularly for more moderate depression, there are very few studies demonstrating the added benefit of combined treatments, and the outcomes vary between studies.[44] Results from studies that have compared antidepressant medications with psychotherapy and from studies of combined treatments for late-life depression have been mixed. Antidepressants seem to be better than IPT for chronic, recurrent, late-life depression, but CBT appears to be as effective as antidepressants.[45,46] Adults with LLD are reluctant to take medications[47,48] and may be prone to drug side effects. Both psychotherapy and pharmacotherapy can be offered as long as there are no contraindications and patient preferences should be considered (**Table 2**).

ALTERNATIVE THERAPEUTIC APPROACHES

In addition to evidence-based treatments, there are also less formal behavioral interventions for LLD, including physical exercise, psychoeducation, and other supportive interventions. Although the effects of these interventions vary by the level of depression severity in the sample, presence of comorbid conditions, and the type of control group used, they seem to have beneficial effects on older adults with less severe depression.[49]

Table 2
Evidence-based treatments and indications

Intervention	Treatment	Indications
CBT	12 sessions. Individual and group	LLD; primary care medicine
PST	4–8 sessions. Individual and group	LLD; LLD+ED; primary care medicine; disabled patients; telephone therapy
IPT	12–16 sessions. Individual	LLD; primary care medicine
SSRIs	Citalopram; escitalopram; fluoxetene; paroxetene; sertraline	LLD; primary care medicine, not indicated for LLD+ED
Serotonin–norepinephrine reuptake inhibitors	Venlafaxine, duloxetine, and milnacipran	LLD; primary care medicine
Antipsychotic augmentation	Aripiprazole; quetiapine	LLD
Mirtazapine	Oral tablets	LLD; primary care medicine
Vortioxetine	Oral tablets	LLD; LLD+ED; primary care medicine
ECT	Recurrent treatments	LLD; LLD+psychosis

Psychoeducation and Bibliotherapy

Providing adults with information about depression, related problems, and ways to overcome the constituent symptoms is effective in helping to manage LLD. Intervention formats include lectures, group discussions, and reading materials (bibliotherapy). One study evaluating a self-management program for adults with age-related macular degeneration found that providing 12 hours of health education and problem-solving skills to a group of older adults over the course of 6 weeks led to the improvement in mood and function and increased confidence in coping abilities and aided in the prevention of depression.[50] The advantages of bibliotherapy are that it is self-paced, more convenient, less costly and does not have the stigma associated with seeing a mental health professional. Bibliotherapy has also been found to be an effective treatment of depression in older adults.[51,52]

Physical Exercise

Because physical activity has been suggested to improve core mood symptoms, exercising has been tested as a means of improving depressive symptoms.[53] Certain forms of exercise, such as Tai Chi, have been found to reduce all categories of depressive symptoms, including somatic, psychological, and interpersonal relations, and improve overall well-being.[54,55] Aerobic exercise also reduces depressive symptoms for adults with low to high symptomatology and leads to longer remission rates over time.[56] In some groups of older adults, exercise has been found to be superior to social intervention in the extent of response in symptoms over a period of 10 weeks.[57]

Supportive Interventions

Supportive interventions include a variety of acts that focus on understanding and supporting an individual's striving toward coping with distress and are less structured and often led by paraprofessionals.[49] There is increasing evidence to suggest that personalized care planning by adequately trained care staff might be an effective intervention for detecting and reducing depression in residential care for older people.[58,59] Furthermore, the delivery of secondary preventative interventions to non-mental health professionals has been linked with improving the quality of care to and reducing clinically significant depression in residential settings.[60]

SELECTING TREATMENT

There are several correlates of response to depression treatment among older adults. Some correlates have clinical utility in selecting treatment, whereas others are important to be aware of, but as of yet cannot inform treatment selection. Discussed here are the correlates that can inform treatment selection and that are easy to measure in a pretreatment clinical interview. **Table 3** lists other predictors of outcome.

Age

A recent meta-analysis indicated that although antidepressants are effective treatment for older adults, age seems to impact these effects. The older the patient, the less likely there is to be a positive response to treatment. Specifically, studies that have set the bar at a lower age of 65 tend not to find significant differences between medications and placebo.[61] This effect has not been found for psychotherapy[62] or ECT.[63]

Executive Dysfunction

Although not listed in the ICD-10 (International Classification of Diseases) or DSM-V (Diagnostic and Statistical Manual), the most prominent subcategory of LLD with

Table 3
Correlates of treatment outcome

	Predictive Value for Treatment Selection		Predictive of Treatment Response in General
Age	Greater age = poorer response to Alzheimer's Disease; behavioral treatment indicated	Late vs early onset	Data are mixed; research finds late onset differs from early,[106] but studies find no association for onset and outcomes[107]
ED	Executive dysfunction = poor response to AD; PST indicated	Personality Dx	Data show poor response to all depression treatment[107,108]
SES	Low SES = poor response to all depression treatment; inclusion of case management indicated	Anxiety	Data are mixed; some indication that posttraumatic stress disorder will reduce effect of all treatment[109]; little evidence that Generalized Anxiety Disorder influences outcome[110]
		Post stroke	Medications have protective effect to prevent depression,[111] but inconclusive as an intervention for LLD
		Heart disease	Caution using antidepressant medications, no clear evidence that any treatment is effective[112]
		Memory impairment	Inconclusive, insufficient data available[113]

predictive value is Late Life Depression with Executive Dysfunction (LLD+ED).[64] LLD+ED is associated with white matter changes on magnetic resonance images (MRIs) of the brain and poor performance on measures of executive functions, cognitive control in particular.[65–68] It is estimated that 50% of older adults with major depression have LLD+ED.[69] LLD+ED has been characterized as major depression (symptoms described above), with these additional clinical characteristics:

- Apathy rather than anhedonia; patients with apathy have difficulty initiating pleasant activities, but once they do, they are able to experience pleasure from them
- Psychomotor slowing
- Lack of insight into their depression
- Poor cognitive control as evidenced by simple cognitive tests (eg, Stroop Color-Word Interference Task) (**Table 4**).

CASE VIGNETTE 1: EXAMPLE OF **LLD** WITH EXECUTIVE DYSFUNCTION (CASE COMPOSITE)

Mrs Y is a 70-year-old Caucasian woman who was referred by her primary care provider for decreased mood and difficulty adhering to her heart medications. Before the doctor's referral, Mrs Y was an active member of her community, but had over the last 6 months dropped all of her activities. A physical examination ruled out any medical reasons for her symptoms. Clinical examination found that Mrs Y had major depression, characterized by sad mood, low energy, sleeping too much, poor appetite (eating too little), feelings of worthlessness, and thoughts of being better off dead. This was her first episode of depression; the only major life event she reported was her 2 adult children returning home to live with her after having lost their jobs. In addition to these symptoms of major depression, Mrs Y also exhibited symptoms of apathy; she had little interest in pursuing pleasant activities, but when her children forced her to go to church or socialize, she reported short-term enjoyment from the activity. She also reported feeling like she was walking through mud during her usual activities and had trouble deciding how to get started on must-do tasks. A brief evaluation of executive dysfunction (eg, Stroop Color-Word Task) revealed a score of 22, indicating mild executive dysfunction.

Several studies have repeatedly found that patients with LLD and ED have a poor and unstable response to SSRI antidepressants, ecitalopram in particular.[70–75] However, behavioral interventions that address executive impairment, namely problem-solving treatment, have significantly positive effects on mood and functioning in older adults with LLD and ED.[12,43]

Assessment of ED is not complex and therefore is an easily identified pretreatment variable that any clinician can measure. The Stroop Color-Word Interference Test is a

Table 4
LLD and LLD + ED

Late Life Depression	LLD with ED
Depression mood × 2 wk	Depressed mood × 2 wk, may lack insight
Anhedonia	Apathy
Trouble sleeping, too little or too much	Trouble sleeping, often too much
Poor appetite (too little or too much)	Poor appetite (too little or too much)
Trouble concentrating/easily distracted	Easily distracted, difficulty making decisions
Low energy	Low energy, trouble getting started
Feelings of guilt or worthlessness	Feelings of guilt or worthlessness
Keyed up or tense/moving more slowly	Moving more slowly
Thoughts of death or suicide	Thoughts of death or suicide
	Poor cognitive control (Stroop<25)

quick and highly predictive measure of this subtype of depression.[65,66] The Stroop is a timed task, taking no more than 2 minutes to complete. There are 3 steps. In the first step, the patient reads word colors (eg, red, blue) that are printed in black. In the second step, the patient identifies the ink color of stimuli (x's or rectangles). In the final step, the patient must identify the color a word is printed in, while ignoring the actual word. The complexity in the last step rests in the fact that the words are colors; for instance, red is printed in blue ink. The patient must read the color of the ink (blue) while ignoring the word itself (red). Each step takes 45 seconds, and the score is based on the number of correct responses given within the 45-second time frame. A score of less than 25 on the final task indicates LLD with ED.

Socioeconomic Factors

Although there is a small pool of data available, both theory and research suggest that depression in the context of poverty and socioeconomic adversity is less responsive to depression treatment alone than in combination with social services like clinical case management.[76] Clinical case management is an intervention whereby patient social needs are assessed (eg, do they need better housing?) and a social worker assists the patient in accessing those services.

Older adults in poverty:

- Overwhelmingly prefer behavioral treatment over pharmacologic treatment[77,78]
- Have a poorer response to medications than higher income older adults[79,80]
- Have a poor response to CBT alone, but significant improvement in outcome when CBT is combined with clinical case management.[76]

CASE VIGNETTE 2: EXAMPLE OF LLD IN THE CONTEXT OF POVERTY AND SOCIOECONOMIC ADVERSITY

Ms T, a 75-year-old African American woman, was living in a low-income senior-housing development in an inner city neighborhood. She had many medical complications, including COPD, hypertension, diabetes, in addition to issues with mobility. She was receiving in-home support services and Meals on Wheels through the county. The social worker in her building referred her for in-home psychotherapy after she repeatedly failed to show up for her medical appointments. A baseline assessment indicated that Ms T met criteria for LLD. She reported experiencing sad mood, low energy and motivation, inability to sleep, feelings of worthlessness, and apathy. She reported feeling this way for a couple of years and that, although her symptoms fluctuated, they were always present. She also reported that she had been homeless before her current living situation and was constantly worried about becoming homeless again. She explained she had missed her medical appointments because she could not always afford the bus fare, was too afraid to wait on the street corners for the bus to arrive, and experienced incontinence from time to time. She found it difficult to manage all the different medications she was on and was not open to the idea of adding medications to her regimen. Because of all the problems in her daily living, Ms T agreed to engage in a problem-solving with a case management treatment program and met with the treating clinician weekly for 12 weeks. At week 4, Ms T was able to generate solutions to problems related to medication. She successfully executed an action plan of calling her doctor and asking for a pillbox. At week 6, Ms T filled out an application for para-transit first with the help of the treating clinician and then with the help of the building social worker. At week 8, Ms T's Patient Health Questionnaire (PHQ)-9 dropped to a 4. She also reported that she had asked her physician to help her attain materials to manage her incontinence, who then referred her to a case manager at the hospital where she was receiving her medical care. By the end of treatment, Ms T was solving problems on her own, was making the most of her medical appointments, and had enrolled in an exercise class at the local senior center.

Although research on targeted treatment of LLD is still in a nascent phase, there is enough evidence to begin to use the process clinically. As detailed above, clinicians may be able to maximize treatment outcomes by considering patient age, income, and executive functions when selecting treatment. It is anticipated that, in the future, the treatment selection model proposed here (**Fig. 1**) will be better specified.

DATA-DRIVEN DECISION-MAKING

Optimizing treatment selection for LLD is only half the battle in promoting recovery from depression. On-going monitoring of treatment response and proactive adjustments and changes in treatment are critical to recovery.[81] Numerous studies found that older adults tend not to take antidepressant medication as prescribed,[82–84] and too often providers fail to change or adjust treatment quickly enough to maximize response to treatment.[16] Several studies point to the importance of regular treatment tracking using symptom measures and regular check-in on patient adherence to treatment.[85–87] The use of algorithms outlining when to expect treatment response can help clinicians make decisions as to when treatment should continue as initiated and when it should be adjusted or changed. Successful data-driven decision-making includes the following:

- Regular use of a symptom tracker (eg, PHQ-9; **Table 5**)
- Implementation of a patient registry to keep track of multiple patients
- Use of a treatment guideline to determine when to expect treatment response (**Fig. 2**)
- Opportunities to provide different treatment options to patients.

CASE VIGNETTE 3: ILLUSTRATION OF DATA-DRIVEN DECISION-MAKING: COMPOSITE CASE

Mr J was a 67-year-old man who had been suffering from major depression for 2 years. Mr J was still employed as a foreman for a construction company, reported he was able to make ends meet, but could not yet retire. Mr J could not identify a precipitating event to his depression, only that 1 day he noticed that he was not enjoying things the way he used to, was easily distracted and moody and had trouble sleeping. The patient also reported trouble getting started on tasks. Mr J indicated that these symptoms were significantly interfering with his ability to work, his relationship with his children, and his ability to enjoy life. Mr J's initial PHQ-9 was 15, and his Stroop Score was a 25. Mr J's response to the 10th item of the PHQ-9 indicated he felt very disabled by his depressive symptoms. He reported no anxiety symptoms, and other than the depression, his health was good. This was his first episode of depression. Based on this assessment, it was determined that Mr J had major depression. He did not appear to suffer from ED. When asked his preference for treatment, he decided to try medication first and was started on 20 mg Citalopram. Mr J's mood was monitored using the PHQ-9 on a monthly basis. After 8 weeks of treatment, his PHQ-9 did drop, but not to the 50% criteria (PHQ-9 at week 8 = 10). The treating clinician and Mr J discussed his progress and potential barriers to improvement. Mr J did report he sometimes forgot to take his medication. He also reported that while he did feel less distracted and could sleep better, his relationship with his wife and children was still strained. Because of his interpersonal struggles, Mr J agreed to add a course of IPT to his treatment program and met with the treating clinician weekly for 8 more weeks. At week 16, Mr J's PHQ-9 dropped to a 5. Although this is still considered symptomatic, Mr J's response to item 10 of the PHQ-9 indicated he no longer felt disabled by the symptoms. He also reported having resolved several conflicts with his wife and oldest son and felt confident he could continue using what he learned in treatment for other interpersonal issues. Mr J was seen 3 more times over 9 months. By the end of treatment, Mr J had made a full recovery.

ACCESS TO CARE AND TREATMENT PREFERENCES

Access to and engagement with depression treatment among older adults continues to be a considerable problem. Studies repeatedly find that older adults do not access

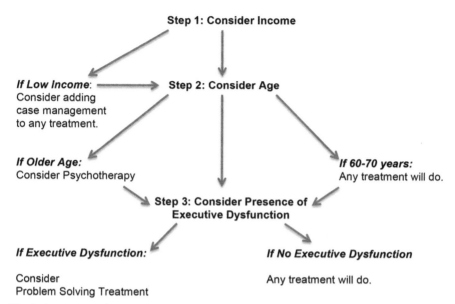

Fig. 1. Treatment selection model.

depression care, despite attempts to make them more available, and that treatment does not seem to be initiated until symptoms become severe.[88] Older minorities are less likely to access care than older whites.[89–91] Several factors have been implicated in underutilization of depression treatment, including the stigma associated with using mental health care, limited availability of preferred treatments, and instrumental access barriers, such as distance to the nearest mental health facility.[92] Integration of depression treatment into primary care medicine seems to improve access to care and engagement with treatment,[93–95] as does the delivery of care into patients' homes, through home health and meals services.[35,36,96,97] Currently, the Affordable Care Act allows for colocation of mental health and primary care services, but costs associated with telephone-based treatment and in-home services for older adults are not covered. Particularly for older adults who live in rural areas with limited access to local treatment and patients with disabilities limiting their ability to make regular visits to primary care or mental health care, inability to reimburse for these services will continue to impact use of depression care.

FUTURE DIRECTIONS FOR IMPROVING TREATMENT OF LLD

Targeted treatment selection based on clinical characteristics known to be associated with treatment outcome is a subject of considerable interest in the mental health field

Table 5 Recommended symptom trackers	
Scale	**Details**
PHQ-9	9 depression items; available in several languages; includes suicide question and disability question
Geriatric Depression Scale	30-, 15-, and 5-item versions; available in several languages
Beck Depression Inventory	21-item scale; available in several languages; includes suicide and hopelessness questions

Step 1:
Select Treatment

Step 2:
Monitor Symptoms for 6-8 weeks

Step 3:
Review progress by 8 weeks

A. Less than 50% response: Re-assess and consider adjusting treatment; Monitor monthly	***B. More than 50% response:*** Monitor monthly

Step 4A: **Step 4B:**
Review Progress by 16 weeks

A1. If no improvement, re-evaluate	***B1:*** If no further improvement, re-evaluate
A2. If response, continue to monitor monthly	***B2:*** If response continues, maintain Treatment to 12 months of treatment.

Fig. 2. Data-driven decision-making.

and is broadly supported by projects such as the National Institute on Mental Health Research Domain Criteria Project.[98,99] With the limited data available, it is possible to maximize the probability of selecting an effective treatment of LLD from the beginning, but we have much work ahead of us before we can target treatments for all presentations of LLD. As detailed elsewhere, the field would benefit from using a line of scientific inquiry consisting of the following:

1. The identification of subtypes of LLD
2. Uncovering the circumstances and processes that underlie those subtypes, and
3. Identifying interventions that appear to address those processes and testing their effectiveness.[23,100]

This line of scientific inquiry was the process used to improve treatment for patients with LLD+ED. By identifying the subtype, describing the underlying correlates, and testing an intervention that had the potential to remediate those correlates, clinicians are now in a position to target treatment of LLD+ED.

It is important that as more is learned about the "flavors" of LLD, the ecological utility of various ways to identify them is also considered. As an example, it is known that patients with LLD+ED have structural abnormalities in the dorsal and rostral anterior cingulate that are associated with both impaired performance on the Stroop Task and poor response to antidepressant medication.[101] Brain MRI as part of the routine clinical workup of LLD is untenable, whereas a 2-minute behavioral task, like the Stroop, has excellent predictive value and is easy to administer in a clinical interview. Efficiencies in identification of LLD subtypes are important for quick deployment of targeted treatment in the field.

As with identification methods, treatment approaches to target the underpinnings of LLD subtypes will also need to be streamlined, particularly in the case of behavioral interventions. A considerable problem with existing evidence-based behavioral interventions is their complexity, which has resulted in too few clinicians being able to deliver them competently.[102] As was described by Alexopoulos and Arean,[100] behavioral interventions can be better streamlined when it is understood what the treatment targets are and the level of complexity of the intervention selected adjusted and delivered.

A chronic problem in LLD treatment is poor access to treatment.[47] With targeted treatment comes the opportunity to leverage technologies to increase identification and intervention for subtypes of LLD. Many older adults use mobile devices and on-line computer programs for health purposes.[103,104] Assessment of depression sub-types and treatment using cognitive training programs could be a potential avenue of targeted assessment and treatment. As Anguera and colleagues[105] recently demonstrated, a computer game targeting specific neural networks underlying a behavioral problem can be a very effective mobile treatment. The authors' research team is in the process of exploring this treatment option for older adults with depression, because it has the potential to both increase access to treatment and individually target treatment to depressive subtypes.

REFERENCES

1. Byers AL, Yaffe K, Covinsky KE, et al. High occurrence of mood and anxiety dis-orders among older adults: the national comorbidity survey replication. Arch Gen Psychiatry 2010;67(5):489–96.
2. Kessler RC, Birnbaum H, Bromet E, et al. Age differences in major depression: results from the national comorbidity survey replication (NCS-R). Psychol Med 2010;40(2):225–37.
3. Unutzer J, Bruce ML, N.A.D. Workgroup. The elderly. Ment Health Serv Res 2002;4(4):245–7.
4. Gallo JJ, Bogner HR, Morales KH, et al. Depression, cardiovascular disease, diabetes, and two-year mortality among older, primary-care patients. Am J Ger-iatr Psychiatry 2005;13(9):748–55.
5. Gildengers AG, Houck PR, Mulsant BH, et al. Trajectories of treatment response in late-life depression: psychosocial and clinical correlates. J Clin Psychophar-macol 2005;25(4 Suppl 1):S8–13.
6. Gallo JJ, Morales KH, Bogner HR, et al. Long term effect of depression care management on mortality in older adults: follow-up of cluster randomized clin-ical trial in primary care. BMJ 2013;346:f2570.
7. Kuo WH, Gallo JJ. Completed suicide after a suicide attempt. Am J Psychiatry 2005;162(3):633.
8. Monin JK, Schulz R, Lemay EP Jr, et al. Spouses' cardiovascular reactivity to their partners' suffering. J Gerontol B Psychol Sci Soc Sci 2010;65B(2):195–201.
9. Martire LM, Schulz R, Reynolds CF, et al. Treatment of late-life depression alle-viates caregiver burden. J Am Geriatr Soc 2010;58(1):23–9.
10. Hunkeler EM, Katon W, Tang L, et al. Long term outcomes from the IMPACT randomised trial for depressed elderly patients in primary care. BMJ 2006; 332(7536):259–63.
11. Arean PA, Ayalon L, Hunkeler E, et al. Improving depression care for older, mi-nority patients in primary care. Med Care 2005;43(4):381–90.
12. Alexopoulos GS, Raue PJ, Kiosses DN, et al. Problem-solving therapy and sup-portive therapy in older adults with major depression and executive dysfunction: effect on disability. Arch Gen Psychiatry 2011;68(1):33–41.
13. Chan D, Fan MY, Unutzer J. Long-term effectiveness of collaborative depression care in older primary care patients with and without PTSD symptoms. Int J Ger-iatr Psychiatry 2011;26(7):758–64.

14. Chan D, Cheadle AD, Reiber G, et al. Health care utilization and its costs for depressed veterans with and without comorbid PTSD symptoms. Psychiatr Serv 2009;60(12):1612–7.
15. Unutzer J, Schoenbaum M, Katon WJ, et al. Healthcare costs associated with depression in medically ill fee-for-service medicare participants. J Am Geriatr Soc 2009;57(3):506–10.
16. Unutzer J, Katon W, Callahan CM, et al. Collaborative care management of late-life depression in the primary care setting: a randomized controlled trial. JAMA 2002;288(22):2836–45.
17. Thorp SR, Ayers CR, Nuevo R, et al. Meta-analysis comparing different behavioral treatments for late-life anxiety. Am J Geriatr Psychiatry 2009;17(2): 105–15.
18. Kvelde T, McVeigh C, Toson B, et al. Depressive symptomatology as a risk factor for falls in older people: systematic review and meta-analysis. J Am Geriatr Soc 2013;61(5):694–706.
19. Krishna M, Honagodu A, Rajendra R, et al. A systematic review and meta-analysis of group psychotherapy for sub-clinical depression in older adults. Int J Geriatr Psychiatry 2013;28(9):881–8.
20. Forsman AK, Schierenbeck I, Wahlbeck K. Psychosocial interventions for the prevention of depression in older adults: systematic review and meta-analysis. J Aging Health 2011;23(3):387–416.
21. Heo M, Papademetriou E, Meyers BS. Design characteristics that influence attrition in geriatric antidepressant trials: meta-analysis. Int J Geriatr Psychiatry 2009;24(9):990–1001.
22. Heo M, Murphy CF, Meyers BS. Relationship between the Hamilton depression rating scale and the Montgomery-Asberg depression rating scale in depressed elderly: a meta-analysis. Am J Geriatr Psychiatry 2007;15(10):899–905.
23. Arean PA. Personalizing behavioral interventions: the case of late-life depression. Neuropsychiatry (London) 2012;2(2):135–45.
24. Gallo JJ, Bogner HR, Morales KH, et al. The effect of a primary care practice-based depression intervention on mortality in older adults: a randomized trial. Ann Intern Med 2007;146(10):689–98.
25. Unutzer J, Katon WJ, Fan MY, et al. Long-term cost effects of collaborative care for late-life depression. Am J Manag Care 2008;14(2):95–100.
26. Schuurmans J, Comijs H, Emmelkamp PM, et al. A randomized, controlled trial of the effectiveness of cognitive-behavioral therapy and sertraline versus a wait-list control group for anxiety disorders in older adults. Am J Geriatr Psychiatry 2006;14(3):255–63.
27. Kraus CA, Kunik ME, Stanley MA. Use of cognitive behavioral therapy in late-life psychiatric disorders. Geriatrics 2007;62(6):21–6.
28. Laidlaw K, Davidson K, Toner H, et al. A randomised controlled trial of cognitive behaviour therapy vs treatment as usual in the treatment of mild to moderate late life depression. Int J Geriatr Psychiatry 2008;23(8):843–50.
29. Arean PA, Mackin S, Vargas-Dwyer E, et al. Treating depression in disabled, low-income elderly: a conceptual model and recommendations for care. Int J Geriatr Psychiatry 2010;25(8):765–9.
30. Arean P, Hegel M, Vannoy S, et al. Effectiveness of problem-solving therapy for older, primary care patients with depression: results from the IMPACT project. Gerontologist 2008;48(3):311–23.
31. Rovner BW, Casten RJ. Preventing late-life depression in age-related macular degeneration. Am J Geriatr Psychiatry 2008;16(6):454–9.

32. Alexopoulos GS, Raue PJ, Kanellopoulos D, et al. Problem solving therapy for the depression-executive dysfunction syndrome of late life. Int J Geriatr Psychiatry 2008;23(8):782–8.

33. Gellis ZD, McGinty J, Horowitz A, et al. Problem-solving therapy for late-life depression in home care: a randomized field trial. Am J Geriatr Psychiatry 2007;15(11):968–78.

34. Choi NG, Wilson NL, Sirrianni L, et al. Acceptance of home-based telehealth problem-solving therapy for depressed, low-income homebound older adults: qualitative interviews with the participants and aging-service case managers. Gerontologist 2013. [Epub ahead of print].

35. Choi NG, Marti CN, Bruce ML, et al. Depression in homebound older adults: problem-solving therapy and personal and social resourcefulness. Behav Ther 2013;44(3):489–500.

36. Choi NG, Hegel MT, Marti N, et al. Telehealth problem-solving therapy for depressed low-income homebound older adults. Am J Geriatr Psychiatry 2014;22:263–71.

37. Miller MD, Frank E, Cornes C, et al. The value of maintenance interpersonal psychotherapy (IPT) in older adults with different IPT foci. Am J Geriatr Psychiatry 2003;11(1):97–102.

38. Dombrovski AY, Mulsant BH. The evidence for electroconvulsive therapy (ECT) in the treatment of severe late-life depression. ECT: the preferred treatment for severe depression in late life. International Psychogeriatr 2007;19(1):10–4, 27–35. [discussion: 24–6].

39. Tew JD Jr, Mulsant BH, Haskett RF, et al. Acute efficacy of ECT in the treatment of major depression in the old-old. Am J Psychiatry 1999;156(12):1865–70.

40. Pinquart M, Duberstein PR, Lyness JM. Treatments for later-life depressive conditions: a meta-analytic comparison of pharmacotherapy and psychotherapy. Am J Psychiatry 2006;163(9):1493–501.

41. Cuijpers P, van Straten A, Smit F. Psychological treatment of late-life depression: a meta-analysis of randomized controlled trials. Int J Geriatr Psychiatry 2006; 21(12):1139–49.

42. Kiosses DN, Teri L, Velligan DI, et al. A home-delivered intervention for depressed, cognitively impaired, disabled elders. Int J Geriatr Psychiatry 2011;26(3):256–62.

43. Arean PA, Raue P, Mackin RS, et al. Problem-solving therapy and supportive therapy in older adults with major depression and executive dysfunction. Am J Psychiatry 2010;167(11):1391–8.

44. Arean PA, Cook BL. Psychotherapy and combined psychotherapy/pharmacotherapy for late life depression. Biol Psychiatry 2002;52(3):293–303.

45. Reynolds CF 3rd, Perel JM, Frank E, et al. Three-year outcomes of maintenance nortriptyline treatment in late-life depression: a study of two fixed plasma levels. Am J Psychiatry 1999;156(8):1177–81.

46. Thompson LW, Coon DW, Gallagher-Thompson D, et al. Comparison of desipramine and cognitive/behavioral therapy in the treatment of elderly outpatients with mild-to-moderate depression. Am J Geriatr Psychiatry 2001;9(3):225–40.

47. Charney DS, Reynolds CF 3rd, Lewis L, et al. Depression and Bipolar Support Alliance consensus statement on the unmet needs in diagnosis and treatment of mood disorders in late life. Arch Gen Psychiatry 2003;60(7):664–72.

48. Wetherell JL, Unutzer J. Adherence to treatment for geriatric Depress Anxiety. CNS Spectr 2003;8(12 Suppl 3):48–59.

49. Pinquart M, Duberstein PR, Lyness JM. Effects of psychotherapy and other behavioral interventions on clinically depressed older adults: a meta-analysis. Aging Ment Health 2007;11(6):645–57.

50. Brody BL, Roch-Levecq AC, Thomas RG, et al. Self-management of age-related macular degeneration at the 6-month follow-up: a randomized controlled trial. Arch Ophthalmol 2005;123(1):46–53.

51. Floyd M, Scogin F, McKendree-Smith NL, et al. Cognitive therapy for depression: a comparison of individual psychotherapy and bibliotherapy for depressed older adults. Behav Modif 2004;28(2):297–318.

52. Scogin F, Jamison C, Gochneaur K. Comparative efficacy of cognitive and behavioral bibliotherapy for mildly and moderately depressed older adults. J Consult Clin Psychol 1989;57(3):403–7.

53. Singh NA, Clements KM, Singh MA. The efficacy of exercise as a long-term antidepressant in elderly subjects: a randomized, controlled trial. J Gerontol A Biol Sci Med Sci 2001;56(8):M497–504.

54. Chou KL, Lee PW, Yu EC, et al. Effect of Tai Chi on depressive symptoms amongst Chinese older patients with depressive disorders: a randomized clinical trial. Int J Geriatr Psychiatry 2004;19(11):1105–7.

55. Li F, Harmer P, McAuley E, et al. An evaluation of the effects of Tai Chi exercise on physical function among older persons: a randomized controlled trial. Ann Behav Med 2001;23(2):139–46.

56. Penninx BW, Rejeski WJ, Pandya J, et al. Exercise and depressive symptoms: a comparison of aerobic and resistance exercise effects on emotional and physical function in older persons with high and low depressive symptomatology. J Gerontol B Psychol Sci Soc Sci 2002;57(2):P124–32.

57. Mather AS, Rodriguez C, Guthrie MF, et al. Effects of exercise on depressive symptoms in older adults with poorly responsive depressive disorder: randomised controlled trial. Br J Psychiatry 2002;180:411–5.

58. Lyne KJ, Moxon S, Sinclair I, et al. Analysis of a care planning intervention for reducing depression in older people in residential care. Aging Ment Health 2006;10(4):394–403.

59. Eisses AM, Kluiter H, Jongenelis K, et al. Care staff training in detection of depression in residential homes for the elderly: randomised trial. Br J Psychiatry 2005;186:404–9.

60. Cuijpers P, van Lammeren P. Secondary prevention of depressive symptoms in elderly inhabitants of residential homes. Int J Geriatr Psychiatry 2001;16(7): 702–8.

61. Tedeschini E, Levkovitz Y, Iovieno N, et al. Efficacy of antidepressants for late-life depression: a meta-analysis and meta-regression of placebo-controlled randomized trials. J Clin Psychiatry 2011;72(12):1660–8.

62. Rojas-Fernandez CH, Miller LJ, Sadowski CA. Considerations in the treatment of geriatric depression: overview of pharmacotherapeutic and psychotherapeutic treatment interventions. Res Gerontol Nurs 2010;3(3):176–86.

63. van der Wurff FB, Stek ML, Hoogendijk WL, et al. The efficacy and safety of ECT in depressed older adults: a literature review. Int J Geriatr Psychiatry 2003; 18(10):894–904.

64. Alexopoulos GS. The vascular depression hypothesis: 10 years later. Biol Psychiatry 2006;60(12):1304–5.

65. Lockwood KA, Alexopoulos GS, van Gorp WG. Executive dysfunction in geriatric depression. Am J Psychiatry 2002;159(7):1119–26.

66. Alexopoulos GS, Kiosses DN, Klimstra S, et al. Clinical presentation of the "depression-executive dysfunction syndrome" of late life. Am J Geriatr Psychiatry 2002;10(1):98–106.

67. Kiosses DN, Klimstra S, Murphy C, et al. Executive dysfunction and disability in elderly patients with major depression. Am J Geriatr Psychiatry 2001;9(3): 269–74.

68. Alexopoulos GS. "The depression-executive dysfunction syndrome of late life": a specific target for D3 agonists? Am J Geriatr Psychiatry 2001;9(1):22–9.

69. Krishnan KR, Hays JC, George LK, et al. Six-month outcomes for MRI-related vascular depression. Depress Anxiety 1998;8(4):142–6.

70. Coffey CE, Figiel GS, Djang WT, et al. White matter hyperintensity on magnetic resonance imaging: clinical and neuroanatomic correlates in the depressed elderly. J Neuropsychiatry Clin Neurosci 1989;1(2):135–44.

71. Kalayam B, Alexopoulos GS, Musiek FE, et al. Brainstem evoked response abnormalities in late-life depression with vascular disease. Am J Psychiatry 1997; 154(7):970–5.

72. Sneed JR, Culang-Reinlieb ME. The vascular depression hypothesis: an update. Am J Geriatr Psychiatry 2011;19(2):99–103.

73. Sneed JR, Culang-Reinlieb ME, Brickman AM, et al. MRI signal hyperintensities and failure to remit following antidepressant treatment. J Affect Disord 2011; 135(1–3):315–20.

74. Sneed JR, Keilp JG, Brickman AM, et al. The specificity of neuropsychological impairment in predicting antidepressant non-response in the very old depressed. Int J Geriatr Psychiatry 2008;23(3):319–23.

75. Sneed JR, Roose SP, Keilp JG, et al. Response inhibition predicts poor antidepressant treatment response in very old depressed patients. Am J Geriatr Psychiatry 2007;15(7):553–63.

76. Arean PA, Gum A, McCulloch CE, et al. Treatment of depression in low-income older adults. Psychol Aging 2005;20(4):601–9.

77. Kasckow J, Ingram E, Brown C, et al. Differences in treatment attitudes between depressed African-American and Caucasian veterans in primary care. Psychiatr Serv 2011;62(4):426–9.

78. Conner KO, Lee B, Robinson D, et al. Attitudes and beliefs about mental health among African American older adults suffering from depression. J Aging Stud 2010;24(4):266–77.

79. Cohen A, Houck PR, Szanto K, et al. Social inequalities in response to antidepressant treatment in older adults. Arch Gen Psychiatry 2006;63(1):50–6.

80. Cohen A, Gilman SE, Houck PR, et al. Socioeconomic status and anxiety as predictors of antidepressant treatment response and suicidal ideation in older adults. Soc Psychiatry Psychiatr Epidemiol 2009;44(4):272–7.

81. Lenze EJ, Sheffrin M, Driscoll HC, et al. Incomplete response in late-life depression: getting to remission. Dialogues Clin Neurosci 2008;10(4):419–30.

82. Wang HR, Song HR, Jung YE, et al. Continuity of outpatient treatment after discharge of patients with major depressive disorder. J Nerv Ment Dis 2013; 201(6):519–24.

83. Kales HC, Nease DE Jr, Sirey JA, et al. Racial differences in adherence to antidepressant treatment in later life. Am J Geriatr Psychiatry 2013;21(10):999–1009.

84. Kennedy J, Tuleu I, Mackay K. Unfilled prescriptions of Medicare beneficiaries: prevalence, reasons, and types of medicines prescribed. J Manag Care Pharm 2008;14(6):553–60.

85. Katon W, Unutzer J. Collaborative care models for depression: time to move from evidence to practice. Arch Intern Med 2006;166(21):2304–6.

86. Katon W, Unützer J, Wells K, et al. Collaborative depression care: history, evolution and ways to enhance dissemination and sustainability. Gen Hosp Psychiatry 2010;32(5):456–64.

87. Katon W, Von Korff M, Lin E, et al. Stepped collaborative care for primary care patients with persistent symptoms of depression: a randomized trial. Arch Gen Psychiatry 1999;56(12):1109–15.

88. Gum AM, Iser L, King-Kallimanis BL, et al. Six-month longitudinal patterns of mental health treatment utilization by older adults with depressive symptoms. Psychiatr Serv 2011;62(11):1353–60.

89. Joo JH, Morales KH, de Vries HF, et al. Disparity in use of psychotherapy offered in primary care between older African-American and white adults: results from a practice-based depression intervention trial. J Am Geriatr Soc 2010;58(1):154–60.

90. Gonzalez HM, Tarraf W, West BT, et al. Research article: antidepressant use among Asians in the United States. Depress Anxiety 2010;27(1):46–55.

91. Quinones AR, Thielke SM, Beaver KA, et al. Racial and ethnic differences in receipt of antidepressants and psychotherapy by veterans with chronic depression. Psychiatr Serv 2014;65(2):193–200.

92. Arean PA, Raue PJ, Sirey JA, et al. Implementing evidence-based psychotherapies in settings serving older adults: challenges and solutions. Psychiatr Serv 2012;63(6):605–7.

93. Arean PA, Gum AM, Tang L, et al. Service use and outcomes among elderly persons with low incomes being treated for depression. Psychiatr Serv 2007;58(8):1057–64.

94. Bartels SJ, Coakley EH, Zubritsky C, et al. Improving access to geriatric mental health services: a randomized trial comparing treatment engagement with integrated versus enhanced referral care for depression, anxiety, and at-risk alcohol use. Am J Psychiatry 2004;161(8):1455–62.

95. Bao Y, Alexopoulos GS, Casalino LP, et al. Collaborative depression care management and disparities in depression treatment and outcomes. Arch Gen Psychiatry 2011;68(6):627–36.

96. Choi NG, Sirey JA, Bruce ML. Depression in homebound older adults: recent advances in screening and psychosocial interventions. Curr Transl Geriatr Exp Gerontol Rep 2013;2(1):16–23.

97. Snowden M, Steinman L, Frederick J. Treating depression in older adults: challenges to implementing the recommendations of an expert panel. Prev Chronic Dis 2008;5(1):A26.

98. Cuthbert BN, Insel TR. Toward new approaches to psychotic disorders: the NIMH research domain criteria project. Schizophr Bull 2010;36(6):1061–2.

99. Insel T, Cuthbert B, Garvey M, et al. Research domain criteria (RDoC): toward a new classification framework for research on mental disorders. Am J Psychiatry 2010;167(7):748–51.

100. Alexopoulos GS, Arean P. A model for streamlining psychotherapy in the RDoC era: the example of 'Engage'. Mol Psychiatry 2014;19(1):14–9.

101. Gunning FM, Cheng J, Murphy CF, et al. Anterior cingulate cortical volumes and treatment remission of geriatric depression. Int J Geriatr Psychiatry 2009;24(8):829–36.

102. Beidas RS, Aarons G, Barg F, et al. Policy to implementation: evidence-based practice in community mental health–study protocol. Implement Sci 2013;8:38.

103. Kerwin M, Nunes F, Silva PA. Dance! Don't Fall - preventing falls and promoting exercise at home. Stud Health Technol Inform 2012;177:254–9.

104. Hughes LD, Done J, Young A. Not 2 old 2 TXT: there is potential to use email and SMS text message healthcare reminders for rheumatology patients up to 65 years old. Health Informatics J 2011;17(4):266–76.

105. Anguera JA, Boccanfuso J, Rintoul JL, et al. Video game training enhances cognitive control in older adults. Nature 2013;501(7465):97–101.

106. Dillon C, Allegri RF, Serrano CM, et al. Late- versus early-onset geriatric depression in a memory research center. Neuropsychiatr Dis Treat 2009;5:517–26.

107. Bukh JD, Bock C, Vinberg M, et al. Differences between early and late onset adult depression. Clin Pract Epidemiol Ment Health 2011;7:140–7.

108. Weber K, Giannakopoulos P, Canuto A. Exploring the impact of personality dimensions in late-life depression: from group comparisons to individual trajectories. Curr Opin Psychiatry 2011;24(6):478–83.

109. Hegel MT, Unützer J, Tang L, et al. Impact of comorbid panic and posttraumatic stress disorder on outcomes of collaborative care for late-life depression in primary care. Am J Geriatr Psychiatry 2005;13(1):48–58.

110. Steffens DC, McQuoid DR. Impact of symptoms of generalized anxiety disorder on the course of late-life depression. Am J Geriatr Psychiatry 2005;13(1):40–7.

111. Mikami K, Jorge RE, Moser DJ, et al. Prevention of poststroke apathy using escitalopram or problem-solving therapy. Am J Geriatr Psychiatry 2013;21(9):855–62.

112. Cowan MJ, Freedland KE, Burg MM, et al. Predictors of treatment response for depression and inadequate social support–the ENRICHD randomized clinical trial. Psychother Psychosom 2008;77(1):27–37.

113. Wilkins CH, Mathews J, Sheline YI. Late life depression with cognitive impairment: evaluation and treatment. Clin Interv Aging 2009;4:51–7.

Suicide in Later Life

Failed Treatment or Rational Choice?

Whitney L. Carlson, MD[a],*, Thuan D. Ong, MD, MPH[b]

KEYWORDS

- Geriatric • Suicide • Depression • Physician-assisted dying • Primary care

KEY POINTS

- Suicide rates in older adults remain high and may continue to increase with the aging of the baby boomer cohort unless more effective suicide prevention interventions are developed.
- Real-world implementation of successful models of depression treatment and suicide prevention offers opportunities to reduce the number of suicides in older adults.
- Hastened death, by suicide or legally sanctioned assistance in dying, can arouse complex emotions in survivors and clinicians that may have lasting impact.
- Investigating feelings of hopelessness, perceived burdensomeness, and thwarted belongingness may help identify older adults who may be thinking about hastening their deaths but do not voice suicidal ideation. All can be symptoms of a depressive illness or a result of deeply held, enduring personal beliefs and values in patients facing insurmountable illness.
- Physicians should explore older adult patients' concerns about dying. Motivations behind a patient's request for physician-assisted dying (PAD) should be explored regardless of a physician's personal attitudes and views.

INTRODUCTION

Suicide is the deliberate act of causing death by self-directed injurious behavior with intent to die as a result.[1] Suicide may be planned or impulsive but by definition involves only personal acts by individuals who intend to end their life, whereas assisted dying (also known as assisted suicide) involves others and usually includes planning to hasten death. PAD specifically refers to receiving the help of a physician who has the means to end life and is subject to strict regulatory protections. All 3 forms of hastening one's own death are used by older adults.

Funding: T.D. Ong, MD, MPH, is supported by Health Resources and Services Administration, Geriatric Academic Career Development Award, Grant: K01HP20463.
Conflict of Interest: None.
[a] Department of Psychiatry and Behavioral Sciences, University of Washington School of Medicine, 325 Ninth Avenue, Seattle, WA 98104-2499, USA; [b] Department of Medicine, Division of Gerontology and Geriatric Medicine, University of Washington School of Medicine, 325 Ninth Avenue, Seattle, WA 98104-2499, USA
* Corresponding author.
E-mail address: cwhitney@u.washington.edu

Older adults generally have higher suicide rates than younger people (**Fig. 1**) and are the group who most often request PAD in the states where it has been legalized for the terminally ill. Age by itself is not as important as contextual factors that may motivate older adults to seek a hastened death. In the following sections, what is known about situational factors and motivations of these older adults and the emotional and psychological effects their decisions can have on survivors are discussed. The clinical implications of suicide and legalized PAD and the impact both have on clinicians also are discussed.

SUICIDE

Suicide can be one of the most emotionally devastating events a family can experience, and it is a deeply troubling event for treating clinicians. Most clinicians who care for older adults face a patient with suicidal ideation at some point in their careers and some encounter a patient who has had a suicide attempt or died by suicide or meet the survivors left behind by suicide. Being aware of the need to face such situations and the complex issues and emotions that surround suicide is important for clinicians who care for older adults and their families.

The following case of Mr. X illustrates one author's personal experience with a patient suicide

Mr X is a 72-year-old retired, married man with hypertension, diabetes, and hyperlipidemia who presents to his long-time primary care provider (PCP) with neuropathic pain and sleep disturbance. He lives with his wife of 47 years and has a son who lives nearby. Mr X drinks an average of 2 drinks per night and has for many years, but has been drinking more lately due to poor sleep and tension in his marriage but does not reveal this to his PCP. He does not report other symptoms of depression and because his presenting concerns seemed related to pain, no depression screen was done at that time. He is prescribed amitriptyline (25 mg) at bedtime for neuropathic pain with the thought that this would also be sedating enough to help him sleep. Three days later, Mr X comes home to find that his wife has unexpectedly, and without explanation, moved out of their home. He learns from his son that he had helped her move out. That night he took a handful of pills, including some amitriptyline, along with his nightly cocktails and that evening is found by his son, who happened to come by to get things for his mother. He was admitted to a monitored bed for 24 hours and showed no signs of arrhythmia. He was seen by a consulting psychiatrist and agreed, with the encouragement of his son, to a voluntary psychiatric admission to address his sleep, poor appetite, and depressed mood. He had no prior history of depression and no history of suicide attempts. He was started on mirtazapine (15 mg) at bedtime and tolerated the medication. He met criteria for major depression because he also acknowledged symptoms of depressed mood, low energy, and weight loss that had been present before the acute stressor. Mirtazapine was titrated to 30 mg every night to target depression. He participated in groups and individual sessions. He met with the inpatient psychiatry team and his son for a family discharge planning meeting and was agreeable to follow-up with his long-time physician in 1 week. Accessing outpatient mental health counseling and psychiatric care was limited by having only Medicare for insurance, a lack of providers accepting this insurance in his geographic area, transportation difficulties, and finances. His son expressed concerns about how his father would do after discharge but agreed to have his father come stay at his home for support after discharge. He was found dead by his son within 48 hours of his discharge. Mr X overdosed on multiple medications while his son was home and asleep.

Older adults have had a higher rate of suicide for decades compared with other demographic groups, particularly in industrialized countries. A recent increased rate of suicide in the 35- to 64-year-old demographic in the United States for the most recent decade suggests that the next cohort of older adults may have an even higher rate of

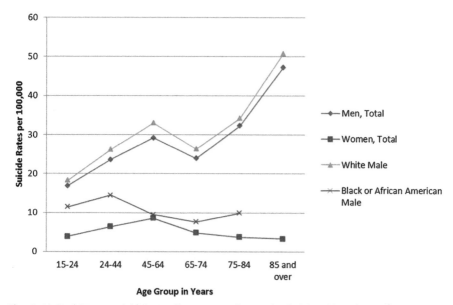

Fig. 1. United States suicide rates by age, gender, and ethnicity, 2010. (*Data from* Centers for Disease Control and Prevention. National Center for Injury Prevention and Control. Web-based Injury Statistics Query and Reporting System (WISQARS) [online]. Available at: www.cdc.gov/injury/wisqars/index.html. Accessed October 19, 2012.)

suicide. In 2010, 5994 adults aged 65 and older killed themselves in the United States. This represents 1 older adult dying by suicide every 1 hour and 28 minutes.[2] Although suicidal ideation is common, suicide attempts and completion are rare events, making the study of risk and proving the efficacy of preventative interventions challenging.

Suicidal Ideation as a Risk Factor for Suicide

Older adults in the United States are less likely than younger adults to report thoughts of suicide to others,[3] but self-reported suicide ideation has been associated with death by suicide within a year.[4] A recent study has demonstrated that more frequent suicidal ideation as measured by item 9 of the Patient Health Questionnaire (PHQ-9) predicts increased individual longitudinal risk of a suicide attempt or death by suicide in both younger and older adults.[5]

Attempts have been made to understand the factors that contribute to suicide through psychological autopsy, a method of look-back analysis of those who die by suicide by assessing potential risk factors and interviewing people who knew the decedent. Moderate to severe depression has been identified as a strong correlate of completed suicide in older adults.[6,7] There are, however, those who experience suicidal ideation that is not related to the syndrome of depressive illness and those who have never expressed or been identified as having suicidal ideation who may attempt or complete suicide. For these individuals, identifying what might have had an impact on their decision and their risk of suicide, and what might have prevented it, is extremely difficult.

The Interpersonal Theory of Suicide

The interpersonal theory of suicide[8,9] has been studied as a model of how older adults develop suicidal ideation and proposes 3 components that contribute to suicide and death ideation, suicide attempts, and death by suicide that have some empiric support. These include feeling disconnected from meaningful social relationships (thwarted belongingness), feeling a burden or a liability to others whether or not others feel burdened (perceived burdensomeness), and the capability of lethal self-injury through repeated exposure to painful experiences leading to habituation to pain and loss of the instincts for self-preservation. The level of perceived burdensomeness—a sense of being a burden to others, especially younger people in their social network—is associated with more severe suicidal ideation. Studies suggest that perceived burdensomeness should be examined in studies of survivors of suicide attempts, in future psychological autopsy studies of decedents of suicide, and in clinical work with patients presenting with suicidal ideation.[10]

Clinician and Family Reactions to Suicide

Inpatient psychiatrist

I learned about the suicide from the medical director and administration of our behavioral health unit within days of his discharge. Although I knew Mr X was at high risk by virtue of a recent suicide attempt, his alcohol use, his wife's recent unexplained departure, and his age, I was not prepared for the feelings I had when faced with knowing he had died by suicide. I felt guilty that I hadn't kept him in the hospital longer. I felt sadness for his son and worry that I would be sued. I felt incompetent—I questioned my skills as a psychiatrist, particularly since it was my first year out of residency; I was a specialist. How did I miss this? I felt ashamed—I didn't want others to know, even though my colleagues assured me that many people had experienced this, too. This is what I was told, but no one offered to tell me who had lost a patient by suicide. I wondered who knew in the hospital system and if my hospitalist colleagues would trust me as a consultant or if my psychiatry colleagues would trust me to care for and discharge their patients. I worried I could be fired for incompetence. I felt I should call the son to express my condolences to him but was advised by administration in a discussion of the medical-legal issues not to contact him but that I could talk to him if he contacted me. I have always regretted the decision not to call him. Since I had met him twice face-to-face and saw his worry and fear about how his father would manage outside the hospital, I can only imagine how he was feeling after his father's death and being the one to find him.

One of the most difficult things about dealing with suicide is the continued stigma and secrecy that are attached to it. Health care providers are trained to diagnose problems, treat them, and hopefully cure disease. There is often less focus on relieving suffering. When someone dies, particularly by suicide, there is frequently a sense of guilt, shame, and failure. Health care providers wonder who will find out and what they will think about them and their knowledge and skills. They worry about being seen as having failed or missed something important, that someone else would have seen the signs and been able to prevent it. They do not know who is safe to talk to or what their reaction will be when they are told. They worry about the reaction of the family and what to say or not to say. Families often expect an explanation for why this happened or how the signs could have been missed. They can express anger and threaten legal action. They want to know how their loved one could do this to them. It can be useful in some cases to acknowledge the unbearable pain that suicide can express and liken it to the physical pain that can be caused by cancer. Patients may have viewed suicide as the only option for relieving the suffering they were experiencing and the only solution to the pain they felt they were causing their families. Many patients truly believe, usually related to a constricted view of their circumstances and often related to depression, that there is no other option and that they truly will help others by being absent from their lives.

It is important to talk to survivors in nonmedical terms and be able to accept that their emotions are likely complex and may not be the same as providers'. Clinicians may need to reduce the distance that they tend to put between themselves and patients and families to be able to discuss how they too are affected by this person's death so that they may also heal. The medical community needs to find a way to make the culture in which it works accepting and supportive of the need to talk about patient losses, including by suicide. Learning from survivors and clinicians who have encountered suicide can provide perspective and comfort to other clinicians.[11]

In cases of older adults, clinicians may struggle with special moral conflicts. On one hand, they can empathize with older patients who, facing increasing physical disability, a shrinking social circle, loss of independence, and financial stresses, wish to limit their suffering by ending their life. On the other hand, their professional training emphasizes preventing harm and saving lives but may not equip clinicians well to deal with the ambiguity inherent in these divergent moral positions. Recognizing their own competing perspectives can be useful—even comforting—in talking with patients who are struggling with suicidal ideation or feelings of hopelessness. When patients see that a clinician can grasp the painfulness of their situation, shared understanding can grow, and real conversation can begin, paving the way to negotiating goals of care and identifying reasons a patient may still have for living.

Inpatient psychiatrist

I am frequently asked when I talk to residents, colleagues, and community audiences if there is anything I would have done differently. I would have spent more time with the patient and his son, really processing the recent events and feelings around his wife's leaving, how he viewed his son's having helped her leave in secrecy while remaining his only social support. Perhaps I felt a false sense of security in sending him home with his son. I think we underestimate the importance of the quality of the relationships of people we identify as supports, particularly for older adults. Mr X likely had many deep feelings toward his son and wife about what had happened that needed to be explored. I did not fully understand the history and the dynamics of his relationships very well. I knew he had no one else in his life besides these two people—who he probably viewed as having betrayed him—and I sent him home with one of them. He had no friends, was socially isolated, and had no structured activities or social contacts to connect to, though we talked about ways to develop some of these. I have wondered if there was a "middle finger" message to his son in having overdosed in his home while his son was there, knowing that he would find him, or if it was only out of complete despair and feeling alone despite another person in the house with him. I believe at the time I felt that because his son showed genuine concern and because he showed up to the hospital that his father would feel loved and that he could tell his son how he was feeling if he felt suicidal again. In retrospect, Mr X never talked a lot about his emotions on the inpatient unit. His affect was not tearful or angry, although he voiced feeling some sadness and anger. He participated in groups and individual visits on rounds but in a somewhat superficial way. He said all the "right" things. He agreed to see his doctor. He was forward thinking in his plans. I don't know if he was just waiting to leave the hospital to do it again or if he genuinely meant he was not suicidal the day he went home. Either could be true and although intellectually I know that, emotionally it still hits me every time I tell the story and I still feel responsible. This was someone I knew for less than a week. I can only imagine the emotions of losing someone I had seen for many years to suicide.

Hope for New Models of Care and Decreased Suicide

Collaborative care research has established that care management of depressed older adults in primary care improves depression outcomes and reduces suicidal ideation over usual care[12,13]; however, there has been no study specifically in older adults to show that any intervention reduces the number of suicides. The spread of comprehensive, integrated approaches to primary care, exemplified in the concept of the medical home and in collaborative models of depression treatment based in primary care, will create more opportunities to develop and evaluate interventions to reduce suicidal ideation and suicide itself. Such approaches are being disseminated into real-world settings through projects, such as the Depression Improvement Across Minnesota—Offering a New Direction (DIAMOND) initiative[14] in Minnesota, that seek to implement evidence-based collaborative depression care in a large number of primary care settings.

Models of depression care, such as the Perfect Depression Care Initiative, have shown success in reducing the suicide rate in large health systems.[15,16] Such models of care involve instilling the belief within the care system that suicide can be prevented and orienting the entire system of care toward the goal of zero suicide.

Assessment of the Patient with Suicidal Ideation

PCPs have a critical role in the assessment and management of older adults who may be at risk of suicide. Many older adults see their PCP shortly before committing suicide; 50% to 75% of older adults who die by suicide see their PCP within 1 month of death and often have multiple visits.[17–19] PCPs can provide a sense of social connectedness for older adults who have regular visits; in some cases, visiting their PCP's office may be older adults' only social contact. Through the strength of their often longstanding relationships, PCPs are in a unique position to be able to have both sensitive and delicate conversations with their patients and a significant influence on their patients' acceptance of recommendations for treatment. PCPs can identify and mitigate many of the factors associated with suicide in older adults, including

- Evaluating for functional impairments that limit the scope of life (eg, falls, incontinence, decreased mobility, vision and hearing deficits, and cognitive deficits) and identifying a treatment plan for support or care
- Aggressively treating pain, particularly when severe
- Identifying alcohol abuse and dependence
- Identifying and adequately treating depression and other mood disorders
- Identifying social factors in need of support from social worker, support staff, or community agencies

The case illustrates a common problem in identifying depression in older adults who often present with somatic symptoms or sleep disturbance rather than reporting depressed mood. In this case, the patient may not have recognized that he was experiencing depression as the reason for some of his symptoms and may or may not have been contemplating suicide in relation to his social stressors. Although the US Preventive Services Task Force does not recommend routine screening for suicidal ideation in primary care unless there is a system of care immediately available to further assess and provide support and treatment of those identified with suicidal ideation,[20] reducing suicide is a priority target for Healthy People 2020 and the Institute of Medicine, among numerous other organizations.[21,22]

When faced with a patient whose symptoms suggest depression, a screen for depression with a scale, such as the PHQ-9, with particular attention to item 9, which asks about suicidal ideation, is appropriate. Any endorsement of suicidal thoughts must be taken seriously; although clinicians often fear asking direct questions about suicidal thoughts and plans, patients do not respond to sensitive questioning with increased impetus to act on their suicidal thoughts. Patients are often relieved about being able to confide how distressed they are feeling and to have someone to whom they can voice their feelings of hopelessness. Clinicians are often ill prepared, however, for the emotions they may experience when a patient reports that they are suicidal and may seem awkward when they want to communicate compassion and empathy. The evaluation that ensues should involve a direct inquiry about whether a plan has been formulated and if so what it entails; actions to limit access to immediate means, such as firearms; identification of potential supports; and a safety plan. Referral for specialty care as needed and close follow-up contact by the provider or nurse with phone calls in the first few days after the visit and a scheduled visit within a week can be useful supports if a patient is able to voice a plan for immediate safety and does not require hospitalization. Once suicide prevention plan is in place, arrangements for mental health treatment must follow.

Psychiatric specialists working with patients with suicidal ideation evaluate several factors in their risk assessment, including talking with the patients about the meaning of their distress, identifying reasons for living as well as the reasons patients think suicide would address their pain and suffering, and detailed evaluation of specific plans, intent, and access to means. Empathizing with and being able to tolerate a patient's level of suffering is extremely important in building a relationship in which trust allows alternatives to suicide to be discussed in detail and a genuine message of hope can be conveyed. A frequent part of developing a safety plan involves identifying potential supports and evaluating the quality of those supports. Particularly for older adults, suicidal ideation is often associated with feeling socially isolated and burdensome to others, either people they are close to (usually spouse or family) or to society. Identifying and aggressively treating depression and other mood disorders, substance use, and psychosis are also important aspects of treating patients who present with suicidal ideation. Continuing to assess for comorbidities that may prevent adequate response to treatment, such as anxiety, cognitive disorders, psychosis, and personality disorders, as well as identifying coping strengths and weaknesses that may be amenable to therapies, such as cognitive behavioral therapy, interpersonal therapy, or problem-solving therapy, are additional aspects of specialty care evaluation and treatment.

It can be anxiety provoking to face patients who are convinced that killing themselves is the only way to relieve their suffering. Clinicians can experience anger at feeling put in a position of saving someone, anxiety about a patient's potential to follow through on their plan, and the role of trying to determine if a patient is going to act now or in the future, fearful of not being able to help identify reasons for living and sometimes feeling incompetent. There can also be pressure from those around patients who express concern and sometimes fears of legal consequences if patients should succeed in killing themselves.

Special Older Adult Populations Vulnerable to Suicidal Ideation and Suicide

Long-term care residents
Suicide is much less common in the nursing home setting than in the general community, which has been proposed related to the close monitoring residents receive as well as relatively low access to the most lethal means.[23] Thoughts of death and suicide have been identified, however, in up to one-third of surveyed residents.[24,25] Older age has been associated with death and suicide thoughts as well as completed suicide.[24,26] Additional factors associated with suicide or suicidal ideation have included

male gender; those recently admitted[27]; history of a mental disorder[28]; and depressive symptoms.[25,29] Predictors of absent suicidal ideation included having an internal locus of control, a sense of self-efficacy, and life satisfaction.[29] Health care leaders in long-term care facilities have identified easy accessibility of mental health consultants as most essential for helping address depression and suicidal ideation in their patients and frequently request education on depression and suicide.[30] In addition to continuing to identify and treat depression and educating caregivers and facility staff about recognizing suicidal ideation, points of intervention might include identifying ways to improve patients' feelings of life satisfaction and self-efficacy, which could potentially mediate suicide risk. Increased access to specialty care could be one way of better identifying and treating this population and educating those who care for them.

Suicide in dementia

Psychiatric symptoms of depression, anxiety, and psychosis are common in dementia, and depression is associated with suicide risk in demented as well as nondemented older people. Results from studies looking at suicide risk among older adults with dementia are mixed.[31–33] A recent review noted that suicide risk in dementia seems equivalent to the age-matched general population but noted that the reviewed studies had many methodological limitations.[34] Predictors of suicide in Veterans Affairs patients with dementia found elevated risk associated with white race, depression, a history of inpatient psychiatric admission, and filled prescriptions of antidepressants or anxiolytics. Most suicides occurred in those newly diagnosed with dementia and of younger age. Firearms were used in 73% of successful suicides. Nursing home admission was associated with lower suicide risk, which was proposed related to lack of access to firearms, the structured nature of a supervised setting, and the increased physical frailty and cognitive impairment that is present in this population that might make formulating and executing a plan for suicide more difficult. The study investigators suggested that those with a new dementia diagnosis with symptoms of anxiety and depression may be at higher suicide risk and that closer monitoring of access to firearms may be particularly important in the population of older male patients with dementia.[23]

Caregivers

Families provide the majority of care for individuals with dementia. This places a significant burden on them financially, emotionally, and physically. Many of those providing this care are older adults themselves or entering into the geriatric demographic. Caregivers are at high risk for depression. One recent pilot study looked at the prevalence of suicidal ideation in caregivers of those with dementia and attempted to look for common elements of risk within those with suicidal ideation. Of 120 caregivers (107 female and 13 male), 26% had contemplated suicide more than once in the previous year and of these, 30% indicated a likelihood that they would attempt suicide in the upcoming year. Only half of those who had contemplated suicide had told anyone about these thoughts. Only depression predicted suicide on multivariate analysis in this study and it was proposed that depression may have mediated many of the differences noted in psychosocial factors (poorer mental health, stronger reactions to behavioral and psychological symptoms, more negative perceptions of social support, lower self-efficacy for using community support services, and using dysfunctional coping strategies) identified between those who had experienced suicidal ideation and those who were not.[35] Identifying and treating depression in this population as well as asking about suicidal ideation may help mediate the potential risk of suicide in caregivers. Understanding the reasons for caregivers' feelings, which may include loss of the intimate relationship (eg, in a spousal relationship), unmet need for increased support for care or an alternative living situation, or a need for increased training and support in dealing with difficult behaviors, may help identify solutions to stresses that may help decrease feelings of hopelessness and increase hope and caregiver well-being. When the PCP of a patient with dementia recognizes symptoms of depression in a caregiver, normalizing this as common in caregivers, considering whether the patient is also depressed, and arranging for suitable referrals and support can be effective interventions.

ASSISTED DYING AND PHYSICIAN-ASSISTED DYING

The wish to die can be driven by many factors and circumstances. Do individuals who are terminally ill have a right to die as they wish? Do individuals suffering from life-limiting diseases, such as many of the current chronic medical conditions, like heart failure, chronic obstructive pulmonary disease, and dementia, have the right to request an end to their lives? Can suicide be considered a rational choice? News headlines about patients who want to end their suffering and advances in palliative medicine and hospice medicine have made the public more aware of the nuances of dying. Discussions of suffering and dying have evolved into substantial efforts toward legalized alternatives for terminally ill patients to choose how and when they will die.

At the core of the ethical pressure to legalize assistance in dying are principles of patient self-determination and the autonomy of individuals to control their own end-of-life care. Patients may proactively choose death rather than live out the natural course of their terminal illness because of physical, emotional, and/or existential suffering. The ethical debate over assisted dying will continue and seems to have been present even since the birth of Western medicine. The Hippocratic oath instructs physicians to "neither give a deadly drug to anybody if asked for it, nor will I make a suggestion to this effect," suggesting it was a contentious issue then too. Advances in medicine and shifts in culture over time have contributed to legalized PAD. A summary of the debate surrounding PAD can be found elsewhere.[36,37] This discussion focuses on legalized PAD practices and refrains from moral arguments for or against it. This discussion reviews the safeguards found in PAD legislation, what is known about patients who request and use it, its impact on families, and its clinical practice.

Definitions

Assisted dying, also known as assisted suicide, is a general term referring to someone dying with the assistance from another person(s). Assistance with dying may come from family members, friends, or advocacy organizations that specifically help with assisted dying and may not specifically involve physicians. PAD, also known as physician-assisted suicide, is defined as the provision, by a physician to a patient, of the means for a patient to end his/her own life. In PAD, the patient performs the act that brings about death. This is distinct from euthanasia, which refers to a physician's direct involvement in a deliberate act that intentionally ends a patient's life, such as administering lethal medication with intent to cause a patient's death. A subtle but important difference between PAD and euthanasia is whether the physician provides means to a patient who acts on his/her own or personally administers the lethal agent. All forms of euthanasia are illegal in the United States.

PAD and euthanasia are distinct from palliative sedation. Palliative sedation is a tool used in palliative medicine and hospice care as a last-ditch effort to treat refractory symptoms, such as pain, dyspnea, or terminal delirium. In palliative sedation, a medical coma is induced with the goal of relieving unbearable symptoms in the final days of a dying patient's life. If death occurs as the secondary result of the process of inducing coma for refractory symptoms, the action of palliative sedation may be considered ethically justifiable, according the ethical principle known as the "rule of double effect."[38] A physician's intent with the action is one important difference between palliative sedation and PAD or euthanasia.

Assisted Dying and Physician-Assisted Dying in the United States

In the United States, 4 states—Oregon, Washington, Montana, and Vermont—have laws allowing doctors to prescribe lethal medication to terminally ill patients. Oregon (in 1998) and Washington (in 2009) enacted their laws, better known as Death with Dignity (DWD), by referendum. In Montana, PAD was legalized by the courts in *Baxter v Montana* in 2009. Vermont, in 2013, was the first state to pass such a law, known as the Patient Choice and Control at End of Life Act, in a process initiated by its legislature. Several other states have similar proposals in varying stages of consideration.[39] PAD laws also exist in some other countries, namely Switzerland and the Netherlands.

In states where PAD laws do not exist, some terminally ill and suffering patients are not waiting for legalization. The specific definition of assisted dying or suicide varies from state to state and is considered a crime in 46 states. Well-publicized cases have brought attention to some physicians, patients, and their families having carried out and continuing to carry out instances of assisted dying without legal sanctioning.[40–42] Some of these cases have included patients suffering from terminal cancer,[41] complications of curative cancer treatment,[43] and functional impairment of moderate dementia.[44] These furtive acts illustrate the desperation and suffering some patients experience and the lengths to which they and/or their families will go to end their protracted illness, where no legalized alternative exist.

Impact on Family and Caregivers

An individual dying with assistance may have significant impact on their remaining families and caregivers. Family members and friends may be charged with manslaughter for assisting someone to die. They may be burdened with the grief of being part of an assisted death and ostracized from the community they live in. Legal and moral dilemmas and feelings of isolation in managing assisted suicide are supported in semistructured interviews of family members involved in assisted dying.[45,46] In a prospective cohort survey of terminally ill patients and their caregivers in the United States, less than 20% of those who deemed euthanasia or PAD to be ethical were willing to personally help their family member end his/her life, reflecting concerns for prosecution, successfully committing these acts reliably, and the emotional burden.[47]

Complicated grief may also be present in cases involving PAD.[48] Research in Oregon has shown no negative impact, however, on mental health outcomes on surviving families. There were no differences in depression, grief, and use of mental health services in family members of those who requested PAD compared with families of individuals dying without PAD. Where PAD was requested, families reported being better prepared for death, accepting of the loved one's death, and being less likely to endorse wanting additional opportunities to care for their loved ones.[49] Quality of death seems no worse and may even be better in some measured domains in those who pursued PAD compared with those who died of terminal illness without requesting PAD. Oregon researchers, using the Quality of Dying and Death Questionnaire, a validated 33-item instrument, showed family members of those choosing PAD had greater symptom control over surroundings, better functioning, better energy, and better control of bowel and bladder.[50]

Family members and friends who are asked to assist in hastening death are often challenged to support their loved one's request while integrating their own personal values and the psychological and legal impacts. A transparent legalized system for PAD seems to not have additional psychological burden on families of patients who request PAD compared with families of patients dying without requesting PAD. Any unresolved family conflict, however, increases the potential for complicated grief no matter the mechanism of death.[51] To the authors' knowledge, direct comparisons between families who participate in secret assisted suicide with those who are involved in legalized PAD do not exist in the medical literature. Further research is needed in measuring the impact of assisted suicides and legalized PAD on families.

D.T. is an 86-year-old Washington state resident with a history of stable depression. A left breast mass is discovered on routine examination with left-sided matted axillary adenopathy. Biopsy shows locally advanced T3, N2 to N3 intermediate-grade invasive ductal carcinoma. D.T.'s goals are to remain as independent and cognitively intact as long as possible and avoid excessive pain. D.T. declines further staging and palliative radiation therapy, electing to enroll in hospice care. Her oncologist supports her decision, noting, "I support her decision and I think that she really has a clear head on her shoulders as to what her goals are." D.T. enrolls in hospice.

D.T. lives in an independent portion of a retirement community where she is well supported by other community residents. She socializes daily in the dining hall and at community events. Over the span of 4 months, she develops progressive weakness with associated functional decline and hires an in-home caregiver to assist her activities of daily living and eventually requires the use of a power chair to get to the main dining hall. Her urge urinary incontinence worsens due to functional limitations. She has no pain, shortness of breath, or nausea. Six months into hospice, D.T. is requesting DWD.

She complains of being fatigued and not being able to have enough energy to tolerate her social events and meetings anymore. Her sleep is unchanged. Her appetite is reduced but she still loves eating seafood. She continues to enjoy her friends' visits, but finds it "hard to have them see me like this." She does not want to "live life like this," referring to her functional dependency, and wants to be in "control." Her "quality of life is declining rapidly" and she feels that her "dignity is slipping." "I don't have any physical pain."

D.T. is widowed with her spouse dying in hospice 15 years earlier from metastatic prostate cancer. She is an only child without any blood relatives. She has a durable power of attorney (DPOA) who is aware and supportive of D.T.'s request for DWD. D.T.'s hospice providers are aware of her plans to pursue DWD. Hospice nurse, social worker, and chaplain are supportive of her wishes, confirming frequent discussions revolving around D.T.'s loss of dignity and control of her own body.

D.T.'s medical history includes depression, psoriatic arthritis, gout, urge urinary incontinence, hypertension, atrial fibrillation, brady-tachy syndrome with a pacemaker, diastolic heart failure, and chronic kidney disease stage III. Her current medications include citalopram, aspirin, allopurinol, diltiazem, hydrochlorothiazide, digoxin, tolterodine, senna, polyethylene glycol (as needed), and morphine (as needed).

On examination, D.T. appears well groomed and developed. D.T. is alert and oriented to person, place, month, and year. She describes her mood as "good, given my circumstances." Her affect is full and congruent. She has picked a day that she would like to take the lethal medication and the people to be present, and has made financial and funeral arrangements. There is no evidence of psychosis. The PHQ-9 score is 4, with 3 points for fatigue and 1 point for suicidal ideation. Her breast mass is larger now compared with 3 months ago and is now fixated to the chest wall.

Physician-Assisted Dying: Assisted-Dying with Physician Involvement

Even before PAD was legalized in Washington, physicians provided aid with dying.[52,53] In a 1996 national stratified probability sample of US physicians in a wide array of specialties, 18% of physicians reported having received a request from a patient for assisted dying and 16% of physicians receiving such a request reported that they had complied with the request to hasten death.[52] Similar results were reported in a random survey in 1994–1995 of physicians practicing in Washington before PAD was legalized in the state. More than one-quarter of physicians had patients explicitly request help to hasten death and, of physicians who had received request, 24% of patient requests for PAD or euthanasia were granted. The investigators also showed that physicians do not consult colleagues about these patient requests.[53] The lack of a second opinion and transparency creates a truncated medical evaluation process and does not allow for an opportunity to potentially relieve patient suffering. Furthermore, an underground PAD system may have significant psychological impact on a physician who elects to participate in PAD because an accepted outlet is not available to discuss the clinical and ethical questions that may arise.

D.T.'s Attending Physician

I've been D.T.'s physician for the past 7 years, and expected this when she was diagnosed with cancer. She has been fiercely independent and has consistently and explicitly expressed her goals of maintaining her independence. This was a woman who ran the show, and her personal experiences of being a nurse, seeing many of her friends at the retirement community become dependent, and caring for her debilitated husband at home on hospice have all influenced her decision. I understood life in her view—what made life worth living and what made it not worth living. Her dignity and life as she previously enjoyed it have been stripped away.

The silence immediately after her request was probably only 1 to 3 seconds but it felt like minutes; emotions came in waves, while I thought of appropriate language to respond to something like this. I felt guilt, failure, honored, and frightened all at the same time. It all gave way to numbness at some point. This was my first patient request for DWD, and I wasn't fully prepared. I'm not sure if I can be fully comfortable in dealing with this.

Psychological effects of Death with Dignity on physicians

Clinicians appreciate the immense emotional burden when a patient requests DWD. The burden is compounded when a pathway is not available to discuss the ethical issues and seek additional guidance from colleagues on how to medically proceed with such requests. Studies on the effects of DWD on physicians are sparse. Anecdotes from physicians describe firsthand the impact DWD has on their practice, professional identity, and the emotional turmoil.[54–56] In structured telephone interviews of randomly selected United States oncologists who reported participating in euthanasia or PAD, 53% received comfort from having helped a patient with euthanasia or PAD, 24% regretted performing it, and 16% reported the emotional burden of performing it adversely affected their medical practice.[57]

Patients choosing physician-assisted dying

Patients using DWD in Oregon and Washington are predominately male, older, white, well educated, and married (**Fig. 2**). End-of-life concerns are similar in citizens of both states (**Table 1**). These end-of-life concerns motivating PAD in patients remain consistent in the medical literature. Through longitudinal semistructured interviews of Washington state patients interested in PAD, Pearlman and colleagues[58] find that the desire

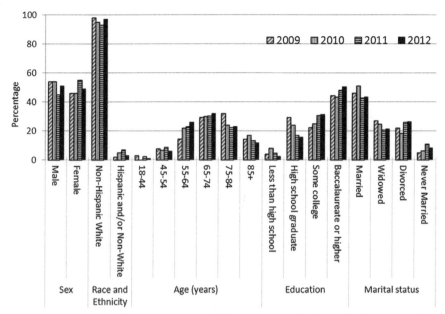

Fig. 2. Characteristics of the participants of the DWD Act who have died in Oregon and Washington. Data for Oregon are from January 1, 2009, through January 14, 2013. Data for Washington are from March 5, 2009, through February 28, 2013. (*Data from* Oregon Health Authority. Death with Dignity Act. Available at: http://public.health.oregon.gov/ProviderPartnerResources/EvaluationResearch/DeathwithDignityAct/Pages/ar-index.aspx. Accessed November 20, 2013; and Washington State Department of Health. Death with Dignity Act. Available at: http://www.doh.wa.gov/YouandYourFamily/IllnessandDisease/DeathwithDignityAct.aspx. Accessed November 23, 2013.)

Table 1 End-of-life concerns of participants in Death with Dignity in Oregon and Washington[a]		
End-of-Life Concerns	**Oregon (%)**	**Washington (%)**
Loss of autonomy	91.2	89.1
Inability to engage in enjoyable activities	88.8	86.5
Loss of dignity	82.0	75.6
Loss of control of bodily functions	51.6	51.8
Burden on family, friends, or caregivers	38.6	45.3
Inadequate pain control or concern about it	23.5	33.1
Financial implications of treatment	2.7	4.1

[a] Data for Oregon are from January 1, 1998, through January 14, 2013. Data for Washington are from March 5, 2009, through February 28, 2013.

Data from Oregon Health Authority. Death with Dignity Act. Available at: http://public.health.oregon.gov/ProviderPartnerResources/EvaluationResearch/DeathwithDignityAct/Pages/pasforms.aspx. Accessed November 20, 2013; and Washington State Department of Health. Death with Dignity Act. Available at: http://www.doh.wa.gov/YouandYourFamily/IllnessandDisease/DeathwithDignityAct/FormsforPatientsProviders.aspx. Accessed November 23, 2013.

for control and self-identity are 2 important themes to why patients choose PAD. The request for PAD is viewed as a means to stop the effects of the terminal illness from unraveling the sense of control and of self-identity.

Table 1 highlights the significance of existential distress to these patients. In semistructured interviews with family members of patients who died from PAD, an emerging theme was the perception that health care professionals lacked awareness of and were unsupportive of a patient's existential suffering. Families perceived health care professionals as uncomfortable and reluctant to discuss existential suffering and moral issues of assisted dying and withdrawing from the situation.[59] Similarly, in structured interviews of Washington state physicians before DWD was legalized, many physicians expressed unwillingness to assess nonphysical suffering.[53] As **Table 1** illustrates, however, these issues illustrate the concerns of patients who request DWD and should not be ignored or made insignificant.

The underlying illness is cancer for more than 75% of patients who die using DWD, which is followed by neurodegenerative diseases, such as amyotrophic lateral sclerosis, respiratory disease, and heart disease. In Oregon and Washington, the numbers of recipients and deaths due to DWD have steadily increased (**Fig. 3**), although the number of people requesting DWD remains a small percentage of each respective total state populations. Most patients who use DWD are also concurrently enrolled in hospice. In 2012, of patients who died using DWD in Oregon and Washington, 97% and 76%, respectively, were enrolled in hospice.[60,61]

Patient requirements for Death with Dignity

Box 1 outlines the required conditions that patients must meet to qualify for DWD. The legal requirements expected for attending physicians are discussed later (see **Box 3**). Age and state of residence are easy to determine. DWD is limited to those who have intact decision-making capacity, hence, not available to those who are unable to dictate their health care decisions, for example, patients with end-stage dementia. DWD is not available to patients who are unable to self-administer the lethal medication, such as patients with advanced neurodegenerative disease or severe functional

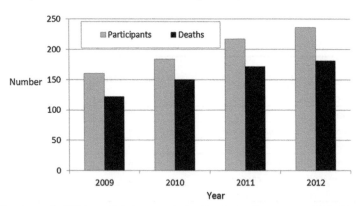

Fig. 3. Number of DWD participants and deaths from Oregon and Washington for 2009–2012. Data for Oregon are from January 1, 2009, through January 14, 2013. Data for Washington are from March 5, 2009, through February 28, 2013. (*Data from* Oregon Health Authority. Death with Dignity Act. Available at: http://public.health.oregon.gov/ProviderPartnerResources/EvaluationResearch/DeathwithDignityAct/Pages/ar-index.aspx. Accessed November 20, 2013; and Washington State Department of Health Death with Dignity Act. Available at: http://www.doh.wa.gov/YouandYourFamily/IllnessandDisease/DeathwithDignityAct.aspx. Accessed November 23, 2013.)

Box 1
Patient requirements of Death with Dignity Acts in Oregon and Washington

The patient is aged 18 years or older.

The patient is a resident of the state of Oregon or Washington.

The patient is capable of making and communicating health care decisions.

The patient is capable of understanding the options of hospice and feasible alternatives to the lethal medication.

The patient is capable of self-administering the lethal medication.

The patient has a terminal illness that would, within reasonable medical judgment, cause death within 6 months.

---

impairment. For example, patients with advanced amyotrophic lateral sclerosis who have the loss the use of their upper extremities are not eligible for DWD because they are unable to self-administer the lethal medication. Lastly, DWD is only available to patients who have a life expectancy of 6 months or less. An attending physician and a consulting physician must certify that a patient, to the best of their medical judgment, has a prognosis of 6 months or less. There is inherent inaccuracy in predicting the course of a patient's illness and time of death based on numerous studies[62,63] and limitations of prognostic tools.[64] Survey results of Oregon physicians showed that among those who were willing to write a lethal prescription and who had received a DWD request from a patient, 27% were not confident they could determine when a patient had less than 6 months to live.[65] Yet clinicians still must use their best medical judgment in making such difficult predictions.

Physician involvement in Death with Dignity in Oregon and Washington

Physicians should reflect on their own personal values and beliefs and determine in advance how they would respond to a patient who requests DWD. Would they be willing to assist and fulfill the attending role? Would they be willing to refer to a colleague? Or would they seek to completely transfer their care? The decision to participate in DWD is voluntary. Physicians, institutions, and health systems have the right to refuse to participate in DWD. Physicians should be aware of and respect the policies of the institutions in which they practice. An active MD or DO degree is required to participate in DWD as an attending or consulting physician. Other providers with prescriptive authority, such as physician assistants and nurse practitioners, are not legalized to participate in DWD as an attending or consultant.

If a physician declines to participate, this should be made clear to the patient. Explicit and open communication is critical in maintaining a therapeutic patient-physician relationship. In structured interviews of patients who were refused PAD and of their physicians, researchers report some physicians deliberately blocking the discussions by telling a patient to stop requesting PAD and other physicians not mentioning PAD themselves anymore, hoping the patient does not resume the subject matter.[66] Physicians may work with patients to find another physician to participate in DWD but remain involved by collaborating with a colleague who is willing to provide the prescription. Alternatively, the attending physician may discuss transferring the care of a patient to another physician who agrees to assume care. If an attending physician has strong ethical objections to participating with DWD and does not want to assist in any way, including making a referral or transfer of care, consideration should be given to referring the patient to the office administrator, hospital or clinic medical director, social worker, or the local medical society. The continuity of patient care should be continued until transfer of care is complete so that abandonment does not occur.

Responding effectively to Death with Dignity requests

Discussions of DWD can be uncomfortable and awkward. Based on analysis of interviews conducted prospectively with patients pursuing PAD and their family members and also retrospectively with family members of deceased patients who pursued PAD, Back and colleagues[67] advise physicians to consider a patient's request for PAD as an invitation to probe for the meaning behind the request. Physicians should explore the patient's concern about dying regardless of their personal views or willingness to participate in DWD. Patient concerns about physical symptoms, loss of control, financial hardship, burden to others, loss of identity, and loss of dignity are common at end-of-life care. Physicians should seek to understand patients' definitions and views of unacceptable suffering. **Box 2** outlines a guideline for responding to patients requesting DWD.

D.T.'s Attending Physician

Assessment/Plan

Enlarging breast mass, with chest wall invasion. D.T. has rapidly declining functional status and is in a power chair now, where she was ambulatory 6 months ago. Her Palliative Performance Scale score is now 40% and was 70% 6 months ago. She is in hospice and continues to derive psychological and physical support from hospice staff. D.T. has a terminal disease and a life expectancy less than 6 months. She has capacity to make this request for DWD. Her chronic mood disorder is well controlled and continues on citalopram. Her mood disorder is not causing impairment in judgment or reasoning. She has asked voluntarily, and no one has encouraged her or pushed her to make the decision to request DWD. She understands her diagnosis and her prognosis and we specifically discussed with her the fact that if she does take the medications prescribed per the DWD Act, that these medications will lead to her death shortly after she ingests them.

We also discussed the fact that should she pursue obtaining these medications, she does not need to take them, and she could change her mind at any point. We discussed alternatives to obtaining the medications to end her life, including living at the assisted or nursing portion of her retirement community when she is no longer able to live alone. She is already currently receiving hospice care. D.T. reports she has considered these options and that they are not acceptable to her; she states that her quality of his life is declining rapidly such that she cannot live independently now and her dignity is loss. She has informed her DPOA of her decision and her DPOA is supportive. She has given me permission to contact her DPOA to discuss her request and help arrange the logistics involved.

D.T. has already selected two people to be present when she takes the medications. She has been counseled about the importance of not taking the medication in a public place.

This is her initial verbal request for DWD. I will proceed with the patient's request and seek additional clinical and administrative support to ensure compliance.

Essential elements and safeguards of Death with Dignity

Oregon and Washington have similar processes and safeguards for DWD (**Box 3**). Both states have official forms and checklists available on their respective departments of health Web sites.[68,69] Health systems electing to participate in DWD may have an interdisciplinary committee review all patient requests and offer guidance. Additionally, some health systems may have a designated individual to ensure adherence to the multistep process. For example, the SCC uses a licensed social worker who assists patients, family, pharmacist, and physicians with the DWD process while ensuring all legal requirements are in compliance.[70]

Box 2
Guidelines for responding to a patient requesting Death with Dignity

Address the DWD request explicitly and openly.

Delve into what is prompting the request by exploring the patient's concerns with end-of-life. Common concerns are physical symptoms, loss of control, financial hardship, burden to others, loss of identity, and loss of dignity.

Inquire what an acceptable death is and what constitutes unacceptable suffering in the patient's view. Ask, "How do you want your death to look?"

Once patient's wishes and expectations are understood, explore treatment options available and how end-of-life concerns can be managed. This may include hospice or other palliative care options.

Assess the patient's perception of the discussion. Ask, "What are you taking away from our talk today?"

Offer follow-up appointments and/or telephone check-ins. Give patients additional opportunity to discuss evolving perceptions and feelings around end-of-life.

Reflect on your own level of involvement and motivations in the physician-patient relationship. Assess the impact of your values and beliefs on decision-making around the patient's end-of-life care.

Adapted from Back AL, Starks H, Hsu C, et al. Clinician-patient interactions about requests for physician-assisted suicide: a patient and family view. Arch Intern Med 2002;162:1257–65; and The Oregon Death with Dignity Act: a guidebook for healthcare professional. The Task Force to Improve the Care of Terminally-Ill Oregonians. 2nd edition. 2008. Available at: http://www.ohsu.edu/xd/education/continuing-education/center-for-ethics-outreach/upload/Oregon-Death-with-Dignity-Act-Guidebook.pdf.

Qualified patients who wish to pursue DWD are required to make an oral and written request. The written request must be signed by 2 witnesses. A 15-day minimum waiting period is required before the second request can be made by the patient. The lethal medication can be prescribed no sooner than 48 hours after receiving the patient's completed and signed written request for DWD. The shortest amount of time from initial verbal request to a patient receiving the medication is 19 days. Patients who are imminently dying may not qualify due to the time required to be in compliance.

Physicians are required to inform patients requesting DWD that they have the right to rescind the request at any time. Physicians are required to recommend to patients who pursue DWD to notify the next of kin or DPOA of their request, although decisions regarding disclosure are respected on the basis of confidentiality. A refusal to do so does not make a patient ineligible. Patients who decline to disclose their intent to pursue DWD with family or friends, because they fear a negative effect on them, should be further counseled.

Psychiatrists and psychologists may have critical roles in DWD. They may be called on to assist in helping to determine a patient's capacity in requesting PAD. Additionally they may be asked to assess the extent to which a mental disorder, such as depression or schizophrenia, might be driving a patient's request. A discussion on capacity determination can be found elsewhere.[71] The distinction between a depressed mood that develops as a response to a terminal illness and clinical depression for which treatment may alter a patient's desire for PAD is subtle and one that is difficult even for experts. Only 6% of surveyed psychiatrists in Oregon were very confident that they could determine whether a mental health disorder is influencing a person's decision to request PAD within a single consultation visit.[72] Additionally, the prevalence of

---

Box 3
Elements and safeguards of the Oregon and Washington Death with Dignity Acts

The patient must make an initial oral request.

The patient must make a written request. The written request requires 2 witnesses. One witness must not be a relative (by blood, marriage, or adoption) of the patient, not be entitled to any portion of the patient's estate on death, and not own, operate, or be employed at a health care facility where the patient is resides. If the patient is an inpatient at a long-term health care facility, one of the witnesses shall be an individual designated by the facility.

After the initial oral request, the patient must wait 15 days to make a second oral request. At the second oral request, the patient must be informed again of the right to rescind the request at any time.

At the initial request, the prescribing physician must

Make a determination of terminal disease with a prognosis of 6 months or less.

Determine the patient's competency and the voluntary nature of the request for lethal medication and, if necessary, referral to a psychiatrist or psychologist to ensure competency and absence of a mental health disorder causing impairment in judgment.

Confirm state residency.

Assess informed consent on the basis of the patient being fully aware of the (1) medical diagnosis, (2) prognosis, (3) potential risks associated with taking the medication to be prescribed, (4) result of taking the medication (death), and (5) the feasible alternatives (palliative care, hospice care, and pain control).

Recommend that the patient (1) has the right to rescind the request at any time, (2) notify next of kin, (3) have someone present at time of medication ingestion, and (4) not take the medication in a public place.

The consulting physician confirms patient's (1) terminal disease with a prognosis of 6 months or less, (2) competency, (3) request for lethal medication is voluntary, and (4) informed consent by assessing complete awareness of the medical diagnosis and prognosis, potential risks associated with taking the medication to be prescribed, the result of taking the medication (death), and feasible alternatives.

Medication can be prescribed no sooner than 48 hours after the patient's written request has been completed, signed, and received.

Immediately prior to writing the prescription, the prescribing physician must

Verify that the patient is making an informed decision at the time of prescription

Immediately after writing the prescription, the prescribing physician must

Deliver the prescription to the pharmacist

The pharmacist dispenses the medication directly to the patient or an identified agent of the patient.

The attending physician completes an after death report. Death certificate indicates the underlying terminal illness as the cause of death.

---

clinical depression, depressive symptoms, or desire to hasten death in terminally ill patients is not negligible.[47,73,74] Rate of clinical depression among patients who request DWD is variable, from zero to 25%, depending on the cohort studied and study methods.[70,75,76] In terminally ill Oregon patients who had requested DWD, the prevalence of clinical depression was 25% diagnosed using the structured clinical interview for American Psychiatric Association *Diagnostic and Statistical Manual of Mental Disorders* (Fourth Edition) axis I disorders, a standard research instrument for diagnosing mental disorders.[76] The experience of the Seattle Cancer Care Alliance

(SCCA), in neighboring Washington, reported that none of their patients who inquired about DWD was found to have current or previous depression. As standard practice, SCCA social workers provide the initial psychological evaluation of all patients using interview-based techniques and standardized assessments (such as the PHQ-9 and the Generalized Anxiety Disorder-7 questionnaire). Physicians retained the responsibility of evaluating and diagnosing depression.[70]

Depression should not in itself invalidate a patient's request for DWD; the question is whether depression might be impairing judgment and rational thought, in which case treatment may alter a patient's choice.[77] In semistructured interviews with Washington state patients and family who plan to or will be taking part in PAD, depressive symptoms when present were not described by subjects and/or family members to be an influential factor in a patient's decision to pursue PAD.[78] Positions for and against mandatory psychiatric evaluations for all patients requesting DWD continue to be debated.[79,80] Current DWD legislation in Oregon and Washington require additional psychiatric evaluation only if the attending or consulting physician determines there is impaired judgment from a psychiatric or psychological disorder. Similar to the practice outlined at the SCCA, it is highly recommended that all patients who request DWD be screened for depression with a validated instrument, such as the PHQ-9 and, if the screening indicates possible depression, the patient should be referred for a psychiatric evaluation.[81]

A barbiturate is usually the prescribed lethal medication used in DWD. Most patients' insurances do not cover the cost of the medication for this purpose. The out-of-pocket cost is substantial and can be variable depending on the pharmacy. Patients should be made aware of the financial costs associated with the lethal medication. Pharmacists and pharmacies may choose to not participate. A pharmacist may assist in finding a willing pharmacist. Physicians should confer with the participating pharmacist prior to writing a prescription to ensure correct dosages are used and instructions are written clearly and to seek additional counsel. An attending physician is required to deliver or mail the prescription to the participating pharmacist. Faxes or verbal orders are not accepted. Patients and families who wish to pursue DWD should be made aware of the additional time required for this step before they receive the lethal medication.

The attending physician should establish with the patient whom he/she would like to be present at the time of self-administration. Depending on the attending physician's comfort, he/she may offer to be present. Physicians should encourage patients to disclose to other health care providers, especially hospice staff, who may be able to provide support to patients, families, and friends. An advance directive and a Physician Orders for Life-Sustaining Treatment document should be completed to avert unwanted emergency interventions. If hospice is involved, it should be contacted once a patient dies from the lethal medication. Otherwise, 9-1-1 should be called when a patient dies. After a patient dies via DWD in Oregon and Washington, the attending physician is required to complete additional follow-up documents to comply with the law. Data are collected and publicly shared annually by each respective state's department of health.[60,61]

D.T.: Conclusion

D.T. selected a date to take her lethal medication. She selected two of her closest friends to be present who were both nurses with experience in palliative care. She declined to have other health care professionals involved. Her attending physician could not be present. D.T. died within 20 minutes after ingesting the lethal medication without complications. According to one of the individuals present, "she died peacefully—and on her own terms."

SUMMARY

Patients seeking PAD share many of the characteristics observed in older persons who are thinking about suicide. The contextual factors and the loss of self-identity are important to both. Hastened deaths, in the forms of suicide, assisted dying, and PAD, lead to complex emotions in survivors and clinicians. Patient stories could shed light on what makes the wish to die so compelling for patients who are thinking about hastening their deaths but have no terminal disease.

REFERENCES

1. Crosby AE, Ortega L, Melonson C. Centers of Disease Control. National Center for Injury Prevention and Control. Self-Directed Violence Surveillance. Uniform definitions and recommended data elements. Atlanta (GA): National Center for Injury Prevention and Control, Centers for Disease Control and Prevention; 2011.
2. American Association of Suicidology. Suicide Data Page 2010. 2012. Available at: www.suicidology.org. Accessed February 7, 2014.
3. Duberstein PR, Conwell Y, Seidlitz L, et al. Age and suicidal ideation in older depressed inpatients. Am J Geriatr Psychiatry 1999;7(4):289–96.
4. Waern M, Beskow J, Runeson B, et al. Suicidal feelings in the last year of life in elderly people who commit suicide. Lancet 1999;354(9182):917–8.
5. Simon GE, Rutter CM, Peterson D, et al. Does response on the PHQ-9 depression questionnaire predict Subsequent suicide attempt or suicide death? Psychiatr Serv 2013;64(12):1195–202.
6. Hawton K, Appleby L, Platt S, et al. The psychological autopsy approach to studying suicide: a review of methodological issues. J Affect Disord 1998; 50(2–3):269–76.
7. Conwell Y, Duberstein PR, Cox C, et al. Relationships of age and axis I diagnoses in victims of completed suicide: a psychological autopsy study. Am J Psychiatry 1996;153(8):1001–8.
8. Joiner T. Why people die by suicide. Cambridge (MA): Harvard University Press; 2005.
9. Van Orden KA, Witte TK, Cukrowicz KC, et al. The interpersonal theory of suicide. Psychol Rev 2010;117(2):575–600.
10. Jahn DR, Cukrowicz KC. The impact of the nature of relationships on perceived burdensomeness and suicide ideation in a community sample of older adults. Suicide Life Threat Behav 2011;41(6):635–49.
11. Myers MF, Fine C. Touched by suicide: bridging the perspectives of survivors and clinicians. Suicide Life Threat Behav 2007;37(2):119–26.
12. Bruce ML, Ten Have TR, Reynolds CF 3rd, et al. Reducing suicidal ideation and depressive symptoms in depressed older primary care patients: a randomized controlled trial. JAMA 2004;291(9):1081–91.
13. Unutzer J, Tang L, Oishi S, et al. Reducing suicidal ideation in depressed older primary care patients. J Am Geriatr Soc 2006;54(10):1550–6.
14. Solberg LI, Crain AL, Jaeckels N, et al. The DIAMOND initiative: implementing collaborative care for depression in 75 primary care clinics. Implement Sci 2013;8(1):135.
15. Coffey CE. Building a system of perfect depression care in behavioral health. Jt Comm J Qual Patient Saf 2007;33(4):193–9.
16. Hampton T. Depression care effort brings dramatic drop in large HMO population's suicide rate. JAMA 2010;303(19):1903–5.

17. Conwell Y, Lyness JM, Duberstein P, et al. Completed suicide among older patients in primary care practices: a controlled study. J Am Geriatr Soc 2000;48(1):23–9.
18. Harwood DM, Hawton K, Hope T, et al. Suicide in older people: mode of death, demographic factors, and medical contact before death. Int J Geriatr Psychiatry 2000;15(8):736–43.
19. U.S. Preventive Services Task Force. Screening for suicide risk: recommendation and rationale. Ann Intern Med 2004;140(10):820–1.
20. US Department of Health and Human Services. Healthy People 2020. Mental Health and Mental Disorders Objectives. Available at: http://www.healthypeople.gov/2020/topicsobjectives2020/objectiveslist.aspx?topicId=28. Accessed February 5, 2014.
21. Goldsmith SK, Institute of Medicine (U.S.), Committee on Pathophysiology & Prevention of Adolescent & Adult Suicide. Reducing suicide: a national imperative. Washington, DC: National Academies Press; 2002.
22. Juurlink DN, Herrmann N, Szalai JP, et al. Medical illness and the risk of suicide in the elderly. Arch Intern Med 2004;164(11):1179–84.
23. Seyfried LS, Kales HC, Ignacio RV, et al. Predictors of suicide in patients with dementia. Alzheimers Dement 2011;7(6):567–73.
24. Scocco P, Fantoni G, Rapattoni M, et al. Death ideas, suicidal thoughts, and plans among nursing home residents. J Geriatr Psychiatry Neurol 2009;22(2):141–8.
25. Wongpakaran N, Wongpakaran T. Prevalence of major depressive disorders and suicide in long-term care facilities: a report from northern Thailand. Psychogeriatrics 2012;12(1):11–7.
26. Mezuk B, Prescott MR, Tardiff K, et al. Suicide in older adults in long-term care: 1990 to 2005. J Am Geriatr Soc 2008;56(11):2107–11.
27. Menghini VV, Evans JM. Suicide among nursing home residents: a population-based study. J Am Med Dir Assoc 2000;1(2):47–50.
28. Scocco P, Rapattoni M, Fantoni G, et al. Suicidal behaviour in nursing homes: a survey in a region of north-east Italy. Int J Geriatr Psychiatry 2006;21(4):307–11.
29. Malfent D, Wondrak T, Kapusta ND, et al. Suicidal ideation and its correlates among elderly in residential care homes. Int J Geriatr Psychiatry 2010;25(8):843–9.
30. Muramatsu RS, Goebert D. Psychiatric services: experience, perceptions, and needs of nursing facility multidisciplinary leaders. J Am Geriatr Soc 2011;59(1):120–5.
31. Erlangsen A, Zarit SH, Conwell Y. Hospital-diagnosed dementia and suicide: a longitudinal study using prospective, nationwide register data. Am J Geriatr Psychiatry 2008;16(3):220–8.
32. Draper B, Peisah C, Snowdon J, et al. Early dementia diagnosis and the risk of suicide and euthanasia. Alzheimers Dement 2010;6(1):75–82.
33. Turvey CL, Conwell Y, Jones MP, et al. Risk factors for late-life suicide: a prospective, community-based study. Am J Geriatr Psychiatry 2002;10(4):398–406.
34. Haw C, Harwood D, Hawton K. Dementia and suicidal behavior: a review of the literature. Int Psychogeriatr 2009;21(3):440–53.
35. O'Dwyer ST, Moyle W, Zimmer-Gembeck M, et al. Suicidal ideation in family carers of people with dementia: a pilot study. Int J Geriatr Psychiatry 2013;28(11):1182–8.
36. Ganzini L, Lee MA. Psychiatry and assisted suicide in the United States. N Engl J Med 1997;336(25):1824–6.
37. Boudreau JD, Somerville MA, Biller-Andorno N. Clinical decisions. Physician-assisted suicide. N Engl J Med 2013;368(15):1450–2.

38. Quill TE, Dresser R, Brock DW. The rule of double effect–a critique of its role in end-of-life decision making. N Engl J Med 1997;337(24):1768–71.
39. Death with dignity national center. Death with dignity around the U.S. Available at: http://www.deathwithdignity.org/advocates/national. Accessed December 2, 2013.
40. Yardley W. For role in suicide, a friend to the end is now facing jail. New York Times 2005.
41. Green R. Assisted suicide in West Hartford shows need for law on difficult decision. Courant 2011.
42. Roig-Franzia M. After the death of Jack Kevorkian, Lawrence Egbert is the new public face of American assisted suicide. The Washington Post 2012.
43. Bethea C. Final Exit. Atlanta (GA): Dell Publishing; 2010.
44. Fein E. Granting Father's Wish, or Manslaughter?, The New York Times Online, October 28, 1994.
45. Gamondi C, Pott M, Forbes K, et al. Exploring the experiences of bereaved families involved in assisted suicide in Southern Switzerland: a qualitative study. BMJ Support Palliat Care 2013. [Epub ahead of print]. http://dx.doi.org/10.1136/bmjspcare-2013-000483.
46. Starks H, Back AL, Pearlman RA, et al. Family member involvement in hastened death. Death Stud 2007;31(2):105–30.
47. Emanuel EJ, Fairclough DL, Emanuel LL. Attitudes and desires related to euthanasia and physician-assisted suicide among terminally ill patients and their caregivers. JAMA 2000;284(19):2460–8.
48. Bascom PB, Tolle SW. Responding to requests for physician-assisted suicide: "These are uncharted waters for both of us...". JAMA 2002;288(1):91–8.
49. Ganzini L, Goy ER, Dobscha SK, et al. Mental health outcomes of family members of Oregonians who request physician aid in dying. J Pain Symptom Manage 2009;38(6):807–15.
50. Smith KA, Goy ER, Harvath TA, et al. Quality of death and dying in patients who request physician-assisted death. J Palliat Med 2011;14(4):445–50.
51. Prigerson HG, Jacobs SC. Perspectives on care at the close of life. Caring for bereaved patients: "All the doctors just suddenly go". JAMA 2001;286(11):1369–76.
52. Meier DE, Emmons CA, Wallenstein S, et al. A national survey of physician-assisted suicide and euthanasia in the United States. N Engl J Med 1998; 338(17):1193–201.
53. Back AL, Wallace JI, Starks HE, et al. Physician-assisted suicide and euthanasia in Washington State. Patient requests and physician responses. JAMA 1996; 275(12):919–25.
54. Kade WJ. Death with dignity: a case study. Ann Intern Med 2000;132(6):504–6.
55. Stevens KR Jr. Emotional and psychological effects of physician-assisted suicide and euthanasia on participating physicians. Issues Law Med 2006;21(3): 187–200.
56. Reagan P. Helen. Lancet 1999;353(9160):1265–7.
57. Emanuel EJ, Daniels ER, Fairclough DL, et al. The practice of euthanasia and physician-assisted suicide in the United States: adherence to proposed safeguards and effects on physicians. JAMA 1998;280(6):507–13.
58. Pearlman RA, Hsu C, Starks H, et al. Motivations for physician-assisted suicide. J Gen Intern Med 2005;20(3):234–9.
59. Gamondi C, Pott M, Payne S. Families' experiences with patients who died after assisted suicide: a retrospective interview study in southern Switzerland. Ann Oncol 2013;24(6):1639–44.

60. Oregon Health Authority. Death with Dignity Act. Available at: http://public. health.oregon.gov/ProviderPartnerResources/EvaluationResearch/Deathwith DignityAct/Pages/index.aspx. Accessed December 12, 2013.

61. Washington State Department of Health. Death with Dignity Act. Available at: http:// www.doh.wa.gov/YouandYourFamily/IllnessandDisease/DeathwithDignityAct. aspx. Accessed December 14, 2013.

62. A controlled trial to improve care for seriously ill hospitalized patients. The study to understand prognoses and preferences for outcomes and risks of treatments (SUPPORT). The SUPPORT Principal Investigators. JAMA 1995;274(20):1591–8.

63. Forster LE, Lynn J. Predicting life span for applicants to inpatient hospice. Arch Intern Med 1988;148(12):2540–3.

64. Lee S, Schonberg M, Widera E, et al. ePrognosis - Estimating Prognosis for Elders. Available at: http://eprognosis.ucsf.edu/faq.php. Accessed February 2, 2014.

65. Ganzini L, Nelson HD, Lee MA, et al. Oregon physicians' attitudes about and experiences with end-of-life care since passage of the Oregon Death with Dignity Act. JAMA 2001;285(18):2363–9.

66. Pasman HR, Willems DL, Onwuteaka-Philipsen BD. What happens after a request for euthanasia is refused? Qualitative interviews with patients, relatives and physicians. Patient Educ Couns 2013;92(3):313–8.

67. Back AL, Starks H, Hsu C, et al. Clinician-patient interactions about requests for physician-assisted suicide: a patient and family view. Arch Intern Med 2002; 162(11):1257–65.

68. Oregon Health Authority. Death with Dignity Act. Available at: http://public. health.oregon.gov/ProviderPartnerResources/EvaluationResearch/Deathwith DignityAct/Pages/pasforms.aspx. Accessed November 20, 2013.

69. Washington State Department of Health. Death with Dignity Act. Available at: http://www.doh.wa.gov/YouandYourFamily/IllnessandDisease/Deathwith DignityAct/FormsforPatientsProviders.aspx. Accessed November 23, 2013.

70. Loggers ET, Starks H, Shannon-Dudley M, et al. Implementing a Death with Dignity program at a comprehensive cancer center. N Engl J Med 2013;368(15): 1417–24.

71. Appelbaum PS. Clinical practice. Assessment of patients' competence to consent to treatment. N Engl J Med 2007;357(18):1834–40.

72. Ganzini L, Fenn DS, Lee MA, et al. Attitudes of Oregon psychiatrists toward physician-assisted suicide. Am J Psychiatry 1996;153(11):1469–75.

73. Chochinov HM, Wilson KG, Enns M, et al. Desire for death in the terminally ill. Am J Psychiatry 1995;152(8):1185–91.

74. Breitbart W, Rosenfeld B, Pessin H, et al. Depression, hopelessness, and desire for hastened death in terminally ill patients with cancer. JAMA 2000;284(22): 2907–11.

75. Ganzini L, Nelson HD, Schmidt TA, et al. Physicians' experiences with the Oregon Death with Dignity Act. N Engl J Med 2000;342(8):557–63.

76. Ganzini L, Goy ER, Dobscha SK. Prevalence of depression and anxiety in patients requesting physicians' aid in dying: cross sectional survey. BMJ 2008; 337:a1682.

77. Quill TE, Cassel CK, Meier DE. Care of the hopelessly ill. Proposed clinical criteria for physician-assisted suicide. N Engl J Med 1992;327(19): 1380–4.

78. Bharucha AJ, Pearlman RA, Back AL, et al. The pursuit of physician-assisted suicide: role of psychiatric factors. J Palliat Med 2003;6(6):873–83.

79. McCormack R, Price A. Psychiatric review should be mandatory for patients requesting assisted suicide. Gen Hosp Psychiatry 2014;36(1):7–9.
80. Ganzini L. Psychiatric evaluations for individuals requesting assisted death in Washington and Oregon should not be mandatory. Gen Hosp Psychiatry 2014;36(1):10–2.
81. The Oregon Death with Dignity Act: a guidebook for Health Care Professionals. The Task Force to Improve the Care of Terminally-Ill Oregonians. 2nd edition. 2008. Available at: http://www.ohsu.edu/xd/education/continuing-education/center-for-ethics-outreach/upload/Oregon-Death-with-Dignity-Act-Guidebook.pdf.

Posttraumatic Stress in Older Adults

When Medical Diagnoses or Treatments Cause Traumatic Stress

Jennifer Moye, PhD[a,b,*], Susan J. Rouse, PMH-CNS-BC[a]

KEYWORDS

- Posttraumatic stress disorder (PTSD) • Geriatric • Cardiac • Cancer

KEY POINTS

- Most older patients adapt after catastrophic medical diagnoses and treatments, but a significant number may develop posttraumatic stress disorder (PTSD) symptoms.
- PTSD symptoms create added burden for the individual, family, and health care system for the patient's recovery.
- Medical-related PTSD may be underdiagnosed by providers who may be unaware that these health problems can lead to PTSD symptoms.
- Treatment research is lacking, but pharmacologic and nonpharmacologic approaches to treatment may be extrapolated and adjusted from the literature focusing on younger adults.
- Additional study is needed.

INTRODUCTION

The Condition

The most familiar form of posttraumatic stress disorder (PTSD) occurs in veterans exposed to combat, and it can recur or worsen in the setting of other stressors in late life, including medical illness. This article draws attention to a different and underappreciated problem of posttraumatic stress symptoms (PTSSs) and PTSD arising from catastrophic medical illness.

In the latest edition of the *Diagnostic and Statistical Manual*,[1] PTSD has 6 components (**Table 1**).

Disclosure: This material is the result of work supported with resources and the use of facilities at the Boston VA Medical Center. Dr J. Moye received funding for research from the Department of Veterans Affairs Rehabilitation Research and Development Service #5I01RX000104-02.
Conflict of Interest: The authors have no conflict of interest relating to this study or this article.
[a] VA Boston Health Care System, MA, USA; [b] Department of Psychiatry, Harvard Medical School, MA, USA
* Corresponding author. Brockton Division, VA Boston Healthcare System, 940 Belmont Street, Brockton, MA 02301.
E-mail address: jennifer.moye@va.gov

Table 1
Diagnostic criteria for PTSD

Criterion	Description
(A) Exposure	Event with actual or threatened death, serious injury, or sexual violation by: Directly experiencing the traumatic event Witnessing in person the traumatic event as it occurred to others Learning that the traumatic event occurred to a close family member/friend Experiencing first-hand repeated or extreme exposure to aversive details of the traumatic event
(B) Reexperiencing	Spontaneous memories of the traumatic event, recurrent distressing dreams, dissociative reactions, intense or prolonged psychological distress or physiologic reaction to cues
(C) Avoidance	Avoidance of distressing memories, thoughts, feelings, or external reminders of the event
(D) Negative cognitions and mood	Persistent and distorted negative beliefs about oneself, others, the world, or causes/consequences of traumatic event; persistent negative emotional state, diminished interest, detachment/estrangement from others; persistent inability to feel positive emotions; inability to remember key aspects of the event
(E) Arousal	Irritable/angry, reckless or self-destructive behavior, hypervigilance, exaggerated startle, problems with concentration or sleep
(F) Duration	More than 1 mo
(G) Functional impairment	Clinically significant distress or impairment in social, occupational, or other important areas of functioning

Risk Factors

Although studies vary as to whether age[2–4] increases risk for medically induced PTSD, several other factors are consistently associated with increased risk (**Box 1**).[2,4–6]

Scope of the Problem

Medically induced PTSD affects the individual, the family, and the health care system. Individuals with PTSD with comorbid depression experience more severe depression,[7] particularly intrusion symptoms, and all-cause mortality.[8] Family and professional caregivers may experience emotional distancing, irritability, and aggression from patients with PTSS,[9] and may also experience increased psychological distress themselves.[10] Older adults with PTSD may have more frequent primary care visits but not receive indicated mental health treatment.[11]

Box 1
Risk factors for medically induced PTSD

- Previous trauma or negative life stressors
- Preexisting psychiatric disorder
- Higher exposure to trauma (eg, longer intensive care unit [ICU] stay; longer duration of cancer treatment)
- Loss of physical functioning as a result of the medical condition
- Pain

Clinical Correlations

Many conditions are associated with risk of PTSD or PTSS (**Box 2**).

DIAGNOSTIC STANDARDS AND DILEMMAS
Process of Eliminating Alternative Diagnoses/Problems

Although anxiety and depression may frequently co-occur with catastrophic medical illness, PTSD can be differentiated from these, especially by the presence of experiences described by the patient as traumatic (criterion A) and intrusive thoughts, memories, and dreams of these events (criterion B). Avoidance is a cardinal component of PTSD but may not be present if the patient is unable to avoid aversive reminders (such as having to return for ongoing health care at the site of the initial diagnosis or subsequent procedures) and even because the body may be a daily reminder (eg, a missing breast). In addition, clinicians should remain alert for PTSS (ie, the presence of symptoms that do not meet criteria for the disorder but still cause clinically significant distress and dysfunction).

Comorbidities

Depression,[12] bipolar disorder,[13] and dementia can occur with PTSD; PTSD conveys an increased risk for developing dementia.[14,15] Although difficult medical experiences may lead to PTSD symptoms, older adults with lifetime PTSD have high rates of physical health conditions, such as of gastritis, angina pectoris, and arthritis.[16] Social changes such as retirement and bereavement may be associated with increased thoughts about military experience earlier in their lives.[17]

CLINICAL FINDINGS
Source of Data

Patient interview and reports of family and professional caregivers provide the key data on PTSD. Patients are most aware of internal signs and often do not tell others

---

Box 2
Conditions associated with medically induced PTSD and PTSD prevalence rates

Diagnoses of life-threatening illness

    Cancer, 0%–35%[34]

    Multiple sclerosis, 16%–75%[35]

Medical events

    Myocardial infarction, 5%[36]–42%[5,37]

    Stroke, 8%–9%[38]

    Delirium, 19%–22%[39]

    Fall, 17%–35%[3]

Surgical procedures

    Cardiac surgery, 17%–20%[40,41]

    Intraoperative awareness, 2%–71%[42,43]

Medical settings

    ICU, 10%–28%[44]

    Long-term care, 9%–22%[45]

about intrusive symptoms. Caregivers are often more aware of external signs such as anger and agitation.

Examination

A clinical interview focusing on symptoms of PTSD is the foundation of the examination. The most important issue is to ask about the occurrence and impact of catastrophic medical events because PTSSs from these are often overlooked. Begin by simply asking about the recent medical experience. For example: "You were recently hospitalized for heart surgery. How was that for you? Some people find themselves having bad memories or dreams of their heart surgery and recovery. Have you found that? Is there anything that happened you wish to discuss? Do you have any questions about your surgery and hospital stay?"

Recommended Rating Scales

Numerous self-report and interview measures can be used to guide PTSD assessment (**Table 2**). These instruments have been validated for use in older adults[18] and can be selected from factors such as brevity versus depth. A lower cut score of 42 (rather than 50) is recommended for older adults on the Posttraumatic Stress Disorder Check List.[19]

INTERVENTIONS: CURRENT EVIDENCE BASE AND WHAT TO DO WHEN EVIDENCE IS LACKING

Treatment of older adults with PTSD, particularly when medically induced, is weakly supported by age-specific and trigger-specific evidence. Although progress has been made on assessment and treatment protocols in the adult population, similar advances have lagged behind for older adults.[20] Therefore, clinical decision making must draw from the literature on younger adults and war or sexual trauma, supplemented with clinical experience.

Many older veterans whom we have seen in our practice at the Veteran's Administration have PTSD related to military trauma. Much of the research available for pharmacologic treatment is based on military-related PTSD or sexual trauma. However, our experience has shown us that elderly patients can have new-onset PTSD symptoms or exacerbation of previously remitted PTSD symptoms in the context of severe medical illness, and may benefit from similar treatment approaches. For example, a 66-year-old Vietnam-era combat veteran had remitted combat PTSD symptoms for

Table 2
Selected assessment scales

Scale	Number of Items	Description
Primary Care PTSD Screen[46]	4	Designed to screen for PTSD in primary care and other medical settings, with an introductory sentence to cue respondents to traumatic events
Posttraumatic Check List–Stressor-specific version[47]	17	Severity rating of 17 PTSD symptoms in relation to a specific stressful experience
Impact of Events Scale - Revised[48]	22	Severity rating of subjective distress caused by traumatic events

many years. He was recently emergently hospitalized for a ventricular tachycardia after his implantable cardioverter defibrillator fired 5 consecutive times while he was alone at the local sanitation station. He sat alone in his vehicle, called 911, and waited to die. Since this retriggering event, the veteran has developed reemerging symptoms of PTSD including hyperarousal, anxiety, nightmares, depressed mood, and ruminative thoughts of death; these thoughts intermix with his earlier trauma and his memories of his cardiac event.

PSYCHOPHARMACOLOGIC TREATMENT

Pharmacologic interventions should target the individual core symptoms of PTSD with attention paid to the medical comorbidities and the risks and benefits of medications. As patients feel threatened, as in the case of the Vietnam veteran during and after his cardiac event, overwhelming fear tends to trigger a typical fight-or-flight response with symptoms of nightmares, insomnia, depressed and anxious mood, and hyperarousal, which is thought to arise from the brain's amygdala. Psychopharmacology in PTSD is focused on restoring balance to the natural inhibitory response of the brain. At present, the US Food and Drug Administration (FDA) has approved only 2 medications for PTSD: the selective serotonin reuptake inhibitors (SSRIs), paroxetine and sertraline. There is currently much research in progress to assess whether these medications are the best available choices for PTSD symptoms. However, first it may be helpful to discuss the use of benzodiazepines, which are widely prescribed for PTSD in medical settings.

Benzodiazepines

Gamma-aminobutyric acid (GABA) is an inhibitory neurotransmitter that, when activated by benzodiazepines (BZDs), is decreases neuronal firing and anxiety. Many clinicians immediately prescribe these drugs without concern for their effects. BZDs can be effective in treating symptoms of anxiety disorders including PTSD and are usually safe. However, in the geriatric population, there are many reasons why these drugs are heavily regulated. Even the BZDs with shorter half-lives (such as alprazolam and lorazepam) must be used with caution in older adults, because of the potential for increased half-life caused by slower hepatic metabolism and decreased renal clearance.[21] Comorbid medical illnesses (cancer, renal and kidney disease, dementia, cardiac disease, vascular disorders) increase risks for adverse drug effects such as gait impairment, falls, confusion, and psychomotor slowing, and intentional or unwitting overuse can also increase risk for motor vehicle and other accidents and unsafe behaviors. Risks of dependency, tolerance, delirium, and withdrawal are also a concern. For all these reasons, BZDs should not be considered drugs of choice in treatment of PTSD, and are best reserved as a last resort.

PREFERRED PHARMACOLOGIC MANAGEMENT OF PTSD SYMPTOMS
Sleep

Patients often report that insomnia is the most distressing PTSD symptom. Lack of sleep can exacerbate other symptoms of PTSD. For these reasons it is useful to treat insomnia first.[22] Sleep disturbances in PTSD are thought to be related to hyperarousal and increased adrenergic activity, which may lead to related symptoms such as nightmares, difficulty initiating sleep, and frequent awakenings. Two medications that decrease nightmares and improve sleep quality are prazosin, and trazodone.[23]

In elderly populations, prazosin (an alpha-1 adrenergic receptor antagonist that crosses blood-brain barrier) is effective but risks of postural hypotension, dizziness, and priapism should be monitored. Risks can be minimized by starting at the lowest possible dosage and titrating slowly. Low-dose trazodone (with activity at 5HT2A, alpha 1, and H1 receptors) is an alternative to prazosin and may help with sleep onset. Because of alpha 1 activity, it also can cause postural hypotension and priapism, especially in combination with prazosin, and patients should be monitored closely. Other medications for sleep include tricyclic antidepressants or sedating atypical antipsychotics (quetiapine). However, a careful individualized review of risks versus benefits is necessary when considering these medications in the elderly.

Hyperarousal, Avoidance, and Reexperiencing

If prazosin and or trazodone are ineffective in treating all the symptoms of PTSD, the next step is to consider a trial of an SSRI. The choice of an antidepressant is crucial. Elderly patients are often nonadherant to medications[24] for several reasons including worry over adverse side effects, costs of medications, fear of addiction, and lack of understanding of the value of medications. Clinical response improves with adherence so when discussing risks and benefits of individual medications with patients there should be clear communication about the patients' conflicting beliefs and preconceived ideas. Addressing these concerns may improve overall compliance. Open communication related to particular side effects of antidepressants can improve knowledge and expectations about the medication in the patient, and thus improve adherence For example, choosing paroxetine (Paxil) for an 85-year-old man already taking oxybutynin for bladder incontinence may potentiate anticholinergic symptoms of dry mouth, sedation, confusion, and ataxia, thus causing the patient to stop the medication prematurely or become delirious. Monitoring comorbid medical conditions, prescribed and nonprescribed over-the-counter medications, as well as having specific target symptoms (sleep, appetite, nightmares, and anxiety) can make this process smoother.

Psychosis

Some geriatric patients experience psychotic symptoms associated with PTSD. In our experience, this is more likely to be the case when PTSD occurs in combination with dementia, and dementia can reveal quiescent PTSD from decades earlier. Low-dose quetiapine, risperidone, and aripiprazole may be helpful in reducing or eliminating psychotic symptoms. The benefits of these medications must be weighed against the risks of side effects such as weight gain, metabolic syndrome, and cardiovascular risk.

   As with all psychiatric medications used in older adults, it is important to start low and go slow, but go. More cautious titration usually results in better tolerance. In contrast, excessive caution can result in failure to reach a therapeutic dose of medication and limited treatment benefit as well as loss of patient confidence resulting in noncompliance. Educate the patient that symptoms can take up to 6 weeks to remit and that consistency of dosing and clinician contact are important in achieving the best results. If the first medication yields only partial response, consider increasing the dosage, augmenting with a second agent, or switching to another medication (**Table 3**).

NONPHARMACOLOGIC TREATMENT
Lifespan Context

In work with older veterans who are experiencing PTSD, often as a resurgence of symptoms late in life, the decision of whether and how to approach the trauma narrative is tempered by the combat trauma having occurred 40 to 60 years ago, being

Table 3
Medications for PTSD

Medication	Target	Notable Side Effects	Geriatric Considerations
First-line Treatment			
Prazosin 1–6 mg PO QHS Titrate by 1 mg weekly until effect or side effects	Hyperarousal Nightmares Fragmented sleep	Orthostatic hypotension Dizziness Headache Slowed heart rate Priapism if taken with trazodone	May only need small dose. (1–3 mg) Titrate cautiously Consider changing BP medication to prazosin Monitor blood pressure or falls
Trazodone 12.5–100 mg PO QHS Titrate by 12.5–25 mg weekly		As for prazosin, and also sedation	Affects serotonin and histamine, and blocks alpha-adrenergic receptors Avoid aggressive dosing
SSRIs in Order of Choice			
Escitalopram 5–10 mg PO daily	Hyperarousal Reexperiencing Depressed mood Sleep disturbance	Sexual side effects Low sodium levels (rare) Usually well tolerated (fewer GI symptoms)	Most effective of the SSRIs Active enantiomer of citalopram; risk for QTC prolongation is lower at dosages of 5–10 mg daily than with equivalent citalopram dose of 20–40 mg Usually well tolerated
Sertraline 12.5–100 mg PO daily Titrate by 12.5 weekly		Diarrhea/nausea Sedation Sexual side effects Hyponatremia (rare)	More effective in women If GI symptoms do not remit, consider change in medication If sedated during the day, switch time of medication to QHS
Fluoxetine 5–40 mg PO daily Titrate by 5 mg every other week		Diarrhea/nausea Sleep interference Potentiates anticoagulants	Many drug-drug interactions caused by CYP450 enzyme system Long half-life Not usually beneficial in elderly patients with PTSD
SNRIs as Next Line of Treatment in Order of Choice			
Venlafaxine SA 37.5–150 mg PO daily Titrate by 37.5 mg every 7–14 d until effect	Depressed mood Avoidance No benefit for insomnia, hyperarousal	Can increase hyperarousal because of noradrenergic activation Hypertension Monitor liver function tests	Reasonable second-line treatment when SSRIs fail SA formula usually better tolerated Discontinuation syndrome: needs slow taper if ineffective

(continued on next page)

Table 3 (continued)			
Medication	**Target**	**Notable Side Effects**	**Geriatric Considerations**
Mirtazapine 7.5–30 mg QHS Titrate by 7.5 mg weekly	Hyperarousal Anxiety Depressed mood Sleep onset	Postural hypotension Dizziness Weight gain Low WBC (rare)	Good choice for cachectic, ill patients if able to tolerate risk of hypotension
Bupropion SR 100–300 mg PO daily Start 100 mg daily for 7 d then increase to 100 mg BID	Fatigue Depressed mood Avoidance	Can cause greater hyperarousal May interfere with sleep	May use with trazodone and or prazosin No sexual side effects, which may be an advantage to some patients Needs more study for PTSD

Abbreviations: BID, twice a day; BP, blood pressure; CYP450, cytochrome P 450; GI, gastrointestinal; PO, orally; QHS, at bedtime; SNRI, serotonin-norepinephrine reuptake inhibitor; WBC, white blood cell count.

interwoven with that individual's lifespan development, and occurring in the context of multiple vulnerabilities such as chronic illness and, potentially, lower cognitive resources. Our research on older veteran cancer survivors suggests a different approach to PTSD symptoms when they arise out of catastrophic medical events rather than war or sexual trauma. We find that younger old veterans (eg, ages 55–65 years) are more likely than older veterans to experience PTSD arising out of the diagnosis and treatment of cancer, and that those with concurrent combat PTSD symptoms are at increased risk for cancer-related PTSD.[25] Older veterans (eg, ages 75–85 years) seem less likely to develop PTSD arising out of medical experience, which may be because of resilience acquired through facing other health and emotional challenges in late life and different normative expectations related to age. These contextual factors influence how we approach the treatment of PTSD symptoms arising out of late-life medical experience.

Eliciting the Trauma Narrative

As with psychopharmacologic treatment, psychotherapy can be used to target specific core symptom groups of PTSD, particularly reexperiencing, numbing, and hyperarousal. Intrusive thoughts, memories, and nightmares are often a signal to patients, families, and health care providers that an individual is having PTSD symptoms that may benefit from treatment. A common starting place in PTSD treatment with psychotherapeutic approaches such as prolonged exposure and cognitive processing therapy (CPT) is a telling and retelling of the trauma story, which individuals often keep to themselves. The telling of the trauma narrative serves several purposes. First, because memory processing during traumatic events is likely to be interrupted, it allows the individual to reconstruct a set of possibly fragmented memories into a coherent narrative from which to build meaning. Second, it desensitizes the individual's psychological and psychophysiologic reaction to the memories as a conditioned stimulus that elicits a fear response, in hopes that it will allow the individual to put less energy into avoiding these and the difficulties that can come with the processes of avoidance. In addition, the process of sharing and allowing another person to bear witness decreases the profound isolation that often accompanies traumatic experience. In contrast with eliciting a combat trauma narrative, our experience is that there is less fragmentation of the memories than commonly occurs in combat and sexual trauma, but, at times, more embarrassment and isolation when the trauma is medical in nature.

Reducing Isolation

The therapeutic process of eliciting and sharing stressful or traumatic medical experiences seems to be useful in reducing intrusive memories and dreams, as well as the numbing symptoms of PTSD, in this case particularly the withdrawal from others. It is our experience that health care providers can become accustomed or sometimes desensitized to the felt responses of patients when performing procedures repeatedly, and that patients, grateful for their care, are reluctant to complain. Because of this, patients may feel alone. For example, some veterans have shared with us that treatments for urologic cancers involved moments of profound embarrassment, fear, or pain (eg, external beam radiation to the prostate, surveillance cystoscopies), all the more so if the veteran has experienced combat trauma as well as childhood sexual trauma.[26] In our clinic's cancer support group, a key intervention is for veterans to be able to share their experiences of treatments and surveillance procedures. In this case, companionship with others who are having similar experiences greatly reduces the burden of isolation, and it is hoped that this will extend to other relationships outside the group.

Managing Hyperarousal

In addition, individual or group psychotherapy can target management of PTSD symptoms of hyperarousal. For example, many cancer survivors find that surveillance imaging causes anxious arousal. Again, this can be worsened in the context of combat trauma. For example, a young veteran has shared that the process of being tied into a magnetic resonance imaging (MRI) cage and placed into an MRI scanner can elicit memories of target searching of tunnels in Vietnam. He finds it useful to ask other veterans to accompany him to scan appointments and to use a combination of benzodiazepine and antihistamine for symptom management. As another example, an older veteran has shared that surveillance scans remind him of hiding beneath floor boards in a French farm house behind German lines, as Germans searched the house. This veteran shared that he approaches scans by clenching his fists and imagining that the MRI sounds are combat sounds, which, for him, provides more mastery than focusing on the present moment. Therefore, in both individual and group psychotherapy it is useful to discuss upcoming medical appointments and procedures, to ensure that the patient is not avoiding these, and also to develop strategies for normalizing and managing any anxiety that may arise. It can also be useful to directly communicate these issues to other health care providers (with the patient's permission) or coach the patient in how to address these with providers (eg, radiology technicians).

Assuaging Worry

However, there are some differences in the psychotherapeutic treatment of PTSD symptoms arising from combat compared with catastrophic or threatening medical experience. The treatment of combat PTSD symptoms focuses on the experiences of combat and how these have, and are, affecting a person's life. The treatment of medical PTSD symptoms may be less retrospective, involving less narrative reconstruction, but more prospective, involving consideration of disease management going forward. For example, for many, a core psychological component is fear of recurrence.[27] In our research we have also found that cancer survivors have other significant worries, including worries about the burden of the disease on family (eg, "Who will take care of my family when I'm gone?"), about long-term side effects (eg, "When will I start to feel better?"), and existential issues (eg, "Am I making the most of the time

I have?").[27] Therefore psychotherapeutic treatment of cancer-related PTSD is likely to involve strategies for managing worries; for example, through mindfulness or acceptance techniques. As an example, in our cancer support group, if a veteran describes getting a worrisome test result, another veteran often reintroduces the idea of waiting to get the information and then making a plan 1 day at a time.

Working from strengths (resilience developed in facing past traumas) is an important component of treating PTSD in older veterans. Posttraumatic growth, the perception of positive benefits arising from trauma, may moderate the association between PTSD symptoms and mental health outcomes following cardiac surgery.[28]

EARLY INTERVENTION

PTSD arising out of medical trauma occurs in or near a health care context, providing the opportunity for early intervention by health care providers. Although early trauma debriefing is not advised,[29] more recent approaches have combined early intervention in the inpatient setting, supplemented with pharmacotherapy and psychotherapy in the weeks after discharge, a so-called stepped collaborative care approach, to reduce PTSD symptoms.[30] Although not tested in older adults, these and other early intervention strategies involving medication[31] or psychotherapy[32] in the acute stage of trauma hold much promise.[33] For example, falling is a common problem in older adults, and is associated with subsequent PTSD symptoms and fear of falling.[3] Screening and early intervention in the emergency or hospital setting could potentially prevent the excess morbidity caused by activity restriction, although these outcomes need to be studied.

Knowledge Needs for Health Care Improvement Going Forward

Although the literature has ample reports of PTSD related to catastrophic medical diagnosis and treatments, and considerable data on the treatment of sexual or combat PTSD, it lacks adequate theoretic and outcome studies of treatment of PTSD in older adults, and there is almost no information about special considerations in treating PTSD arising out of medical experience in older adults. Randomized treatment trials of psychopharmacologic and/or psychotherapeutic approaches to reducing PTSD symptoms are needed, but so are qualitative studies that systematically describe the varieties of PTSD symptoms that develop after accidents, injuries, and medical illness in older patients. In addition, further inquiry into the role of the health care team in recognition; early intervention; and, in situations in which medical events and care can traumatize patients, prevention is also badly needed.

REFERENCES

1. American Psychiatric Association. Diagnostic and statistical manual of mental disorders. 5th edition. Arlington (VA): American Psychiatric Association; 2013.
2. Boer KR, van Ruler O, Emmerik AA, et al. Factors associated with posttraumatic stress symptoms in a prospective cohort of patients after abdominal sepsis: a nomogram. Intensive Care Med 2008;34(4):664–74.
3. Man Cheung C, McKee KJ, Austin C, et al. Posttraumatic stress disorder in older people after a fall. Int J Geriatr Psychiatry 2009;24(9):955–64.
4. Whitehead DL, Perkins-Porras L, Strike PC, et al. Post-traumatic stress disorder in patients with cardiac disease: predicting vulnerability from emotional responses during admission for acute coronary syndromes. Heart 2006;92(9):1225–9.
5. Wilder Schaaf KP, Artman LK, Peberdy MA, et al. Anxiety, depression, and PTSD following cardiac arrest: a systematic review of the literature. Resuscitation 2013; 84:873–7.

6. French-Rosas L, Moye J, Naik A. Improving the recognition and treatment of cancer-related posttraumatic stress disorder. J Psychiatr Pract 2011;17:270–6.

7. Chan D, Fan MY, Unützer J. Long-term effectiveness of collaborative depression care in older primary care patients with and without PTSD symptoms. Int J Geriatr Psychiatry 2011;26(7):758–64.

8. Edmondson D, Rieckmann N, Shaffer JA, et al. Posttraumatic stress due to an acute coronary syndrome increases risk of 42-month major adverse cardiac events and all-cause mortality. J Psychiatr Res 2011;45(12):1621–6.

9. So SS, La Guardia JG. Matters of the heart: patients' adjustment to life following a cardiac crisis. Psychol Health 2011;26:83–100.

10. Bunzel B, Roethy W, Znoj H, et al. Psychological consequences of life-saving cardiac surgery in patients and partners: measurement of emotional stress by the impact of event scale. Stress Health 2008;24(5):351–63.

11. Van Zelst WH, De Beurs E, Beekman AT, et al. Well-being, physical functioning, and use of health services in the elderly with PTSD and subthreshold PTSD. Int J Geriatr Psychiatry 2006;21(2):180–8.

12. Ginzburg K. Comorbidity of PTSD and depression following myocardial infarction. J Affect Disord 2006;94(1–3):135–43.

13. Sajatovic M, Blow FC, Ignacio RV. Psychiatric comorbidity in older adults with bipolar disorder. Int J Geriatr Psychiatry 2006;21(6):582–7.

14. Qureshi SU, Kimbrell T, Pyne JM, et al. Greater prevalence and incidence of dementia in older veterans with posttraumatic stress disorder. J Am Geriatr Soc 2010;58(9):1627–33.

15. Kristine Yaffe K, Vittinghoff E, Lindquist K, et al. Posttraumatic stress disorder and risk of dementia among US veterans. Arch Gen Psychiatry 2010;67:608–13.

16. Pietrzak RH, Goldstein RB, Southwick SM, et al. Physical health conditions associated with posttraumatic stress disorder in U.S. older adults: results from wave 2 of the National Epidemiologic Survey on Alcohol and Related Conditions. J Am Geriatr Soc 2012;60(2):296–303.

17. Davison EH, Pless AP, Gugliucci MR, et al. Late-life emergence of early-life trauma. Res Aging 2006;28(1):84–114.

18. Thorp SR, Sones HM, Cook JM. Posttraumatic stress disorder among older adults. In: Sorocco KH, Lauderdale S, editors. Cognitive behavior therapy with older adults: innovations across care settings. New York: Springer Publishing Company; 2011. p. 189–218.

19. Cook JM, Thompson R, Coyne JC, et al. Algorithm versus cut-point derived PTSD in ex-prisoners of war. J Psychopathol Behav Assess 2003;25:267–71.

20. Cook JM, O'Donnell C. Assessment and psychological treatment of posttraumatic stress disorder in older adults. J Geriatr Psychiatry Neurol 2005;18(2): 61–71.

21. Salzman C. Clinical geriatric psychopharmacology. Philadelphia: Lippincott Williams & Wilkins; 2005.

22. Bajor LA, Ticlea AN, Osser DN. Psychopharmacology Algorithm Project at the Harvard South Shore program: an update on PTSD. Harv Rev Psychiatry 2011; 19:240–58.

23. Stahl SM. Stahl's essential psychopharmacology. 3rd edition. New York: Cambridge University Press; 2009.

24. Vik SA, Maxwell CJ, Hogan DB. Measurement, correlates, and health outcomes of medication adherence among seniors. Ann Pharmacother 2004;38:303–12.

25. Moye J, Gosian J, Snow R, et al, Vetcares Research Team. Emotional health following diagnosis and treatment of oral-digestive cancer in military veterans.

119th Annual Meeting of the American Psychological Association. Washington, DC, August 4–7, 2011.

26. Hilgeman M, Moye J, Archambault E, et al. In the veterans voice. Fed Pract 2012; 29(Suppl):51S–9S.

27. Moye J, Wachen JS, Mulligan EA, et al. Assessing multidimensional worry in cancer survivors. Psychooncology 2014;23:237–40.

28. Bluvstein I, Moravchick L, Sheps D, et al. Posttraumatic growth, posttraumatic stress symptoms and mental health among coronary heart disease survivors. J Clin Psychol Med Settings 2013;20(2):164–72.

29. Rose S, Bisson J, Churchill R, et al. Psychological debriefing for preventing post traumatic stress disorder (PTSD). Cochrane Database Syst Rev 2002;(2): CD000560.

30. Zatzick D, Roy-Byrne P, Russo J, et al. A randomized effectiveness trial of stepped collaborative care for acutely injured trauma survivors. Arch Gen Psychiatry 2004;61:498–506.

31. Schelling G, Roozendaal B, Krauseneck T, et al. Efficacy of hydrocortisone in preventing posttraumatic stress disorder following critical illness and major surgery. Ann N Y Acad Sci 2006;1071:46–53.

32. Rothbaum BO, Houry D, Heekin M, et al. A pilot study of an exposure-based intervention in the ED designed to prevent posttraumatic stress disorder. Am J Emerg Med 2008;26:326–30.

33. Kearns MC, Ressler KJ, Zatzick D, et al. Early interventions for PTSD: a review. Depress Anxiety 2012;29:833–42.

34. Kangas M, Henry JL, Bryant RA. Posttraumatic stress disorder following cancer: a conceptual and empirical review. Clin Psychol Rev 2002;22(4):499–524.

35. Chalfant AM, Bryant RA, Fulcher G. Posttraumatic stress disorder following diagnosis of multiple sclerosis. J Trauma Stress 2004;17(5):423–8.

36. O'Reilly SM, Grubb N, O'Carroll RE. Long-term emotional consequences of in-hospital cardiac arrest and myocardial infarction. Br J Clin Psychol 2004;43(1): 83–95.

37. Chung MC, Berger Z, Jones R, et al. Posttraumatic stress and co-morbidity following myocardial infarction among older patients: the role of coping. Aging Ment Health 2008;12(1):124–33.

38. Sembi S, Tarrier N, O'Neill P, et al. Does post-traumatic stress disorder occur after stroke: a preliminary study. Int J Geriatr Psychiatry 1998;13(5):315–22.

39. Dimartini A, Dew MA, Kormos R, et al. Posttraumatic stress disorder caused by hallucinations and delusions experienced in delirium. Psychosomatics 2007;48: 436–9.

40. Parmigiani G, Tarsitani L, De Santis V, et al. Attachment style and posttraumatic stress disorder after cardiac surgery. Eur Psychiatry 2013;28:S1.

41. Rothenhäusler HB, Stepan A. The effects of cardiac surgery on health-related quality of life, and emotional status outcomes: a follow-up study. Eur Psychiatry 2010;25:515.

42. Bruchas R, Kent C, Wilson H, et al. Anesthesia awareness: narrative review of psychological sequelae, treatment, and incidence. J Clin Psychol Med Settings 2011;18(3):257–67.

43. Mashour GA, Wang LY, Turner CR, et al. A retrospective study of intraoperative awareness with methodological implications. Anesth Analg 2009;108:521–6.

44. Davydow DS, Gifford JM, Desai SV, et al. Posttraumatic stress disorder in general intensive care unit survivors: a systematic review. Gen Hosp Psychiatry 2008;30: 421–34.

45. Carlson EB, Lauderdale S, Hawkins J, et al. Posttraumatic stress and aggression among veterans in long-term care. J Geriatr Psychiatry Neurol 2008;21(1):61–71.
46. Prins A, Ouimette P, Kimerling R, et al. The primary care PTSD screen (PC-PTSD): development and operating characteristics. Prim Care Psychiatr 2004;9(1):9–14.
47. Weathers FW, Litz BT, Herman DS, et al. The PTSD checklist (PCL-C): reliability, validity, and diagnostic utility. Annual Convention of the International Society for Traumatic Stress Studies. San Antonio (TX), November, 1993.
48. Weiss DS, Marmar CR. The impact of event scale - revised. In: Keane JW, editor. Assessing psychological trauma and PTSD. New York: Guilford; 1996. p. 399–411.

Sleep in Older Adults

Normative Changes, Sleep Disorders, and Treatment Options

Nalaka S. Gooneratne, MD, MSc[a,b,*], Michael V. Vitiello, PhD[c]

KEYWORDS

- Sleep apnea • Positive airway pressure • Insomnia
- Cognitive-behavioral therapy (CBT) • Sedative-hypnotic • Polysomnography
- Depression • Dementia

KEY POINTS

- Insomnia symptoms, although present in 20% to 40% of older adults, meet the clinical criteria for an insomnia diagnosis (ie, significant daytime symptoms and duration criteria) in only approximately 5%.
- Sleep apnea, as defined by an apnea-hypopnea index 15 or more events per hour, meeting Medicare treatment guidelines, is present in up to 20% of older adults, with a markedly increased prevalence in certain conditions, such as congestive heart failure or dementia (approximately 50%–70%).
- A high index of suspicion is particularly important for the diagnosis of sleep apnea.
- Effective treatment exists for most sleep disorders, such as positive airway pressure therapy for sleep apnea and cognitive-behavioral therapy/pharmacotherapy for insomnia.

INTRODUCTION

Overview of Sleep

With the advent of new technologies to measure sleep, such as nocturnal polysomnography and frequent biomarker sampling, the medical community has gained an increasing appreciation of the significant influence that sleep disorders have on a

Conflicts of Interest: There are no author conflicts of interest related to this article.
[a] Division of Geriatric Medicine, Department of Medicine, University of Pennsylvania, 3615 Chestnut Street, Philadelphia, PA 19104, USA; [b] Division of Sleep Medicine, Center for Sleep and Circadian Neurobiology, School of Medicine, University of Pennsylvania, Philadelphia, PA, USA; [c] Department of Psychiatry and Behavioral Sciences, School of Medicine, University of Washington, Seattle, WA, USA
* Corresponding author. Division of Geriatric Medicine, Center for Sleep and Circadian Neurobiology, School of Medicine, University of Pennsylvania, 3615 Chestnut Street, Philadelphia, PA 19104.
E-mail address: ngoonera@mail.med.upenn.edu

Clin Geriatr Med 30 (2014) 591–627
http://dx.doi.org/10.1016/j.cger.2014.04.007
0749-0690/14/$ – see front matter © 2014 Elsevier Inc. All rights reserved.

geriatric.theclinics.com

broad range of medical and psychiatric diseases. This appreciation is particularly relevant for older adults because of their increased prevalence of medical comorbidities and age-related changes in sleep. This review provides an overview of sleep and its assessment and then focuses on 2 of the most common sleep disorders that geriatricians are likely to encounter, insomnia and sleep apnea, along with a brief discussion of less prevalent sleep disorders that may also be relevant for the clinical care of older adults.

Sleep stages

Sleep is divided into non–rapid eye movement sleep (NREM) and rapid eye movement sleep (REM). NREM sleep is further subdivided into stage 1, 2, and 3 based on unique electroencephalographic (EEG) and electromyographic (EMG) criteria. Stage 3 is of particular importance because it is a period of slow-wave EEG activity that correlates with the release of growth hormone. Selective experimentally induced deprivation of stage 3 sleep has been associated with increased insulin resistance.[1] REM sleep is characterized by the presence of rapid eye movements as noted on electrooculography (EOG) and is commonly referred to as dream sleep. Most individuals have a progression through these stages, starting with stage 1 and ultimately reaching REM sleep. Most individuals will cycle through this progression 4 to 5 times per night. Thus, they may have 3 to 5 REM (dream) episodes but may not recall any of them. Nocturnal arousals, as defined by episodes lasting at least 3 seconds characterized by acute changes in EEG activity, are also common during sleep, with an average of 27 arousals per hour noted in healthy older adults without sleep complaints as compared with 10 to 20 arousals per hour in younger age groups.[2]

Before the modern era, nighttime sleep generally occurred in 2 major intervals, which were bridged by a period of wakefulness that may have lasted for up to an hour.[3] This natural sleep pattern has been described as split sleep, and these sleep episodes were frequently referred to historically as first sleep and second sleep.[3] This has been confirmed in clinical research studies whereby study participants were allowed to sleep for longer than the typical contemporary 7- to 8-hour sleep period.[4] This research suggests that the loss of the natural split sleep pattern is in part a result of the condensed (restricted) sleep window that characterizes the modern era with its access to 24-hour lighting caused by electricity.[3]

In addition to growth hormone release during slow wave sleep, there are several other key hormonal changes that occur during sleep, which highlight the importance of sleep in physiologic homeostasis. Cortisol tends to be highest shortly before awakening.[5] Melatonin levels generally have a significant increase at sleep onset, with a decrease in melatonin levels before awakening.[6] Several other hormones related to energy balance and metabolism also vary considerably as a function of the sleep-wake cycle.[7]

Changes with sleep with age

As with many other physiologic processes, there are several age-related changes in sleep that occur across the lifespan. Total sleep time decreases considerably from 10 to 14 hours a night in the pediatric age range to 6.5 to 8.5 hours a night as a young adult, then decreases at a slower rate into older ages, whereby average values may range from 5 to 7 hours a night.[8] When provided up to 16 hours a day to sleep, maximal sleep capacity, as indicated by total sleep time, also decreases with age, averaging 8.9 hours in younger subjects and 7.4 hours in older subjects.[9] Assuming good health is maintained, the trend for total sleep time to continue to decrease with age tends to cease after 60 years of age, at which point the total sleep time plateaus.[8]

Other elements of sleep architecture also change with age, including time spent awake at night. Although anecdotally we might expect sleep latency (the time it takes to fall asleep at the beginning of the night) to also increase with age, this is generally not the case.[8] Instead, we see prominent increases in wakefulness after sleep onset (WASO, or the tendency to be awake in the middle of the night or early morning).[8] The sleep stages also tend to change with advancing age such that there is less time spent in slow wave sleep (stage 3 sleep).[8] Understanding these physiologic reductions in sleep need with aging are important, especially in the context of helping older adults with insomnia complaints to adjust their normative expectations of sleep.

Subjective changes These objective sleep/wake changes give rise to the common perception that sleep becomes more difficult with age. Although there is indeed an objective deterioration of sleep as measured using polysomnography, there is a decoupling of subjective perception of sleep quality such that many older adults are less likely to complain of sleep problems than younger age groups. One population-based study in the United States found that the generic complaint of sleep disturbances, after controlling for covariates, such as general health and depression, was highest in the 18- to 24-year-old age group, peaked again in the 45- to 54-year-old age group (for women only) but otherwise declined with age, with the lowest rates of subjective sleep disturbance in older adults.[10] The American Insomnia Survey of 10,094 individuals also noted that self-reported insomnia rates were lower in older adults relative to young/middle-aged cohorts.[11]

What might explain this decoupling between objective and subjective sleep quality in older adults? The impact of general health status on sleep quality may be a key component. The odds of having sleep disturbance are markedly increased with poor health, suggesting that poor health is a major driver of subjective sleep problems and that older adults with good health are less likely to have subjective sleep problems.[10] Ohayon,[12] in his landmark review of epidemiologic research on insomnia, concluded that "healthy elderly sleep as well as younger subjects." In addition, there are profound changes in an older adult's perception of acceptable health status compared with younger adults. That is, although many older adults note objective sleep problems, they nonetheless perceive their sleep as acceptable.[13] This age-related adjustment of health expectations was noted by Brouwer and colleagues[14] in a study in which individuals across the age spectrum were asked if it would be acceptable to live with extreme pain or severe impairment. More than 10% of adults aged 75 years or older thought this was acceptable, as compared with 5% or less of adults younger than 65 years (**Fig. 1**).[14] Similar findings have been noted for sleep complaints,[15] with only weak correlations between objective and subjective sleep in older adults.[16] A final consideration is the phenomenon of sleep debt, that is, the difference between the actual amounts of sleep an individual obtains as compared with the amount of sleep that they need. Older adults may have fewer daytime symptoms from fragmented nocturnal sleep because increased flexibility caused by retirement allows time for daytime naps. The fragmented nocturnal sleep may then be perceived as less of a problem.

Cultural Perspectives on Sleep

The multiracial nature of the US population means that many older adults may be immigrants or have close ties to cultures outside of the United States. This idea has important ramifications within the context of sleep medicine in terms of reporting sleep

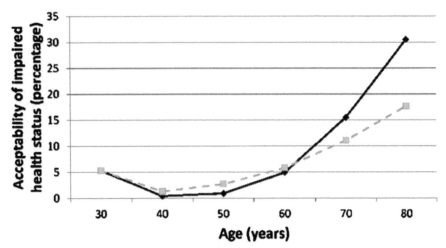

Fig. 1. Adjustment of perception of acceptable health with aging. Black line indicates acceptability of severe impairment with usual activities. Gray line indicates acceptability of extreme pain or discomfort. (*Data from* Brouwer WB, van Exel NJ, Stolk EA. Acceptability of less than perfect health states. Soc Sci Med 2005;60(2):237–46.)

complaints. Members of certain cultures and ethnic groups may be more or less likely to complain of poor sleep. For example, one study comparing the prevalence of insomnia symptoms in Europe, the United States, and Japan noted that the prevalence was 37.2%, 27.1%, and 6.6%, respectively.[17] Another study of older American women found that the prevalence of general insomnia symptoms also varied considerably by ethnic group, ranging from approximately 70% in African Americans and European Americans to 35% for English-speaking Caribbeans or Haitians; race/ethnicity explained up to 20% of the variance of insomnia symptom prevalence.[18] Although there may be biologic factors underlying this difference, the large range suggests that cultural aspects that influence symptom perception may lead patients with a specific cultural background to either report or not report sleep problems.

Coping with Sleep Problems

There is a general tendency to think that sleep disruption in older adults results in significant cognitive and functional consequences. Research examining psychomotor performance, however, suggests that older adults may actually be more tolerant of sleep deprivation than younger age groups. Stenuit and Kerkhofs[19] measured psychomotor vigilance task (PVT) performance after several nights of sleep restriction in women aged 20 to 30 years compared with older women aged 55 to 65 years. They noted that both groups had similar PVT performance initially but that the younger women had more prominent impairments with sleep deprivation than the older women by the third night of sleep restriction.[19] Another sleep restriction study that examined performance on a driving simulator noted similar findings.[20] One limitation of this literature is that the research study participants were restricted to a fixed number of hours each night, such as 5 hours. For a younger adult, this could result in 3 to 4 hours of sleep debt; but for an older adult, who has a lower average total sleep time, the sleep debt may only be 2 to 3 hours. Further research is, thus, needed to clarify whether older adults are actually more resistant to the effects of sleep loss than younger adults and whether this underlies the age differences in sleep complaints.

Measuring Sleep

The past several years have seen a significant growth in sleep assessment tools available for clinical practice. This growth has been largely the result of changes in the Medicare guidelines in 2008, which now allow for reimbursement of portable at-home sleep studies. A typical in-laboratory sleep study records EEG, EOG, EMG, chest/abdominal movement, airflow, and oxygen saturation, among other physiologic parameters. Portable sleep studies generally record a more limited set of physiologic signals, usually respiratory effort, airflow, heart rate, and oxygen saturation. This approach is generally more convenient for the patients but has several important limitations. First, because many portable sleep studies do not include EEG, devices have limited ability to determine if the patients are awake or asleep. Patients with insomnia can, thus, have artificially low sleep apnea indexes because the sleep apnea severity is calculated as the number of apnea or hypopnea events divided by the time spent asleep. Most portable devices start recording from the time the patients press the start button on the device and stop based on patient input in the morning. They generally count this entire period as asleep and use it to calculate the apnea-hypopnea index for sleep apnea severity. If the patients were awake during much of this time, however, they will not have any sleep apnea; this will artificially lower their apnea-hypopnea index. Second, patients must demonstrate adequate cognitive capacity or have a caregiver available throughout the night to assist with the device. Third, the patients must have the physical capacity in terms of upper arm strength and mobility, as well as adequate visual acuity, to use the device. Fourth, portable sleep studies are generally only useful for diagnosing or excluding sleep apnea and are of minimal benefit for assessing other sleep disorders.

Sleep Disorders

Sleep disorders can be broadly categorized into insomnias, hypersomnias, circadian rhythm disorders, sleep-breathing disorders, narcolepsy, parasomnias, and sleep movement disorders. A symptom-based diagnostic algorithm for sleep complaints is shown in **Fig. 2**. This review focuses on the 2 most common sleep disorders seen in older adults, insomnia and sleep-breathing disorders, and provides a much briefer discussion of several other sleep disorders, including restless legs syndrome (RLS), periodic limb movement disorder (PLMD), REM behavior disorder (RBD), and the hypersomnias.

INSOMNIA
Insomnia Disorder Description

Insomnia is broadly defined as dissatisfaction with sleep. Insomnia as a diagnostic entity appears in numerous nosologies, including the *International Classification of Sleep Disorders* (Second Edition) (*ICSD-2*), the *International Classification of Diseases, Tenth Revision* (ICD-10), and the *Diagnostic and Statistical Manual of Mental Disorders* (Fifth Edition) (*DSM-V*). Research examining the concordance across nosologies has found that the prevalence of insomnia varies considerably depending on the diagnostic nosology: insomnia prevalence is approximately 15% (across all adult age groups) for the *ICSD-2*, whereas it is only 4% when using the *ICD-10* criteria. This variation is largely caused by differences in the definition. All of the diagnostic approaches generally include symptoms of difficulty falling asleep at bedtime, waking up in the middle of the night with difficulty going back to sleep, or waking up too early in the morning again with difficulty returning to sleep. Of note, the perception that sleep is nonrestorative is no longer an accepted diagnostic symptom for the *DSM-V* definition

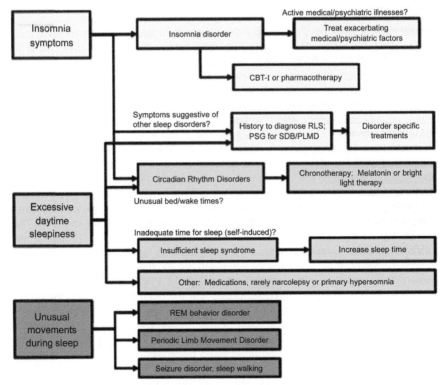

Fig. 2. Diagnostic and treatment approach for sleep disorders in older adults. CBT-I, cognitive-behavioral therapy for insomnia; PLMD, periodic limb movement disorder; PSG, polysomnogram; RLS, restless legs syndrome; SDB, sleep-disordered breathing. (*Adapted from* Bloom HG, Ahmed I, Alessi CA, et al. Evidence-based recommendations for the assessment and management of sleep disorders in older persons. J Am Geriatr Soc 2009;57(5):761–89.)

because it is thought to be too broad of a complaint, but it remains in the *ICD-10* criteria. In addition, the nosologies usually require a frequency of at least 3 nights per week. Duration requirements vary, with the *ICD-10* requiring a duration of 1 month, whereas the recently revised *DSM-V* proposed a symptom duration of at least 3 months.[21] The major reason for the lower prevalence using the *ICD-10* is the requirement that the diagnosis of insomnia be associated with a "preoccupation with the sleeplessness and excessive concern over its consequences at night and during the day and the unsatisfactory quantity and/or quality of sleep either causes marked distress or interferes with ordinary activities in daily living."[22]

Because the *ICD-10* is used commonly in clinical practice and will be mandatory for billing and reimbursement after October 2014, the authors focus on this diagnostic schema. The *ICD-10* defines insomnia as either organic insomnia (G47.–) or nonorganic insomnia (F51.–), with the former referring to insomnia that occurs as a result of another medical condition/substance and the latter being independent of any known substance or medical condition. Within these categories, the most common *ICD-10* diagnoses are shown in **Table 1**. It is important to highlight that the recently released *DSM-V* has collapsed several of these categories in favor of a more streamlined, symptom-based diagnostic approach.[21] In particular, the *DSM-V* emphasizes the concept of a more general insomnia disorder as opposed to requiring delineation

Table 1
Commonly used *ICD-10* codes for insomnia

Diagnosis	*ICD-10* Code	Notes
Primary insomnia	F51.01	Does not occur in the context of any other sleep disorder and is not linked to any other substance or medical condition; often has a childhood or young-adult onset
Adjustment insomnia	F51.02	Transient insomnia, usually less than 1 mo in duration
Paradoxic insomnia	F51.03	Also known as sleep-state misperception
Psychophysiological insomnia	F51.04	Chronic, conditioned insomnia
Insomnia caused by other mental disorder	F51.05	Often related to anxiety or depression
Other insomnia not caused by a substance or known physiologic condition	F51.09	Generally refers to persistent insomnia
Insomnia, unspecified	G47.00	Suspected insomnia caused by other conditions but not definitive (not otherwise specified)
Insomnia caused by medical condition	G47.01	Attempt to code the medical condition if possible
Alcohol-related insomnia	F10.182	Although alcohol has an initial soporific effect, it can increase the rate of arousals as blood alcohol levels decrease, usually after about 2 h
Drug-related insomnia	Multiple	Different *ICD-10* codes depending on drug

of causal attribution.[23] This emphasis was motivated in part because of low rates of diagnostic concordance when attempting to classify insomnia into specific categories, such as primary insomnia or insomnia caused by other conditions.[24]

Scope of the Problem

The overall prevalence of insomnia depends in large part on how it is defined. Most epidemiologic studies note a prevalence of 20% to 40% for nocturnal insomnia complaints, such as difficulty initiating/maintaining sleep or unrefreshing sleep.[11,12] When including daytime symptoms of fatigue or impaired concentration, the prevalence decreases to 10% to 20%.[12] When diagnostic nosologies such as the *ICD-10* are applied, the prevalence is approximately 2% to 5%.[11] A key factor driving the prevalence of insomnia is the rate of incidence, remission, and relapse. A study of 6899 older adults observed an incidence rate for insomnia symptoms of approximately 5% per year.[25] Of note, this study extrapolated the 1-year incidence rate based on a 3-year follow-up interview. Research using a 1-year follow-up noted a yearly incidence rate of 7.97% in older adults.[26] Recent research (across all age groups) that used a more frequent sampling period of 1 and 3 months extrapolated an annual incidence rate of 31.2%.[27] Approximately half of the patients with insomnia symptoms will have remission during the follow-up period, with higher remission rates in older adult men relative to women.[26,28] Another study across all age groups that used the *DSM-V* criteria for insomnia noted that although the majority (78.6%) would have remission of their insomnia, a sizable minority of 21.4% developed chronic insomnia[27] and that insomnia is more likely to be persistent in older adults.[29]

A commonly used framework for understanding the cause and persistence of insomnia is the 3-factor model (**Fig. 3**), as conceptualized by Spielman and colleagues,[30] which identifies predisposing, precipitating, and perpetuating factors. These factors combine to increase the likelihood of insomnia above the insomnia threshold as shown in **Fig. 3**. Examples of predisposing factors are demographic characteristics. Women older than 45 years are approximately 1.7 times more likely to have insomnia than men.[12] Individuals who are divorced, separated, or widowed are also more likely to have insomnia.[12] Lower levels of education attainment or income have also been linked to higher rates of insomnia in some but not all studies.[12,31] Smoking and alcohol use are also associated with higher rates of insomnia.[12] Reduced physical activity has been linked to higher rates of insomnia in older adults.[32] Recent research suggests that there may also be genetic variants in clock genes that can influence sleep parameters in older adults.[33]

Precipitating factors are generally acute life stressors or medical conditions that may disrupt sleep. Individuals with respiratory symptoms, physical disability, and fair to poor perceived health are at an increased risk of developing insomnia.[25] Medications may be one of the factors that contribute to developing insomnia in patients with multiple medical conditions. Examples of such medications include beta-blockers, glucocorticoids, nonsteroidal antiinflammatory drugs, decongestants, and antiandrogen agents. Depression was also a major risk factor for incident and persistent insomnia.[25,28] Another study of 1814 patients (mean age of 57 years) that completed a 2-year follow-up assessment noted that the presence of major or subthreshold depression, even when adjusting for baseline insomnia, was associated with an odds ratio of 1.7 and 2.4, respectively, for developing insomnia.[34] High rates of insomnia also occur in patients with generalized anxiety disorder, with up to 90% reporting insomnia symptoms.[35] These studies, along with several others, highlight the profound role that mental illness and medical conditions have on disrupting sleep.

Perpetuating factors result in a persistence of insomnia. Once patients with predisposing and precipitating factors have developed acute insomnia, this acute insomnia will not necessarily develop into chronic insomnia unless these perpetuating factors

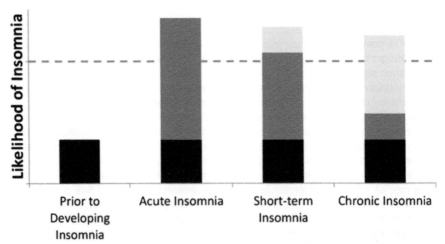

Fig. 3. The 3-factor model of insomnia.[30] The dashed line indicates the threshold above which clinically significant insomnia occurs. (*Data from* Spielman AJ, Caruso LS, Glovinsky PB. A behavioral perspective on insomnia treatment. Psychiatr Clin North Am 1987;10(4): 541–53.)

are present. These perpetuating factors are often behavioral or cognitive changes that arise as a result of the acute insomnia. For example, patients may develop increased presleep anxiety because of a fear of having another night of insomnia (conditioning), or they may use television or radio to help relax or occupy their time while waiting to fall asleep. Others may start to have variable bed times to deal with insomnia or take daytime naps; although naps are generally not recommended for patients with insomnia, for older adults without insomnia complaints, it is important to note that naps have minimal side effects[36] and improve vigilance/performance after naps.[37] Addressing these perpetuating factors is an important goal of nonpharmacologic insomnia treatment as discussed further later.

Insomnia Clinical Correlations

As noted earlier, although the prevalence of objective changes in sleep with aging is high, many older adults do not complain of significant sleep problems. An important clinical ramification of this is that when older adults do complain of insomnia symptoms that are causing significant daytime distress and meet criteria for insomnia disorder, the clinician should take this complaint seriously. Clinicians should, therefore, ask themselves what is prompting their patients to bring forward this complaint and seek assistance when most older adults do not have significant distress from age-related objective changes in sleep.

If left untreated, insomnia can be associated with significant morbidity across a variety of domains. The strongest level of evidence entails mental illness. Older adults with insomnia symptoms have a 23% increase in their risk of developing depression symptoms.[38] Several other studies have also suggested an increased risk for depression in older adults, especially those with persistent insomnia.[39] Cole and Dendukuri,[40] in a meta-analysis of risk factors for depression in the elderly, noted that sleep disturbance had an odds ratio of 2.6, higher than that of prior depression or disability. Furthermore, data from the Improving Mood-Promoting Access to Collaborative Treatment (IMPACT) study of older adults with depression noted that 44% of patients with persistent insomnia continued to have depression at the 6-month time point as compared with only 16% of those without insomnia.[41] Depression recurrence is also markedly increased in older adults with persistent sleep disturbances, with one study noting an adjusted hazard ratio of 16.1.[42] Of particular concern, insomnia may be a risk factor for suicide; however, research studies have had conflicting findings in this area, with some showing an increased risk of suicide,[43] whereas others found no increased risk in older adults.[44]

Understanding the relationship between insomnia and mental disorders is complex because they may have a bidirectional relationship.[45] That is, patients with insomnia at baseline have higher risks of developing anxiety or depression, and those with anxiety or depression at baseline have a higher risk of developing insomnia.[45] The insomnia symptoms most strongly associated with subsequent depression risk are poor sleep quality and difficulty initiating and maintaining sleep, whereas early morning awakening is not a risk factor.[38] When exploring the pathway through which insomnia may increase the risk of depression, Sadler and colleagues[46] postulated that hopelessness and maladaptive sleep beliefs were important components. Another aspect of the insomnia-depression association is that insomnia is one of the defining symptoms of depression; thus, many of the assessment tools used to identify depression include questions related to insomnia. Furthermore, patients with depression will often endorse insomnia questionnaires that inquire about daytime fatigue or impairment. Research studies that have removed sleep-related items from depression scales, however, continue to show evidence of bidirectional links between insomnia and depression.[42]

In addition to mental health effects, older adults with insomnia may be at a higher risk for other medical conditions and impaired quality of life. A meta-analysis of insomnia symptoms and their association with heart disease, after adjusting for age and other cardiovascular risk factors, found that risk ratios for heart disease from insomnia symptoms ranged from 1.47 to 3.90.[47] Recent research suggests that the insomnia symptoms may lead to increased rates of cancer, such as prostate cancer.[48]

Although many older adults with insomnia complain of next-day neurocognitive difficulties, research examining daytime neuropsychological or cognitive performance has shown no evidence of significant impairments.[49,50] Long-term insomnia complaints may be associated with an increased risk of cognitive impairment,[51] although this has not been noted in all studies.[52] Recent research using wrist-activity monitors to identify objective sleep fragmentation (as opposed to self-reported insomnia symptoms) observed that study participants in the highest 10% bracket of sleep fragmentation had a 50% increased risk of developing Alzheimer disease compared with those in the lowest 10% bracket over an average 3.3 years of follow-up.[53]

Older adults with insomnia also tend to have lower quality-of-life assessment scores.[54] However, this is generally not associated with significant impairments in self-reported overall functional status.[55] When considering objective measures, such as wrist-activity monitoring of activity, next-day increases in physical activity with reduced sleep fragmentation were noted, although the overall effects were small. (The researchers estimated that a 10% increase in sleep efficiency, which is a large change, was associated with only a 3.2% increase in next day activity.)[56] Furthermore, the data linking insomnia to mortality are equivocal, with several studies finding no strong link between insomnia symptoms and mortality.[57–59]

Diagnostic Standards and Dilemmas for Insomnia Disorder

As noted earlier, one of the main challenges in evaluating insomnia symptoms is determining if they are related to another condition, such as chronic pain or depression, or whether they exist as a primary diagnosis. To minimize this diagnostic dilemma, the revised *DSM-V* guidelines use the term insomnia disorder to avoid the need to differentiate insomnia into specific subtypes such as those in the *ICD-10*.[23] There remain, however, several important alternative diagnoses that should be considered. These diagnoses include the presence of other sleep disorders, such as sleep apnea or PLMD (see **Fig. 2**).[60,61] Older adults with both insomnia and sleep apnea may be at a particularly increased risk of functional impairments.[62]

Another important category of sleep disorders that is often associated with insomnia complaints is that of circadian rhythm disorders. Although there is a general perspective that older adults experience advanced sleep phase (ie, a tendency to go to sleep early and wake early), this may not necessarily be the case for older adults with insomnia symptoms. Youngstedt and colleagues[63] noted that older adults with insomnia complaints were more likely to have a delayed circadian phase than an advanced circadian phase and had significant circadian dispersion and malsynchronization compared with young, healthy subjects. Understanding this distinction is important because circadian rhythm disorders generally respond well to chronotherapy using appropriately timed melatonin and light therapy, thus, avoiding the need for sedative hypnotics; detailed clinical practice guidelines for circadian rhythm disorders are available.[64]

Insomnia Disorder Clinical Findings

It is important to emphasize that the diagnosis of insomnia is a clinical one that relies on history obtained from the patients. In cases when patients are not reliable informants, history may be obtained from a proxy caregiver. Although specific cut points for sleep onset latency (18–30 minutes) or WASO (21–60 minutes) have been proposed, they generally should not be used as diagnostic clinical criteria but instead as general treatment goals.[65,66] As is the case with many other mental health disorders, there is no objective test used to diagnose insomnia; there are not any specific physical examination findings.

Examination
When evaluating patients with insomnia symptoms, a variety of tests may be useful to rule out possible alternate diagnoses. Possible laboratory tests that may be worthwhile depending on the presence of other associated clinical symptoms are listed in **Table 2**.

Recommended rating scales
There are several insomnia rating scales available that are useful both for cataloging baseline symptoms and for gauging treatment progress. A list of the more useful evaluation scales appears in the adjacent box enclosure (**Box 1**).

Diagnostic modalities
In addition to the medical and sleep history, the essential diagnostic tool for evaluating insomnia is the sleep diary. This diary is a nightly record of sleep patterns and disruptions as well as attempted treatments and sleep hygiene factors. Recently, a consensus sleep diary has been proposed that incorporates the recommended measures of bedtime, sleep onset latency, nocturnal awakenings, WASO, terminal wakefulness, total sleep time, final awakening time, sleep efficiency, sleep medication use, daytime napping and caffeine and alcohol consumption.[67,68] The recommended duration of a sleep diary is ideally 2 weeks in order to provide a comprehensive perspective on a patient's sleep patterns because of day-to-day variability. Several organizations, such as the National Sleep Foundation, provide free on-line sleep diaries that can

Table 2
Additional tests and evaluations for an insomnia work-up

Condition	Test	Other Clinical Symptoms
Autoimmune disorders	Erythrocyte sedimentation rate, antinuclear antibody, rheumatoid factor	Joint pain, rash, neurologic symptoms
Fibromyalgia	Presence of at least 11 tender points on examination and history of at least 3 mo of chronic pain	Muscle/joint pain, fatigue
Hyperthyroid	Thyroid stimulating hormone	Palpitations, weight loss, diaphoresis
Parkinson disease	Clinical examination	Tremor, gait instability
Circadian rhythm disorders/insufficient sleep opportunity	Wrist-activity monitor (actigraphy) + sleep diary	Abnormal sleep times
PLMD/RLS	Polysomnography	Leg or arm movement that interferes with sleep onset (RLS) or that wakes patients from sleep (PLMD)
Sleep apnea	Polysomnography	Snoring, witnessed apneas, nocturnal choking/gasping

Box 1
Recommended insomnia and sleep apnea evaluation scales

Condition	Scale	Notes
Insomnia	Sleep diary	Consensus sleep diary available[67]
	Insomnia Severity Index	Values of 15 or more consistent with clinical insomnia
	Pittsburgh Sleep Quality Index	A global measure of sleep quality that is not limited to insomnia symptoms
	Multidimensional Fatigue Inventory or Fatigue Severity Scale	Used to measure daytime fatigue, which is more common in patients with insomnia than daytime sleepiness
Sleep Apnea	STOP-BANG	Primarily used for preoperative screening for sleep apnea risk
	Epworth Sleepiness Scale	Measure of daytime sleepiness; older adults may not respond to all items, thus under-reporting sleepiness severity

be printed and provided to patients (http://www.sleepfoundation.org/sleep-diary/SleepDiaryv6.pdf).

In addition to the sleep diary, other diagnostic modalities that can be used include wrist activity monitoring (actigraphy, a portable accelerometer worn on the wrist).[60,68,69] Although not required for the diagnosis of insomnia, actigraphy can be used to monitor the response to therapy and to screen for circadian rhythm disorders.[69] Of note, the specific parameters used for the actigraphy analysis can significantly influence the findings, especially in older adults with intellectual impairments,[70] research attempting to define actigraphy cut points for insomnia diagnosis has been unsuccessful[66]; there can be considerable discordance between self-report sleep diaries and actigraphy in older adults.[71]

Polysomnography is not required for the evaluation of insomnia and is generally not recommended for routine cases.[72] However, polysomnography is warranted in certain specific situations, such as when sleep apnea or another sleep disorder is suspected (ie, a history of limb movements, loud snoring/witness apneas/nocturnal choking, or violent behavior is obtained) or the insomnia persists despite treatment.[72] Other sleep diagnostic tests, such as the Multiple Sleep Latency Test (MSLT) and Maintenance of Wakefulness Test, are not indicated for the evaluation or management of patients with insomnia unless there are potential occupational safety risks from daytime fatigue.[73]

Insomnia Disorder Management

Effective management of insomnia requires setting realistic goals with patients. Insomnia can be a chronic condition that can be significantly improved, but patients may not ultimately achieve an idealized version of sleep characterized by rapid sleep onset and sustained sleep with the complete absence of next-day fatigue. Furthermore, patients may relapse or have occasional nights of poor sleep. Helping patients to adjust their expectations to fit the natural course of sleep changes with aging can, thus, be crucial in coping with insomnia.

Interventions/Current Evidence Base

A summary of the recommendations for the treatment of insomnia is presented in **Table 3**. Treatment can be divided into nonpharmacologic and pharmacologic approaches. Because of the risks of side effects with pharmacologic approaches

Table 3
Evidence-based recommendations for insomnia evaluation and treatment

Recommendation	Quality of Evidence	Strength of Evidence
A sleep diary is an essential component of an insomnia evaluation.[68]	III	A
Polysomnography is not routinely required for insomnia evaluation.[72]	III	A
CBT-I is effective in older adults and is associated with minimal side effects.[60,80,181]	I	A
Nonbenzodiazepine hypnotics can improve insomnia symptoms but can be associated with side effects, such as tolerance and neurocognitive effects.[60,80]	I	A
Melatonin-receptor agonists can improve sleep-onset insomnia symptoms.[60]	I	A
Concurrent CBT-I and pharmacotherapy can be efficacious.[79]	II	A
Doxepin at subantidepressant doses can be efficacious.[137]	I	B
Antihistamines, anticonvulsants, and antipsychotics are not recommended for the chronic treatment of insomnia.[60]	II	B
Exercise and bright-light therapy may improve sleep.[80]	II	B

Quality of evidence: I: at least one properly designed randomized controlled trial; II: substantial evidence from nonrandomized trials; III: expert committee reports.
Strength of evidence: A: good evidence to support the use of a recommendation; B: moderate evidence; C: poor evidence (clinicians may elect to not follow the recommendation).
Abbreviation: CBT-I, cognitive-behavioral therapy for insomnia.
Adapted from Bloom HG, Ahmed I, Alessi CA, et al. Evidence-based recommendations for the assessment and management of sleep disorders in older persons. J Am Geriatr Soc 2009;57(5):761–89.

and the potential for benefits to attenuate over time in comparison to nonpharmacologic approaches, older adults should first receive nonpharmacologic treatment for several months before implementing pharmacologic therapy.[74,75]

Nonpharmacologic
Although there are numerous nonpharmacologic options, the most commonly used include sleep hygiene and cognitive-behavioral therapy for insomnia (CBT-I). Several of these behavior-based approaches have been found to be effective even in patients with cognitive impairment.[76]

Sleep hygiene Sleep hygiene consists of several interventions that promote a stable sleep pattern and nondisruptive environment. It is not realistic to expect patients to engage in all of these sleep hygiene practices at once; one approach is to prioritize the most relevant sleep hygiene practices based on the patients' sleep history and implement changes in a serial fashion. Sleep hygiene practices grouped by general category are summarized in the adjacent boxed text (**Box 2**). Although sleep hygiene is often used as an initial step in the treatment of insomnia, the evidence suggesting that it is effective as monotherapy is limited.[77]

CBT-I When sleep hygiene alone is not effective, CBT-I is a reasonable next step. CBT-I generally consists of 6 to 10 sessions with a trained therapist that address counterproductive behaviors and cognitive beliefs that perpetuate insomnia. It has been found to be effective in older adults across multiple studies.[78–80] The core elements of CBT-I are shown in the boxed text (**Box 3**).

Box 2
Sleep hygiene interventions for insomnia

Create a stable sleep pattern

1. Maintain a regular sleep/wake schedule. It is most important to keep the same rise time every day; bedtime is also important but it can be more difficult for patients to have a consistent bedtime because of day-to-day demands of work/family. Advise patients to set their alarm to get up at the same time each morning, regardless of how much sleep they got during the night, in order to maintain a consistent sleep/wake schedule.

2. Do not attempt to make up for lost sleep on weekends or holidays.

3. Refrain from taking naps during the day.

Encourage a nondisruptive sleep environment

4. Keep the bedroom dark and at a temperature that is comfortable.

5. Block out noises that can disturb sleep with sponge earplugs or white noise made by fans, air conditioners, or a white noise machine.

Reduce presleep tension

6. Do not watch the alarm clock and worry about the time or lost sleep.

7. Develop a sleep ritual. Do the same things each evening before retiring for the night to give your body cues (signals) that it is time to settle down.

8. Plan evening activities that promote relaxation. Before going to the bedroom, make a list of things to deal with tomorrow and make a list of things to do before bedtime.

Dietary/Lifestyle modifications

9. Maintain a healthy diet. Going to bed hungry or eating a large meal before bedtime can worsen sleep. If hungry at bedtime, eat a light snack. Eat meals at approximately the same time each day, every day.

10. Avoid or minimize the use of caffeine. It is recommended not to drink coffee, tea, or soda after lunch. If patients continue to have difficulty falling asleep, avoid drinking caffeinated beverages after breakfast.

11. Avoid alcohol. Although it may temporarily lead to somnolence, for most people it causes awakenings as well as poor sleep later in the night. Alcohol can make snoring and sleep apnea worse.

12. Maintain a regular exercise schedule. Walking is an excellent form of exercise. The best time is in the late morning or midday (9 AM–1 PM). For some people, strenuous exercise before bedtime can be too stimulating and may prevent them from falling asleep. Light stretching can be done on rainy days.

Although most research has been conducted with up to 8 sessions of CBT-I, a growing body of evidence suggests that brief behavioral treatment or computerized/Internet-based CBT-I can also be effective.[81,82] CBT-I can also be useful to taper patients off of pharmacologic therapy, but maximal effects may take months to manifest.[83] In addition to primary insomnia, it may also be effective in patients with insomnia and chronic pain,[84] comorbid psychiatric conditions,[85] or cancer.[86]

Other nonpharmacologic interventions for insomnia with limited evidence include bright-light therapy and exercise.[80]

Pharmacologic

Pharmacotherapy options are benzodiazepine sedatives, nonbenzodiazepine sedatives, melatonin-receptor agonists, and antidepressants. A listing of the available Food and Drug Administration (FDA)–approved compounds, their doses, and key

---

Box 3
Components of CBT-I

Address maladaptive sleep cognitions: Patients with insomnia may have exaggerated perceptions of how sleep impacts their life and how much sleep they need. These inaccurate beliefs lead to increased worry and unrealistic expectations.

Sleep hygiene: Promote regular sleep-wake patterns and minimize nocturnal disruptions.

Stimulus control therapy: Chronic insomnia can condition negative associations between the bed and sleep such that patients find it difficult to relax in bed; stimulus control therapy seeks to reassociate the bed with sleep. Patient instructions include avoiding sleep-incompatible behaviors (do not use the bed as a place to read, watch television, or catch up on work), go to bed only when sleepy, and get out of the bed if unable to sleep and patients are beginning to feel anxious.

Sleep restriction therapy: Many patients with insomnia attempt to overcompensate for their insomnia by spending excessive time in bed. Although seeming counterintuitive, sleep restriction induces partial sleep deprivation, which in turn increases the likelihood that patients with insomnia will actually sleep when they are in bed. The ultimate goal is to break the cycle of insomnia.

Relaxation techniques: These techniques include progressive muscle relaxation or guided imagery.

---

side effects are listed in **Table 4**. Both benzodiazepine and nonbenzodiazepine sedatives bind to γ-aminobutyric acid A (GABA-A) receptors, with the main difference being that the nonbenzodiazepine sedatives are more selective for the alpha-1 subclass, which is closely linked to sedation, but has minimal anxiolytic effects. Risks associated with sedative-hypnotics include next-day sedation, confusion, falls, and worsening depression/suicide; these have been identified by the FDA as warnings/precautions on many of the package inserts. Although concerns have been raised regarding long-term mortality risks from sedatives, a recently published 12-year observational study that controlled for multiple covariates found no evidence of an increased mortality rate in sedative users and noted that comorbid psychiatric disorders may be important confounders.[87] One option to reduce the risk of habituation or dependence is to adopt an intermittent dosing approach in which patients are given 10 to 15 tablets for the entire month and are allowed to use them on an as-needed basis.[88] Other FDA-approved agents include melatonin-receptor agonists, such as ramelteon, which have shown efficacy in older adults for sleep initiation insomnia.[89] It is not associated with dependence or nocturnal gait instability, but there are conflicting results regarding next-day morning sedation.[90–92]

Diverse categories of antidepressants have also been used for insomnia, including tricyclic antidepressants (TCA), phenylpiperazine compounds (trazodone), and noradrenergic/specific-serotonergic antidepressants (ie, mirtazapine); of these, only low-dose doxepin, a TCA, is FDA approved for insomnia. Uncertainty exists regarding the role of other agents because of the paucity of randomized clinical trials in older adults.[93] In general, antidepressants may be appropriate for insomnia symptoms when there is a diagnosis of depression or subthreshold depression.[93] Clinically, trazodone is widely used for insomnia in older adults at doses ranging from 50 to 100 mg at bedtime, which are less than the dose range for antidepressant effects, despite limited clinical trial evidence.[94] It is also important to note that serotonin-specific reuptake inhibitors tend to worsen insomnia initially.[95] However, antidepressants with strong 5-hydroxytryptamine-2 (5-HT2) antagonism, such as mirtazapine or trazodone, may improve insomnia and may be preferred to agents that create sedative effects

Table 4
FDA-approved medications for insomnia

Category	Generic (Trade) Name	Indication	Geriatric Dose (mg)	Half-life in Older Adults (h)	Comments
Benzodiazepines[a]	Temazepam (Restoril)	Short-term treatment of insomnia (7-10 d)	7.5-15.0	10-15	Long half-life carries increased risk of next-day drowsiness; adverse event (AE) 5%-10%: drowsiness, headache,* nervousness*,b
	Triazolam (Halcion)	Short-term treatment of insomnia (7-10 d)	0.0625-0.25	1.7-5.0	Risk of confusion, daytime anxiety, anterograde amnesia; AE 10%-15%: drowsiness, headache AE 5%-9%: dizziness, nervousness, light-headedness, ataxia, nausea[b]
Nonbenzodiazepine	Eszopiclone (Lunesta)[e]	No short-term limitation for use	1-2	9	AE 10%-15%: headache,* unpleasant taste; AE 5%-9%: dry mouth, dyspepsia, pain, dizziness[b]
	Zolpidem (Ambien, Edluar [sublingual form])[e]	Short-term treatment of insomnia (up to 35 d)	5	2.9-3.7	AE 5%-10%: drowsiness, dizziness[b,c]
	Zolpidem ER (Ambien CR)[e]	Sleep initiation or sleep maintenance insomnia	6.25	1.9-7.3	AE 10%-20%: headache; AE 5%-9%: dizziness, nausea, somnolence, nasopharyngitis[b,c]
	Zolpidem, low-dose sublingual (Intermezzo)[e]	Sleep maintenance with at least 4 h of sleep time remaining	1.75	1.4-3.6	AE 2%-5%: headache[b,c]
	Zolpidem, oral spray (Zolpimist)[e]	Sleep initiation insomnia	5	2.5-3.1	AE 5%-10%: drowsiness, dizziness[b,c]
	Zaleplon (Sonata)	Short-term treatment of insomnia (up to 30 d)	5	1	AE 30%-40%: headache*; AE 5%-9%: dizziness,* nausea,* asthenia,* abdominal pain,* somnolence*,b

| Melatonin receptor agonist | Ramelteon (Rozerem) | Sleep imitation insomnia; no short-term limitation for use | 8 | 1.0–2.6 | AE 2%–5%: dizziness, somnolence, nausea, insomnia exacerbation[b], not a schedule IV drug |
| Antidepressants | Doxepin | Sleep maintenance insomnia | 3 | 15.3 | CI: untreated narrow angle glaucoma or severe urinary retention; AE 5%–10%: somnolence; AE 2%–4%: upper respiratory tract infection, nausea/emesis[d] |

Data obtained from FDA prescribing information (package inserts) and literature review. Available at: www.accessdata.fda.gov.

All side effects listed were more common in the medication group than in the placebo group except when indicated with an asterisk. (In this case, the occurrence of the side effect was similar in both the medication and placebo arm.)

[a] The following benzodiazepines are FDA approved for insomnia but should generally be avoided in older adults because of their long half-life: flurazepam (Dalmane), quazepam (Doral), and estazolam (ProSom).

[b] Warnings/precautions: anaphylaxis, abnormal thinking/behavior changes, complex behaviors while not fully awake (sleep-driving, and so forth), central nervous system depressant effects, worsening of depression, or suicidal thinking.

[c] Concomitant administration with antidepressants, such as sertraline or fluoxetine, may increase zolpidem levels.

[d] Warnings/precautions: abnormal thinking/behavior changes, complex behaviors while not fully awake (sleep-driving and so forth), central nervous system depressant effects, worsening of depression, or suicidal thinking.

[e] Can cause next-day impairment of driving and other activities that require alertness, based on the FDA warnings. Available at: http://www.fda.gov/drugs/drugsafety/ucm334033.htm; http://www.fda.gov/Drugs/DrugSafety/ucm397260.htm.

Data from Bloom HG, Ahmed I, Alessi CA, et al. Evidence-based recommendations for the assessment and management of sleep disorders in older persons. J Am Geriatr Soc 2009;57(5):761–89; and Krystal AD, Durrence HH, Scharf M, et al. Efficacy and safety of doxepin 1 mg and 3 mg in a 12-week sleep laboratory and outpatient trial of elderly subjects with chronic primary insomnia. Sleep 2010;33(11):1553–61.

solely through histamine receptor antagonism.[95,96] Mirtazapine should not be used solely for the treatment of insomnia in the absence of depression symptoms because of conflicting evidence.[97] Additional treatment options for insomnia in the setting of depression are available.[98] Potential future pharmacologic agents for insomnia include orexin-receptor agonists, although as of 2013, none have yet been FDA approved. For postmenopausal women, hormone replacement therapy can lead to objective reductions in nocturnal awakenings and WASO.[99]

A variety of alternative medicine options are also available for insomnia, but there is a relative paucity of data demonstrating clinical efficacy in older adults.[100] One exception is melatonin whereby one randomized clinical trial demonstrated efficacy in older adults for up to 6 months.[101] An important aspect of this particular trial is that the melatonin was taken approximately 2 hours before bedtime, suggesting that circadian phase aspects of the melatonin may have led to observed treatment benefits rather than any direct effect on sleep per se.

Combination Therapies

CBT-I can be used in combination with pharmacotherapy. In one study, concomitant CBT-I and temazepam use was associated with reduced temazepam use as compared with the temazepam-only arm.[102] Another study examining combination therapy noted that the maximal sleep benefits were noticed in the combination-therapy arm but that patients who completed combination therapy with CBT-I/pharmacotherapy and then tapered off of pharmacotherapy had improved remission rates compared with those that did not taper off of their pharmacotherapy and continued to use pharmacotherapy.[103]

Treating Insomnia Disorder in Institutionalized Settings and in Cognitively Impaired Patients

Institutionalized older adult patients are at risk of insomnia because of the increased prevalence of comorbid conditions and medications that can exacerbate insomnia as well as environmental factors related to the institutional setting. Loud noises, for example, may be common in institutional environments. However, it is important to note that most of these loud noises are not from patient vocalizations but instead from equipment and staff and that incontinence care frequently contributes to nocturnal awakenings.[104] Interventions to reduce noise and other environmental disruptions, however, have had minimal benefit and should be combined with behavioral approaches.[105] Low levels of light exposure and other circadian rhythm cues in institutional settings can also increase the risk of developing circadian rhythm disorders that may manifest with symptoms suggestive of insomnia. Bright-light therapy and melatonin have been effective in institutionalized settings for these circadian rhythm sleep disorders.[106] CBT-I can also be effective: an open-label noncontrolled study of CBT-I in nursing home elderly patients demonstrated improvements in sleep quality.[107] For community-dwelling older adults with cognitive impairment, a combined intervention that included sleep hygiene, increased activity (walking), and light therapy has been effective in reducing time awake at night and nighttime awakenings.[108] Pharmacotherapy, as discussed previously, can also be used for treating insomnia in institutionalized patients or cognitively impaired elders. However, there are little data regarding safety and efficacy in these populations; thus nonpharmacologic approaches should be implemented first.[76,109]

Caregiver Perspectives for Insomnia Disorder

Caregivers for patients with dementia frequently identify nocturnal awakenings by their care recipient to be significantly distressing behaviors that adversely impact the caregivers' quality of life.[110] These nocturnal sleep difficulties can be a contributing factor in the decision by a caregiver to institutionalize an older adult with cognitive impairment.[111] Caregivers' personal appraisal of their situation, which is influenced by their coping skills, affect, and social support network, can be important mediators of the disruption the caregivers perceive from their care recipients' nocturnal awakenings.[110] CBT-I and exercise therapy for caregivers have both been shown to improve caregiver sleep quality.[112,113]

SLEEP APNEA
Sleep Apnea Description

Sleep apnea, also referred to as sleep-disordered breathing and sleep-related breathing disorder, is a condition in which respiration ceases or decreases considerably in volume during sleep. It can be caused by either obstruction of the upper airway (obstructive sleep apnea), dysfunction in the neurologic drive to breath (central sleep apnea, Cheyne-Stokes breathing, medications/substance abuse), or their combination (mixed apnea, complex apnea, or obesity-hypoventilation syndrome). It is generally defined by the apnea-hypopnea index (AHI), which measures the number of apneas (cessation of breathing for at least 10 seconds) or hypopneas (reduction in the volume of breathing with associated evidence of neurologic arousal or oxyhemoglobin desaturations).

The range for sleep apnea severity as a function of the AHI is as follows: 5 or more up to less than 15 events per hour is mild; 15 or more up to less than 30 events per hour is moderate; and 30 or more events per hour is severe.[114] Medicare guidelines will cover sleep apnea treatment if the AHI is 15 or more events per hour or if it is 5 or more events per hour and patients have clinical symptoms of excessive daytime sleepiness, impaired cognition, mood disorders, or insomnia or a medical history of hypertension, ischemic heart disease, or stroke. Most clinical research studies on sleep apnea use an AHI of 15 or more events per hour (independent of symptoms) as the diagnostic criteria; the authors use these criteria for the remainder of this review unless otherwise mentioned.

Scope of the Problem

The prevalence of sleep apnea can vary considerably based on the AHI criteria. Using a criterion of 5 or more events per hour, the prevalence of sleep apnea in older adults is approximately 50%, whereas at a criterion of 15 or more, it is approximately 20%.[115] There is a clear age-related increase in the prevalence of sleep apnea because only 10% of young adults have an AHI of 15 or more events per hour.[115] The prevalence of sleep apnea is increased in certain medical conditions, most notably congestive heart failure, atrial fibrillation, cerebrovascular disease, and dementia, whereby prevalence rates for an AHI of 15 or more events per hour may be as high as 50% to 80%.[116,117] The likelihood of having central sleep apnea variants is also increased in cardiovascular/cerebrovascular disease.[116] Sleep apnea is more common in Asians than in Caucasians by an odds ratio of 2.1, whereas most data suggest that African Americans have prevalence rates similar to Caucasians.[118] Thus, the overall prevalence of sleep apnea is high, and it should be considered in the evaluation of a broad range of conditions as discussed further later. Unfortunately, it is frequently underdiagnosed; for example, sleep apnea was diagnosed and treated in only 2% of patients with incident congestive heart failure, though, as previously noted, the prevalence of sleep apnea in congestive heart failure is greater than 50%.[119]

Sleep Apnea Clinical Correlations

Risk factors for sleep apnea are shown in **Table 5**. In general, these risk factors are similar to those for younger age groups with 4 important differences. First, although obesity is a risk factor for older adults, it decreases in importance with age. This point is likely because older adults have increased upper airway collapsibility relative

Table 5 Risk factors for sleep apnea in older adults		
	Mehra et al,[118] Osteoporotic Fractures in Men Sleep Study[a]	Ancoli-Israel et al,[182] San Diego Cohort Community-Dwelling Elderly[b]
Risk Factor	**Odds Ratio (Confidence Intervals)**	**Coefficient (P Value)**
Female sex (reference: male)	Study sample all male	0.52 (.025)
Snoring (>3–5 times/wk)	2.01 (1.62–2.49)	—
Age (per 5-year increase)	1.24 (1.15–1.34)	—
Race (reference: Caucasian)		
African American	1.05 (0.66–1.68)	—
Asian	2.14 (1.33–3.45)	—
Hispanic	1.38 (0.85–2.22)	—
Obesity (BMI>30 kg/m^2)	2.54 (2.09–3.09)	0.087 (.0067)
Neck circumference (per 5-cm increase)	2.19 (1.88–2.56)	—
Waist circumference (per 5-cm increase)	1.24 (1.19–1.29)	—
Socioeconomic status (range 1–10, per 1 unit increase)	0.95 (0.90–1.00)	—
Current smoker	0.63 (0.31–1.29)	—
Alcohol (per category increase)	1.01 (0.96–1.06)	—
Daytime sleepiness		
Excessive daytime somnolence (Epworth Sleepiness Scale score >10)	1.41 (1.11–1.79)	—
Napping	—	0.41 (.033)
Falling asleep reading	—	0.102 (.046)
Comorbid factors (self-report)		
Hypertension	1.26 (1.06–1.50)	—
Diabetes mellitus	1.18 (0.93–1.51)	—
Cardiovascular disease	1.24 (1.03–1.48)	—
Heart failure	1.81 (1.31–2.51)	—
Stroke	0.86 (0.55–1.37)	—

Abbreviation: BMI, body mass index.

[a] Logistic regression with Respiratory Disturbance Index greater than 15 events per hour as outcome. Study sample male. Data presented as adjusted odds ratios (confidence intervals), with models adjusted for race, age, and body mass index except for race, age, and obesity indices—these were adjusted for other subject characteristics. Alcohol categories were drinks per week defined as follows: 0, less than 1, 1 to 2, 3 to 5, 6 to 13, and 14 or more.

[b] Logistic regression coefficients of dependent variables with Respiratory Disturbance Index of 10 or more events per hour as outcome.

to younger subjects, and other factors that are not obesity dependent play a role in older adults.[120,121] Second, although sleep apnea is more common in young/middle-aged males than females, for older adults there is an equal prevalence by sex, which starts after the menopause transition.[122] Third, the diagnosis can be challenging because the clinical presentation can be subtle. For example, although snoring is a common complaint of partners of younger patients, many older adults will not endorse snoring as a symptom because they may not have a bed partner.[122] In these cases, it can be helpful to inquire if snoring was noted during vacations or when napping. Fourth, the edentulous state markedly increases the risk of having sleep apnea.[123]

As noted previously, sleep apnea is common in patients with cognitive impairment, with one study of institutionalized patients with severe Alzheimer's Disease observing a 63% prevalence.[117] One mechanism for this is found in Alzheimer disease–related reductions in cholinergic neural activity: cholinergic neurons play a role in upper airway motor regulation and thalamic cholinergic neurons influence respiratory drive; thus, damage to these neurons could increase the risk of sleep apnea in patients with Alzheimer disease.[124]

In addition to cognitive impairment potentially increasing the likelihood of sleep apnea, it is also highly likely that sleep apnea increases the likelihood of cognitive impairment. A prospective observational study of 298 women, with average age of 82.3 years and without dementia at baseline followed for an average of 4.4 years, found that those with sleep apnea had a striking 85% increase in the risk of developing mild cognitive impairment or dementia, even after adjusting for other risk factors.[125] Furthermore, oxyhemoglobin desaturation, likely related to sleep apnea, was a particularly important risk factor, suggesting that oxyhemoglobin desaturation is a major mediator of neurocognitive consequences of sleep apnea.[125] Further evidence of the importance of sleep apnea in the context of cognitive impairment can be seen in positive airway pressure (PAP) treatment studies, which have shown preliminary signs of improvements in cognitive status in older adults with dementia[126] and in neuroimaging in nondemented/nonelderly patients,[127] although many cognitive deficits persist and may be irreversible.[128]

Several research studies, mostly in younger cohorts, have shown links between sleep apnea and depression,[129,130] with one longitudinal study demonstrating an odds ratio of 2.6 for developing depression in those with moderate or worse sleep apnea over 4-year follow-up intervals.[131] Others have noted that it is not the severity of sleep apnea as measured by the apnea-hypopnea index but rather daytime sleepiness and fatigue that are correlated with depression.[132–135] Sex and type of depression symptoms may also be a factor: somatic depression complaints were associated with sleep apnea severity in males only.[136] Treatment with armodafinil, a stimulant, improved sleepiness but not depression.[137] CBT for depression in patients after myocardial infarction was less beneficial in those who had sleep apnea as compared with those without sleep apnea.[138] Attempts to use continuous PAP (CPAP) for treating sleep apnea in depression have had more success, with improvements in depression scores that may be attributed to reduced daytime sleepiness.[139] The relationship between anxiety and sleep apnea is unclear, with some research finding no significant associations.[140,141]

Sleep apnea has also been found to increase the risk of other medical conditions. A longitudinal study of incident congestive heart failure found that each 10-unit increase in the AHI led to a 13% increase in heart failure in men but not in women.[142] Similarly, the rate of incident stroke was increased in subjects with sleep apnea, especially at higher AHI levels.[143,144] In one cross-sectional research study, sleep apnea was associated with the frailty syndrome only in older women but not in older men.[145] Sleep apnea has also been linked to higher rates of postoperative delirium.[146] Because of the potential increased perioperative risk, screening for sleep apnea by history and examination is recommended before surgery, with subsequent polysomnography evaluation and treatment if necessary.[147]

Despite the increased rate of various comorbidities as a result of sleep apnea, research examining sleep apnea and long-term mortality in older adults has had conflicting findings. One of the largest epidemiologic studies, the Sleep Heart Health Study, noted an increased mortality rate for an AHI of 15 or more events per hour only in study participants younger than 70 years.[148] Several factors may explain this observation. First, it is possible that a higher AHI criteria, such as greater than 30 or greater than 40 events per hour, may be appropriate for older adults as several studies have noted an increased mortality rate in older adults in the setting of sleep apnea at these higher cut points.[149,150] Second, the inclusion of symptoms, such as sleepiness, as part of the diagnostic criteria for sleep apnea can markedly impact findings; one study noted that in the absence of symptoms of daytime sleepiness, older adults with only an elevated AHI (AHI$\geq$20 events per hour) had mortality rates similar to those with an AHI of less than 20 events per hour (approximately 35% at 10 years) as compared with older adults with an AHI of 20 or more events per hour and daytime sleepiness complaints who had a markedly increased mortality rate of approximately 70% at 10 years.[151] Third, because older adults are at an increased risk for mortality from their other comorbid medical conditions, these competing risks for mortality may reduce the impact of sleep apnea alone.[152,153] Of note, a recent long-term quasi-experimental study that compared older adults with treated sleep apnea with older adults with untreated sleep apnea noted markedly improved survival rates with treatment.[154]

Diagnostic Standards and Dilemmas for Sleep Apnea

The diagnosis of sleep apnea requires overnight polysomnography. As noted earlier, this previously necessitated an overnight stay at an in-laboratory sleep facility; however, the Centers for Medicare and Medicaid Services has approved portable at-home testing. Although portable testing provides several additional options for convenient diagnosis of suspected sleep apnea that can shorten the time to diagnosis and treatment, it is important to keep in mind the potential limitations discussed earlier (see "Measuring Sleep").[155–157] Before ordering the polysomnography, a face-to-face physician evaluation is necessary, during which key history and physical elements must be documented as outlined in "Sleep Apnea Clinical Findings" later; this is necessary to help ensure that Medicare will cover the costs of treatment. A repeat polysomnography may be warranted if there is a high clinical suspicion of sleep apnea in the setting of a negative initial polysomnography; AHI variability of greater than 10 events per hour has been noted in 18% of older adults.[158]

There are 3 major diagnoses within the category of sleep apnea. Obstructive sleep apnea is characterized primarily by obstructive apneas (complete cessation of breathing with evidence of upper thoracic respiratory effort as detected by abdominal or respiratory belts), whereas in central sleep apnea, there are at least 5 central apneas per hour (cessation of breathing with absence of thoracic effort indicating a central origin). Obesity-hypoventilation syndrome (also known as sleep-related hypoventilation) is diagnosed by increasing hypercapnia with sleep.[159] There are also often daytime hypercapnia (Paco$_2$>45 mm Hg) and obstructive/central apneas.[159] It is generally thought to be caused by extreme obesity and/or neuromuscular/chest wall disorders, such as kyphosis.

Sleep Apnea Clinical Findings

The clinical history physical examination for sleep apnea is similar for older adults as it is for younger age groups. Important questions include asking about the presence of snoring, witnessed apneas, or nocturnal choking, gasping, or dyspnea. While many clinicians assess daytime sleepiness, less well recognized is the fact that insomnia is another possible diagnostic symptom of sleep apnea.[159] The physical examination should include a cardiopulmonary examination and a head and neck examination to confirm that there is no asymmetry suggestive of a mass effect that may compress the upper airway, such as a goiter or enlarged lymph nodes. For suspected central sleep apnea, the examination should also include a detailed cardiovascular, neurologic, and chest/back musculoskeletal assessment as these may all contribute to the pathophysiology. Unique aspects relevant to older adults are presented in **Table 6**. At present, there is no laboratory or radiographic tests that can be used to diagnose sleep apnea.

Sleep Apnea Management

Interventions/Current evidence base

The treatment of sleep apnea in older adults has several similarities to younger age groups. The major difference relates to the recommendation for weight loss, which is commonly suggested for younger patients for whom obesity is often a major risk factor. For older adults, the link between obesity and sleep apnea is attenuated; thus, it is possible to have older adults at an ideal body weight who have sleep apnea. Furthermore, weight loss, even for overweight or obese older adults, can be problematic. Epidemiologic studies have noted that overweight older adults have improved survival rates relative to those at ideal body weight, with one study noting that every unit increase in the body mass index (BMI) led to an improvement in the survival rate of 1% to 8% even after controlling for other mortality risk factors.[160] This finding is possibly caused by increased amounts of physiologic reserve (in terms of nutrition and so forth) in overweight older adults that allow them to tolerate acute illnesses. Clinical trials are few; however, observational studies have noted improvement in sleep apnea in morbidly obese older adults after bariatric surgery.[161,162] For these reasons, weight loss, although often a universal recommendation for younger patients with sleep apnea, may not be appropriate for many older adults, and a more nuanced approach may be warranted.

Sleep apnea is frequently worse when supine because it is easier for the tongue to prolapse backwards and obstruct the upper airway in this position. Therefore, advising patients to sleep on their side (lateral position) can be effective in some cases. The potential utility of this positional therapy can be determined from polysomnography, which records sleep apnea severity in the supine and lateral positions. There are several commercial aids/pillows that can be used by patients to help keep them in the lateral position while sleeping.

If positional therapy is not an option, PAP (also referred to as CPAP) therapy is an appropriate initial treatment recommendation. It is highly effective when used consistently. One concern is that some older adults have upper extremity weakness that may interfere with their ability to apply a PAP mask.[153] Cognitive impairment can also limit adherence; however, the active assistance of a caregiver can help promote adherence even in those cases.[163] The appropriate PAP settings are usually determined either during an in-laboratory titration sleep study or by an auto-titrating PAP device used at home for several weeks. Although auto-titrating PAP can be more convenient, it is not recommended for patients with severe congestive heart failure, chronic

Table 6
Unique aspects of sleep apnea assessment for older adults

Component	Domain	Specific Considerations
History	Daytime symptoms of sleepiness	Existing scales, such as the Epworth Sleepiness Scale, may under-report sleepiness in older adults because they may not drive and so forth. Naps (clarify if voluntary or involuntary): Increased voluntary napping may be a result of a loss of daily social rhythms and not necessarily a sign of excessive sleepiness.
	Sleep signs and symptoms when visiting family/friends	For witnessed apneas, nocturnal choking or gasping, and loud snoring, symptom reporting may under-report symptoms in older adults who do not have a bed partner.
	Additional history suggestive of sleep apnea	These include nocturia, gait problems/falls at night, and/or nocturnal confusion.
	Caregiver aspects	Consider the concerns of patients' caregivers. If patients are caregivers themselves, how feasible is diagnosis/treatment of their own sleep disorder in the context of their caregiving duties.
	Medical history	Atrial fibrillation, congestive heart failure, cerebrovascular events, dementia, hypertension, and chronic obstructive pulmonary disease/asthma may influence pretest probability of sleep apnea or complicate management.
	Differential considerations	Rule out atypical depression in an older adult, polypharmacy effects, and hypothyroidism.
Physical examination	Dentition	Edentulous/missing teeth: Sleep apnea may worsen when dentures are removed.
	Upper extremity function	Arthritis may also affect hand dexterity. Can they apply portable polysomnography sensors? Perform the drop arm test to screen for rotator cuff tears and assess shoulder range of motion. Can they apply a CPAP mask themselves?
	Cognitive status	Screen for memory impairment (eg, animal naming test: patients should be able to name at least 14 different animals in 1 min).

obstructive pulmonary disease, or central sleep apnea.[164] If patients are initially treated with an auto-titrating PAP device, but do not experience symptom improvement, an in-laboratory titration study may be warranted.

The major limiting factor for PAP use is patient adherence: approximately 40% to 50% are adherent.[165] However, overall adherence to PAP in older patients is similar to younger ones.[166] PAP therapy can also be used effectively in patients with dementia with good adherence rates, especially if there is caregiver involvement and patients do not have significant levels of depression.[163] Several strategies can be used to help patients adjust to PAP, including trying alternate masks, heated humidification, and short daytime trials to encourage habituation. The cost can also be an important consideration. The first year of PAP therapy obtained through a durable medical equipment provider can generate charges of up to $1500 to $2000; although the majority is covered by Medicare, for older adults with copays, the cost for the first year could still be several hundred dollars. For Medicare to cover PAP therapy in the long-term, patients must use the PAP device for a minimum of 4 hours a night on 70% of the nights for at least a 1-month period during the initial 3-month trial. In addition, they must have a face-to-face encounter with the ordering physician to document the clinical response at some time between months 1 and 3.

Despite these challenges, when used consistently, PAP therapy can be highly effective in older adults, even in those with diminished cognitive capacity. A landmark quasi-experimental study that examined the outcomes of PAP treatment in older adults found that those who were adherent had overall survival rates that were similar to patients without sleep apnea.[154] The mortality rate over a median follow-up of 5.75 years was 16.7% for older adults without significant sleep apnea, 16.1% for those with sleep apnea that were adherent to PAP, and 34.1% for those with severe untreated sleep apnea.[154]

Oral appliances are another option for the treatment of sleep apnea that is primarily obstructive. These devices resemble a mouth guard and move the lower mandible forward by several centimeters. Because the tongue is attached to the lower mandible, this has the effect of opening up the retroglossal space, a key site of obstructive apneas and hypopneas. Although PAP is more effective than an oral appliance in decreasing the AHI into the normal range, the improved adherence to oral appliances leads to similarities in average outcomes across all study participants.[167] For patients with more severe sleep apnea, though, PAP may be more effective.[168] Approximately 25% will experience temporomandibular joint discomfort in the initial treatment period; fortunately, these were not associated with any permanent consequences.[169] Oral appliances are custom manufactured, usually by dentists, and adjusted over a several month period. They are generally not covered by Medicare, and costs can range from $1000 to $2500.

Additional treatment options for sleep apnea include oral pressure therapy, which creates a negative pressure in the mouth to move the tongue forward,[170] and upper-airway surgery.[114] A limited amount of data is available on oral pressure therapy, and further research is necessary to examine long-term outcomes. Upper airway surgery, such as an uvulopalatopharyngoplasty, involves the removal of the tonsils, adenoids, posterior tongue, and soft palate. One retrospective review found no evidence of increased risk with advancing age.[171] However, dysphagia remains a concern, with up to 29% of patients having dysphagia at 1-year postoperatively.[172] Supplemental oxygen via nasal cannula (not using PAP) has also been attempted. Because sleep apnea often has an obstructive component, delivering supplemental oxygen alone may not be able to overcome the upper airway obstruction without the presence of PAP. Research comparing supplemental oxygen with PAP suggests that the former does not reduce the AHI significantly but that supplemental oxygen resulted in similar average nocturnal oxygen levels to PAP.[173] Adherence rates were similar to PAP.[173] In addition, it may be particularly effective for patients with predominantly central sleep apnea and congestive heart failure; for these patients, research has shown improvements in exercise capacity and cardiac function with PAP therapy.[174] There are at present no pharmacologic options for the treatment of sleep apnea.

OTHER SLEEP DISORDERS

In addition to insomnia and sleep apnea, other sleep disorders that may be encountered in clinical practice include RLS, PLMD, RBD, and the hypersomnias. A detailed discussion of these conditions and others from a geriatric medicine perspective was recently conducted by Bloom and colleagues[60]; they are briefly reviewed here.

RLS is characterized by significant discomfort in the legs or arms before sleep that progressively worsens over the course of the evening and is relieved by movement. It is distinct from arthritis pain or fibromyalgia in that pain is usually not present in RLS. It is present in approximately 10% of older adults and is twice as common in women as men.[175,176] Furthermore, it is frequently underdiagnosed, with one study noting that only 9 of 103 patients who met the criteria for RLS had been diagnosed.[175] Low ferritin levels and end-stage renal disease may exacerbate RLS.[175] RLS may be even more common in dementia; up to 24% of community-dwelling patients with dementia were noted to have RLS in one study.[177] Of particular interest, the presence of RLS was associated with higher rates of nocturnal agitation in these community-dwelling older adults with dementia.[177] The diagnosis of RLS is based on clinical history. Treatment involves the use of dopaminergic agents, such as levodopa.

Patients with PLMD experience frequent (at least 5 per hour) sleep-related extremity movements that are often associated with increased brain activity (arousals). Many patients are not aware of the limb movements, but their bed partner may endorse them. Patients may instead complain of frequent nocturnal awakenings and daytime sleepiness. The prevalence of PLMD is 4% to 11% in older adults and is more common in patients undergoing dialysis.[176] PLMD often accompanies RLS. The diagnosis of PLMD requires a polysomnography with EEG and EMG signal acquisition (usually an in-laboratory polysomnogram). Treatment frequently involves dopaminergic agents or sedative-hypnotics.

REM behavior disorder is a condition in which patients act out their dreams because of a loss of physiologic atonia during sleep. Although rare, it can be associated with significant injuries because patients are not aware of their surroundings. In addition, there is a growing body of evidence to suggest that many patients with REM behavior disorder will subsequently develop Parkinson disease or other neurologic disorders.[178] Diagnosis requires an in-laboratory polysomnography with EEG and EMG to confirm the presence of increased muscle tone during REM sleep. Treatment centers around patient education and safety, with pharmacotherapy consisting of clonazepam or melatonin.[179]

Insufficient sleep syndrome refers to habitual patient behaviors that result in self-induced sleep deprivation. This syndrome may either be work/social related or caused by frequent use of electronics or television watching at night. A sleep diary is often useful to elucidate this history. Effective treatment can be difficult as patients are often resistant to changing their lifestyle. It is imperative in these cases to avoid using stimulant therapy.

Other rare sleep disorders in older adults include narcolepsy and primary hypersomnia. Narcolepsy is characterized by the presence of significant hypersomnia as well as nocturnal sleep fragmentation. It may or may not be associated with sleep attacks (cataplexy). Generally, it is diagnosed in younger adults, but delayed diagnosis with initial identification in older adults can occur. Accurate diagnosis requires an MSLT, which will show rapid entry into REM sleep (sleep-onset REM). If patients demonstrate rapid sleep onset without sleep-onset REM episodes, and they do not have any other underlying sleep disorder or medication cause, then a diagnosis of primary hypersomnia may be appropriate. Treatment of either condition relies on the use of stimulant therapy with dopamine modulators, such as modafinil, or methamphetamines.

SUMMARY

Significant changes occur in sleep with advancing age. There is a reduction in total sleep time from an average of 8.9 hours per day in young adults to 7.4 hours per day in older adults.[9] In addition, there is an increase in nocturnal awake time, with older adults spending 30 to 60 minutes awake after sleep onset.[8] Despite these objective changes and a 20% to 30% prevalence of insomnia complaints, the actual prevalence of clinically significant insomnia disorder is approximately 5%[12]; older adults may be less likely than younger adults to meet *ICD-10* diagnostic criteria for insomnia disorder because it requires an associated daytime impairment.[11] The evaluation of insomnia relies on a self-report history and a sleep diary. Treatment options include the following: sleep hygiene, which, although helpful, has not been found to be effective when used as monotherapy[180]; CBT-I, which requires multiple sessions but can have sustained benefit; and pharmacotherapy with sedative-hypnotics, melatonin agonists, or antidepressants. Patients with chronic insomnia that is resistant to treatment may benefit from a polysomnography to screen for other sleep disorders.[72] If left untreated, insomnia can increase the risk of depression.

Sleep apnea is characterized by recurrent cessation or reduction in breathing, with 5 to 15 events per hour considered mild, 15 to 30 considered moderate, and 30 or more considered severe. It may lead to hypoxia or increased nocturnal sleep arousal and fragmentation. It is present in approximately 20% of older adults, a high prevalence that is double that of young adults.[115] It can increase the risk of cardiovascular disease and may nearly double the risk of cognitive impairment over a 5-year period.[125] Diagnosis requires a polysomnography; however, Medicare guidelines now allow for coverage of portable at-home polysomnography in most cases. Effective diagnosis requires a high clinical suspicion because many older adults lack a bed partner to report classic symptoms, such as snoring or witnessed apneas. Furthermore, an increased BMI is not as prominent a risk factor in older adults as in younger ones.[115] Treatment with PAP can be highly effective if patients are adherent. Other treatment options include an oral appliance, weight loss or surgery in select patients, and oral pressure therapy. Treatment with PAP has been shown to improve survival in older adults.[154]

Finally, in addition to insomnia and sleep apnea, geriatricians need to be aware of the possibility of the presence of other sleep disorders in their patients, such as RLS, PLMD, REM behavior disorder, and the hypersomnias, for all of which efficacious treatments are available.

REFERENCES

1. Herzog N, Jauch-Chara K, Hyzy F, et al. Selective slow wave sleep but not rapid eye movement sleep suppression impairs morning glucose tolerance in healthy men. Psychoneuroendocrinology 2013;38(10):2075–82.
2. Boselli M, Parrino L, Smerieri A, et al. Effect of age on EEG arousals in normal sleep. Sleep 1998;21(4):351–7.
3. Ekirch AR. Sleep we have lost: pre-industrial slumber in the British Isles. Am Hist Rev 2001;106(2):343–86.
4. Wehr TA. In short photoperiods, human sleep is biphasic. J Sleep Res 1992; 1(2):103–7.

5. Elder GJ, Wetherell MA, Barclay NL, et al. The cortisol awakening response - applications and implications for sleep medicine. Sleep Med Rev 2013;18(3): 195–204.

6. Gooneratne NS, Edwards AY, Zhou C, et al. Melatonin pharmacokinetics following two different oral surge-sustained release doses in older adults. J Pineal Res 2012;52(4):437–45.

7. Kalsbeek A, Fliers E. Daily regulation of hormone profiles. Handb Exp Pharmacol 2013;(217):185–226.

8. Ohayon MM, Carskadon MA, Guilleminault C, et al. Meta-analysis of quantitative sleep parameters from childhood to old age in healthy individuals: developing normative sleep values across the human lifespan. Sleep 2004;27(7):1255–73.

9. Klerman EB, Dijk DJ. Age-related reduction in the maximal capacity for sleep– implications for insomnia. Curr Biol 2008;18(15):1118–23.

10. Grandner MA, Martin JL, Patel NP, et al. Age and sleep disturbances among American men and women: data from the U.S. Behavioral Risk Factor Surveillance System. Sleep 2012;35(3):395–406.

11. Roth T, Coulouvrat C, Hajak G, et al. Prevalence and perceived health associated with insomnia based on DSM-IV-TR; International statistical classification of diseases and related health problems, tenth revision; and research diagnostic criteria/international classification of sleep disorders, second edition criteria: results from the America Insomnia Survey. Biol Psychiatry 2011;69(6): 592–600.

12. Ohayon MM. Epidemiology of insomnia: what we know and what we still need to learn. Sleep Med Rev 2002;6(2):97–111.

13. Malakouti SK, Foroughan M, Nojomi M, et al. Sleep patterns, sleep disturbances and sleepiness in retired Iranian elders. Int J Geriatr Psychiatry 2009;24(11): 1201–8.

14. Brouwer WB, van Exel NJ, Stolk EA. Acceptability of less than perfect health states. Soc Sci Med 2005;60(2):237–46.

15. Vitiello MV, Larsen LH, Moe KE. Age-related sleep change: gender and estrogen effects on the subjective-objective sleep quality relationships of healthy, noncomplaining older men and women. J Psychosom Res 2004;56(5):503–10.

16. Gooneratne NS, Bellamy SL, Pack F, et al. Case-control study of subjective and objective differences in sleep patterns in older adults with insomnia symptoms. J Sleep Res 2011;20(3):434–44.

17. Leger D, Poursain B. An international survey of insomnia: under-recognition and under-treatment of a polysymptomatic condition. Curr Med Res Opin 2005; 21(11):1785–92.

18. Jean-Louis G, Magai C, Casimir GJ, et al. Insomnia symptoms in a multiethnic sample of American women. J Womens Health (Larchmt) 2008;17(1):15–25.

19. Stenuit P, Kerkhofs M. Age modulates the effects of sleep restriction in women. Sleep 2005;28(10):1283–8.

20. Filtness AJ, Reyner LA, Horne JA. Driver sleepiness-comparisons between young and older men during a monotonous afternoon simulated drive. Biol Psychol 2012;89(3):580–3.

21. American Psychiatric Association. Diagnostic and statistical manual of mental disorders, 5th edition: DSM-V. Washington, DC: American Psychiatric Association; 2013.

22. World Health Organization. The ICD-10 classification of mental and behavioural disorders: diagnostic criteria for research. Geneva, Switzerland: World Health Organization; 1993.

23. Reynolds CF 3rd, Redline S, DSM-V Sleep-Wake Disorders Workgroup and Advisors. The DSM-V sleep-wake disorders nosology: an update and an invitation to the sleep community. Sleep 2010;33(1):10–1.

24. Buysse DJ, Reynolds CF 3rd, Hauri PJ, et al. Diagnostic concordance for DSM-IV sleep disorders: a report from the APA/NIMH DSM-IV field trial. Am J Psychiatry 1994;151(9):1351–60.

25. Foley DJ, Monjan A, Simonsick EM, et al. Incidence and remission of insomnia among elderly adults: an epidemiologic study of 6,800 persons over three years. Sleep 1999;22(Suppl 2):S366–72.

26. Gureje O, Oladeji BD, Abiona T, et al. The natural history of insomnia in the Ibadan study of ageing. Sleep 2011;34(7):965–73.

27. Ellis JG, Perlis ML, Neale LF, et al. The natural history of insomnia: focus on prevalence and incidence of acute insomnia. J Psychiatr Res 2012;46(10): 1278–85.

28. Foley DJ, Monjan AA, Izmirlian G, et al. Incidence and remission of insomnia among elderly adults in a biracial cohort. Sleep 1999;22(Suppl 2):S373–8.

29. Morin CM, Belanger L, LeBlanc M, et al. The natural history of insomnia: a population-based 3-year longitudinal study. Arch Intern Med 2009;169(5): 447–53.

30. Spielman AJ, Caruso LS, Glovinsky PB. A behavioral perspective on insomnia treatment. Psychiatr Clin North Am 1987;10(4):541–53.

31. Patel NP, Grandner MA, Xie D, et al. "Sleep disparity" in the population: poor sleep quality is strongly associated with poverty and ethnicity. BMC Public Health 2010;10:475.

32. Morgan K. Daytime activity and risk factors for late-life insomnia. J Sleep Res 2003;12(3):231–8.

33. Evans DS, Parimi N, Nievergelt CM, et al. Common genetic variants in ARNTL and NPAS2 and at chromosome 12p13 are associated with objectively measured sleep traits in the elderly. Sleep 2013;36(3):431–46.

34. Katz DA, McHorney CA. Clinical correlates of insomnia in patients with chronic illness. Arch Intern Med 1998;158(10):1099–107.

35. Brenes GA, Miller ME, Stanley MA, et al. Insomnia in older adults with generalized anxiety disorder. Am J Geriatr Psychiatry 2009;17(6):465–72.

36. Dautovich ND, McCrae CS, Rowe M. Subjective and objective napping and sleep in older adults: are evening naps "bad" for nighttime sleep? J Am Geriatr Soc 2008;56(9):1681–6.

37. Batejat DM, Lagarde DP. Naps and modafinil as countermeasures for the effects of sleep deprivation on cognitive performance. Aviat Space Environ Med 1999; 70(5):493–8.

38. Jaussent I, Bouyer J, Ancelin ML, et al. Insomnia and daytime sleepiness are risk factors for depressive symptoms in the elderly. Sleep 2011;34(8):1103–10.

39. Perlis ML, Smith LJ, Lyness JM, et al. Insomnia as a risk factor for onset of depression in the elderly. Behav Sleep Med 2006;4(2):104–13.

40. Cole MG, Dendukuri N. Risk factors for depression among elderly community subjects: a systematic review and meta-analysis. Am J Psychiatry 2003; 160(6):1147–56.

41. Pigeon WR, Hegel M, Unutzer J, et al. Is insomnia a perpetuating factor for late-life depression in the IMPACT cohort? Sleep 2008;31(4):481–8.

42. Lee E, Cho HJ, Olmstead R, et al. Persistent sleep disturbance: a risk factor for recurrent depression in community-dwelling older adults. Sleep 2013;36(11): 1685–91.

43. Suh S, Kim H, Yang HC, et al. Longitudinal course of depression scores with and without insomnia in non-depressed individuals: a 6-year follow-up longitudinal study in a Korean cohort. Sleep 2013;36(3):369–76.

44. Bjorngaard JH, Bjerkeset O, Romundstad P, et al. Sleeping problems and suicide in 75,000 Norwegian adults: a 20 year follow-up of the HUNT I study. Sleep 2011;34(9):1155–9.

45. Jansson-Frojmark M, Lindblom K. A bidirectional relationship between anxiety and depression, and insomnia? A prospective study in the general population. J Psychosom Res 2008;64(4):443–9.

46. Sadler P, McLaren S, Jenkins M. A psychological pathway from insomnia to depression among older adults. Int Psychogeriatr 2013;25(8):1375–83.

47. Schwartz S, McDowell Anderson W, Cole SR, et al. Insomnia and heart disease: a review of epidemiologic studies. J Psychosom Res 1999;47(4):313–33.

48. Sigurdardottir LG, Valdimarsdottir UA, Mucci LA, et al. Sleep disruption among older men and risk of prostate cancer. Cancer Epidemiol Biomarkers Prev 2013; 22(5):872–9.

49. Lovato N, Lack L, Wright H, et al. Working memory performance of older adults with insomnia. J Sleep Res 2013;22(3):251–7.

50. Sivertsen B, Hysing M, Wehling E, et al. Neuropsychological performance in older insomniacs. Neuropsychol Dev Cogn B Aging Neuropsychol Cogn 2013;20(1):34–48.

51. Cricco M, Simonsick EM, Foley DJ. The impact of insomnia on cognitive functioning in older adults. J Am Geriatr Soc 2001;49(9):1185–9.

52. Tworoger SS, Lee S, Schernhammer ES, et al. The association of self-reported sleep duration, difficulty sleeping, and snoring with cognitive function in older women. Alzheimer Dis Assoc Disord 2006;20(1):41–8.

53. Lim AS, Kowgier M, Yu L, et al. Sleep fragmentation and the risk of incident Alzheimer's disease and cognitive decline in older persons. Sleep 2013;36(7): 1027–32.

54. Xiang YT, Weng YZ, Leung CM, et al. Prevalence and correlates of insomnia and its impact on quality of life in Chinese schizophrenia patients. Sleep 2009;32(1): 105–9.

55. Hidalgo JL, Gras CB, Garcia YD, et al. Functional status in the elderly with insomnia. Qual Life Res 2007;16(2):279–86.

56. Lambiase MJ, Pettee Gabriel K, Kuller LH, et al. Temporal relationships between physical activity and sleep in older women. Med Sci Sports Exerc 2013;45(12): 2362–8.

57. Phillips B, Mannino DM. Does insomnia kill? Sleep 2005;28(8):965–71.

58. Ohayon MM. Insomnia: a dangerous condition but not a killer? Sleep 2005; 28(9):1043–4.

59. Mallon L, Broman JE, Hetta J. Relationship between insomnia, depression, and mortality: a 12-year follow-up of older adults in the community. Int Psychogeriatr 2000;12(3):295–306.

60. Bloom HG, Ahmed I, Alessi CA, et al. Evidence-based recommendations for the assessment and management of sleep disorders in older persons. J Am Geriatr Soc 2009;57(5):761–89.

61. Al-Jawder SE, Bahammam AS. Comorbid insomnia in sleep-related breathing disorders: an under-recognized association. Sleep Breath 2012;16(2):295–304.

62. Gooneratne NS, Gehrman PR, Nkwuo JE, et al. Consequences of comorbid insomnia symptoms and sleep-related breathing disorder in elderly subjects. Arch Intern Med 2006;166(16):1732–8.

63. Youngstedt SD, Kripke DF, Elliott JA, et al. Circadian abnormalities in older adults. J Pineal Res 2001;31(3):264–72.
64. Morgenthaler TI, Lee-Chiong T, Alessi C, et al. Practice parameters for the clinical evaluation and treatment of circadian rhythm sleep disorders. An American Academy of Sleep Medicine report. Sleep 2007;30(11):1445–59.
65. McCall WV. Setting quantitative thresholds for detecting insomnia in older persons. J Clin Sleep Med 2013;9(2):133–4.
66. Levenson JC, Troxel WM, Begley A, et al. A quantitative approach to distinguishing older adults with insomnia from good sleeper controls. J Clin Sleep Med 2013;9(2):125–31.
67. Carney CE, Buysse DJ, Ancoli-Israel S, et al. The consensus sleep diary: standardizing prospective sleep self-monitoring. Sleep 2012;35(2):287–302.
68. Buysse DJ, Ancoli-Israel S, Edinger JD, et al. Recommendations for a standard research assessment of insomnia. Sleep 2006;29(9):1155–73.
69. Morgenthaler T, Alessi C, Friedman L, et al. Practice parameters for the use of actigraphy in the assessment of sleep and sleep disorders: an update for 2007. Sleep 2007;30(4):519–29.
70. van Dijk E, Hilgenkamp TI, Evenhuis HM, et al. Exploring the use of actigraphy to investigate sleep problems in older people with intellectual disability. J Intellect Disabil Res 2012;56(2):204–11.
71. Van Den Berg JF, Van Rooij FJ, Vos H, et al. Disagreement between subjective and actigraphic measures of sleep duration in a population-based study of elderly persons. J Sleep Res 2008;17(3):295–302.
72. Littner M, Hirshkowitz M, Kramer M, et al. Practice parameters for using polysomnography to evaluate insomnia: an update. Sleep 2003;26(6):754–60.
73. Littner MR, Kushida C, Wise M, et al. Practice parameters for clinical use of the multiple sleep latency test and the maintenance of wakefulness test. Sleep 2005;28(1):113–21.
74. Riemann D, Perlis ML. The treatments of chronic insomnia: a review of benzodiazepine receptor agonists and psychological and behavioral therapies. Sleep Med Rev 2009;13(3):205–14.
75. National Institute of Health. National Institutes of Health State of the Science Conference statement on manifestations and management of chronic insomnia in adults, June 13-15, 2005. Sleep 2005;28(9):1049–57.
76. Shub D, Darvishi R, Kunik ME. Non-pharmacologic treatment of insomnia in persons with dementia. Geriatrics 2009;64(2):22–6.
77. McCurry SM, Logsdon RG, Teri L, et al. Evidence-based psychological treatments for insomnia in older adults. Psychol Aging 2007;22(1):18–27.
78. Montgomery P, Dennis J. A systematic review of non-pharmacological therapies for sleep problems in later life. Sleep Med Rev 2004;8(1):47–62.
79. Morin CM, Colecchi C, Stone J, et al. Behavioral and pharmacological therapies for late-life insomnia: a randomized controlled trial. JAMA 1999;281(11):991–9.
80. Alessi C, Vitiello MV. Insomnia (primary) in older people. Clin Evid (Online) 2011; 2011. pii:2302.
81. Buysse DJ, Germain A, Moul DE, et al. Efficacy of brief behavioral treatment for chronic insomnia in older adults. Arch Intern Med 2011;171(10):887–95.
82. Cheng SK, Dizon J. Computerised cognitive behavioural therapy for insomnia: a systematic review and meta-analysis. Psychother Psychosom 2012;81(4):206–16.
83. Morin CM, Bastien C, Guay B, et al. Randomized clinical trial of supervised tapering and cognitive behavior therapy to facilitate benzodiazepine discontinuation in older adults with chronic insomnia. Am J Psychiatry 2004;161(2):332–42.

84. Jungquist CR, O'Brien C, Matteson-Rusby S, et al. The efficacy of cognitive-behavioral therapy for insomnia in patients with chronic pain. Sleep Med 2010;11(3):302–9.

85. Sanchez-Ortuno MM, Edinger JD. Cognitive-behavioral therapy for the management of insomnia comorbid with mental disorders. Curr Psychiatry Rep 2012; 14(5):519–28.

86. Espie CA, Fleming L, Cassidy J, et al. Randomized controlled clinical effectiveness trial of cognitive behavior therapy compared with treatment as usual for persistent insomnia in patients with cancer. J Clin Oncol 2008;26(28): 4651–8.

87. Jaussent I, Ancelin ML, Berr C, et al. Hypnotics and mortality in an elderly general population: a 12-year prospective study. BMC Med 2013;11(1):212.

88. Perlis ML, McCall WV, Krystal AD, et al. Long-term, non-nightly administration of zolpidem in the treatment of patients with primary insomnia. J Clin Psychiatry 2004;65(8):1128–37.

89. Roth T, Seiden D, Sainati S, et al. Effects of ramelteon on patient-reported sleep latency in older adults with chronic insomnia. Sleep Med 2006;7(4):312–8.

90. Zammit G, Wang-Weigand S, Rosenthal M, et al. Effect of ramelteon on middle-of-the-night balance in older adults with chronic insomnia. J Clin Sleep Med 2009;5(1):34–40.

91. Zammit G, Erman M, Wang-Weigand S, et al. Evaluation of the efficacy and safety of ramelteon in subjects with chronic insomnia. J Clin Sleep Med 2007; 3(5):495–504.

92. Mets MA, de Vries JM, de Senerpont Domis LM, et al. Next-day effects of ramelteon (8 mg), zopiclone (7.5 mg), and placebo on highway driving performance, memory functioning, psychomotor performance, and mood in healthy adult subjects. Sleep 2011;34(10):1327–34.

93. Wiegand MH. Antidepressants for the treatment of insomnia: a suitable approach? Drugs 2008;68(17):2411–7.

94. Walsh JK. Drugs used to treat insomnia in 2002: regulatory-based rather than evidence-based medicine. Sleep 2004;27(8):1441–2.

95. Wilson S, Nutt D. Management of insomnia: treatments and mechanisms. Br J Psychiatry 2007;191:195–7.

96. Winokur A, DeMartinis NA 3rd, McNally DP, et al. Comparative effects of mirtazapine and fluoxetine on sleep physiology measures in patients with major depression and insomnia. J Clin Psychiatry 2003;64(10):1224–9.

97. Vande Griend JP, Anderson SL. Histamine-1 receptor antagonism for treatment of insomnia. J Am Pharm Assoc (2003) 2012;52(6):e210–9.

98. Buysse DJ. Insomnia, depression and aging. Assessing sleep and mood interactions in older adults. Geriatrics 2004;59(2):47–51 [quiz: 52].

99. Tranah GJ, Parimi N, Blackwell T, et al. Postmenopausal hormones and sleep quality in the elderly: a population based study. BMC Womens Health 2010; 10:15.

100. Sarris J, Byrne GJ. A systematic review of insomnia and complementary medicine. Sleep Med Rev 2011;15(2):99–106.

101. Wade AG, Ford I, Crawford G, et al. Nightly treatment of primary insomnia with prolonged release melatonin for 6 months: a randomized placebo controlled trial on age and endogenous melatonin as predictors of efficacy and safety. BMC Med 2010;8:51.

102. Morin CM, Bastien CH, Brink D, et al. Adverse effects of temazepam in older adults with chronic insomnia. Hum Psychopharmacol 2003;18(1):75–82.

103. Morin CM, Vallieres A, Guay B, et al. Cognitive behavioral therapy, singly and combined with medication, for persistent insomnia: a randomized controlled trial. JAMA 2009;301(19):2005–15.
104. Schnelle JF, Ouslander JG, Simmons SF, et al. The nighttime environment, incontinence care, and sleep disruption in nursing homes. J Am Geriatr Soc 1993;41(9):910–4.
105. Schnelle JF, Alessi CA, Al-Samarrai NR, et al. The nursing home at night: effects of an intervention on noise, light, and sleep. J Am Geriatr Soc 1999;47(4):430–8.
106. Mishima K, Okawa M, Hozumi S, et al. Supplementary administration of artificial bright light and melatonin as potent treatment for disorganized circadian rest-activity and dysfunctional autonomic and neuroendocrine systems in institutionalized demented elderly persons. Chronobiol Int 2000;17(3):419–32.
107. El Kady HM, Ibrahim HK, Mohamed SG. Cognitive behavioral therapy for institutionalized elders complaining of sleep disturbance in Alexandria, Egypt. Sleep Breath 2012;16(4):1173–80.
108. McCurry SM, Gibbons LE, Logsdon RG, et al. Nighttime insomnia treatment and education for Alzheimer's disease: a randomized, controlled trial. J Am Geriatr Soc 2005;53(5):793–802.
109. Paniagua MA, Paniagua EW. The demented elder with insomnia. Clin Geriatr Med 2008;24(1):69–81, vii.
110. McCurry SM, Gibbons LE, Logsdon RG, et al. Insomnia in caregivers of persons with dementia: who is at risk and what can be done about it? Sleep Med Clin 2009;4(4):519–26.
111. Pollak C, Perlick D. Sleep problems and institutionalization of the elderly. J Geriatric Psych Neurology 1991;4(4):204–10.
112. McCurry SM, Logsdon RG, Vitiello MV, et al. Successful behavioral treatment for reported sleep problems in elderly caregivers of dementia patients: a controlled study. J Gerontol B Psychol Sci Soc Sci 1998;53(2):122–9.
113. King AC, Baumann K, O'Sullivan P, et al. Effects of moderate-intensity exercise on physiological, behavioral, and emotional responses to family caregiving: a randomized controlled trial. J Gerontol A Biol Sci Med Sci 2002;57(1):M26–36.
114. Epstein LJ, Kristo D, Strollo PJ Jr, et al. Clinical guideline for the evaluation, management and long-term care of obstructive sleep apnea in adults. J Clin Sleep Med 2009;5(3):263–76.
115. Young T, Shahar E, Nieto FJ, et al. Predictors of sleep apnea in community-dwelling adults: the Sleep Heart Health Study. Arch Intern Med 2002;162(8):893–900.
116. Herrscher TE, Akre H, Overland B, et al. High prevalence of sleep apnea in heart failure outpatients: even in patients with preserved systolic function. J Card Fail 2011;17(5):420–5.
117. Gehrman PR, Martin JL, Shochat T, et al. Sleep apnea and agitation in institutionalized adults with Alzheimer disease. Am J Geriatr Psychiatry 2003;11(4):426–33.
118. Mehra R, Stone KL, Blackwell T, et al. Prevalence and correlates of sleep apnea in older men: osteoporotic fractures in men sleep study. J Am Geriatr Soc 2007;55(9):1356–64.
119. Javaheri S, Caref EB, Chen E, et al. Sleep apnea testing and outcomes in a large cohort of Medicare beneficiaries with newly diagnosed heart failure. Am J Respir Crit Care Med 2011;183(4):539–46.
120. Eikermann M, Jordan AS, Chamberlin NL, et al. The influence of aging on pharyngeal collapsibility during sleep. Chest 2007;131(6):1702–9.

121. Oliven A, Carmi N, Coleman R, et al. Age-related changes in upper airway muscles morphological and oxidative properties. Exp Gerontol 2001;36(10): 1673–86.

122. Young T, Finn L, Austin D, et al. Menopausal status and sleep apnea in the Wisconsin Sleep Cohort Study. Am J Respir Crit Care Med 2003;167(9):1181–5.

123. Bucca C, Cicolin A, Brussino L, et al. Tooth loss and obstructive sleep apnoea. Respir Res 2006;7:8.

124. Gilman S, Chervin RD, Koeppe RA, et al. Obstructive sleep apnea is related to a thalamic cholinergic deficit in MSA. Neurology 2003;61(1):35–9.

125. Yaffe K, Laffan AM, Harrison SL, et al. Sleep apnea, hypoxia, and risk of mild cognitive impairment and dementia in older women. JAMA 2011;306(6): 613–9.

126. Ancoli-Israel S, Palmer BW, Cooke JR, et al. Cognitive effects of treating obstructive sleep apnea in Alzheimer's disease: a randomized controlled study. J Am Geriatr Soc 2008;56(11):2076–81.

127. Canessa N, Castronovo V, Cappa SF, et al. Obstructive sleep apnea: brain structural changes and neurocognitive function before and after treatment. Am J Respir Crit Care Med 2011;183(10):1419–26.

128. Kotterba S, Rasche K, Widdig W, et al. Neuropsychological investigations and event-related potentials in obstructive sleep apnea syndrome before and during CPAP-therapy. J Neurol Sci 1998;159(1):45–50.

129. Wheaton AG, Perry GS, Chapman DP, et al. Sleep disordered breathing and depression among U.S. adults: National Health and Nutrition Examination Survey, 2005-2008. Sleep 2012;35(4):461–7.

130. Harris M, Glozier N, Ratnavadivel R, et al. Obstructive sleep apnea and depression. Sleep Med Rev 2009;13(6):437–44.

131. Peppard PE, Szklo-Coxe M, Hla KM, et al. Longitudinal association of sleep-related breathing disorder and depression. Arch Intern Med 2006;166(16): 1709–15.

132. Jackson ML, Stough C, Howard ME, et al. The contribution of fatigue and sleepiness to depression in patients attending the sleep laboratory for evaluation of obstructive sleep apnea. Sleep Breath 2011;15(3):439–45.

133. Asghari A, Mohammadi F, Kamrava SK, et al. Severity of depression and anxiety in obstructive sleep apnea syndrome. Eur Arch Otorhinolaryngol 2012;269(12): 2549–53.

134. Ishman SL, Cavey RM, Mettel TL, et al. Depression, sleepiness, and disease severity in patients with obstructive sleep apnea. Laryngoscope 2010;120(11): 2331–5.

135. Castro LS, Castro J, Hoexter MQ, et al. Depressive symptoms and sleep: a population-based polysomnographic study. Psychiatry Res 2013;210(3): 906–12.

136. Aloia MS, Arnedt JT, Smith L, et al. Examining the construct of depression in obstructive sleep apnea syndrome. Sleep Med 2005;6(2):115–21.

137. Krystal AD, Harsh JR, Yang R, et al. A double-blind, placebo-controlled study of armodafinil for excessive sleepiness in patients with treated obstructive sleep apnea and comorbid depression. J Clin Psychiatry 2010;71(1):32–40.

138. Freedland KE, Carney RM, Hayano J, et al. Effect of obstructive sleep apnea on response to cognitive behavior therapy for depression after an acute myocardial infarction. J Psychosom Res 2012;72(4):276–81.

139. Habukawa M, Uchimura N, Kakuma T, et al. Effect of CPAP treatment on residual depressive symptoms in patients with major depression and coexisting sleep

apnea: contribution of daytime sleepiness to residual depressive symptoms. Sleep Med 2010;11(6):552–7.

140. Kjelsberg FN, Ruud EA, Stavem K. Predictors of symptoms of anxiety and depression in obstructive sleep apnea. Sleep Med 2005;6(4):341–6.

141. Macey PM, Woo MA, Kumar R, et al. Relationship between obstructive sleep apnea severity and sleep, depression and anxiety symptoms in newly-diagnosed patients. PLoS One 2010;5(4):e10211.

142. Gottlieb DJ, Yenokyan G, Newman AB, et al. Prospective study of obstructive sleep apnea and incident coronary heart disease and heart failure: the sleep heart health study. Circulation 2010;122(4):352–60.

143. Redline S, Yenokyan G, Gottlieb DJ, et al. Obstructive sleep apnea-hypopnea and incident stroke: the sleep heart health study. Am J Respir Crit Care Med 2010;182(2):269–77.

144. Munoz R, Duran-Cantolla J, Martinez-Vila E, et al. Severe sleep apnea and risk of ischemic stroke in the elderly. Stroke 2006;37(9):2317–21.

145. Endeshaw YW, Unruh ML, Kutner M, et al. Sleep apnea and frailty in the Cardiovascular Health Study Cohort. Am J Epidemiol 2009;170(2):193–202.

146. Flink BJ, Rivelli SK, Cox EA, et al. Obstructive sleep apnea and incidence of postoperative delirium after elective knee replacement in the nondemented elderly. Anesthesiology 2012;116(4):788–96.

147. American Society of Anesthesiologists Task Force on Perioperative Management of patients with obstructive sleep apnea. Practice guidelines for the perioperative management of patients with obstructive sleep apnea: an updated report by the American Society of Anesthesiologists Task Force on Perioperative Management of Patients with Obstructive Sleep Apnea. Anesthesiology 2014; 120(2):268–86.

148. Punjabi NM, Caffo BS, Goodwin JL, et al. Sleep apnea and mortality: a prospective cohort study. PLoS Med 2009;6(8):e1000132.

149. Ancoli-Israel S, Kripke DF, Klauber MR, et al. Morbidity, mortality and sleep apnea in community dwelling elderly. Sleep 1996;19(4):277–82.

150. Gami AS, Howard DE, Olson EJ, et al. Day-night pattern of sudden death in obstructive sleep apnea. N Engl J Med 2005;352(12):1206–14.

151. Gooneratne N. Insomnia in the elderly. In: Forciea MA, Lavizzo-Mourey R, Schwab EP, editors. Geriatric secrets. 2nd edition. Philadelphia: Hanley and Belfus; 2000. p. 44–9.

152. Welch HG, Albertsen PC, Nease RF, et al. Estimating treatment benefits for the elderly: the effect of competing risks. Ann Intern Med 1996;124(6):577–84.

153. Gooneratne NS, Pien G, Gurubhagavatula I. Sleep-related breathing disorders in the elderly. In: Kushida CA, editor. Encyclopedia of sleep, vol. 3. Philadelphia, PA: Elsevier, Inc; 2013. p. 547–54.

154. Martinez-Garcia MA, Campos-Rodriguez F, Catalan-Serra P, et al. Cardiovascular mortality in obstructive sleep apnea in the elderly: role of long-term continuous positive airway pressure treatment: a prospective observational study. Am J Respir Crit Care Med 2012;186(9):909–16.

155. Polese JF, Santos-Silva R, de Oliveira Ferrari PM, et al. Is portable monitoring for diagnosing obstructive sleep apnea syndrome suitable in elderly population? Sleep Breath 2013;17(2):679–86.

156. Agency for Healthcare Research and Quality. Obstructive Sleep Apnea-Hypopnea Syndrome: Modeling different diagnostic strategies. 2010. Available at: http://www.cms.hhs.gov/determinationprocess/downloads/id50TA.pdf. Accessed January 2014.

157. Centers for Medicare and Medicaid Services. Decision memo for continuous positive airway pressure (CPAP) therapy for obstructive sleep apnea (OSA) (CAG-00093R2) [HTML]. March, 2008. Available at: http://www.cms.hhs.gov/mcd/viewdecisionmemo.asp?id=204. Accessed February 2010.

158. Bliwise DL, Benkert RE, Ingham RH. Factors associated with nightly variability in sleep apnea in the elderly. Chest 1991;100(4):973–6.

159. American Academy of Sleep Medicine. International classification of sleep disorders, 2nd edition: diagnostic and coding manual. Westchester (IL): American Academy of Sleep Medicine; 2005.

160. Stessman J, Jacobs JM, Ein-Mor E, et al. Normal body mass index rather than obesity predicts greater mortality in elderly people: the Jerusalem longitudinal study. J Am Geriatr Soc 2009;57(12):2232–8.

161. van Rutte PW, Smulders JF, de Zoete JP, et al. Sleeve gastrectomy in older obese patients. Surg Endosc 2013;27(6):2014–9.

162. Busetto L, Angrisani L, Basso N, et al. Safety and efficacy of laparoscopic adjustable gastric banding in the elderly. Obesity (Silver Spring) 2008;16(2):334–8.

163. Ayalon L, Ancoli-Israel S, Stepnowsky C, et al. Adherence to continuous positive airway pressure treatment in patients with Alzheimer's disease and obstructive sleep apnea. Am J Geriatr Psychiatry 2006;14(2):176–80.

164. Morgenthaler TI, Aurora RN, Brown T, et al. Practice parameters for the use of autotitrating continuous positive airway pressure devices for titrating pressures and treating adult patients with obstructive sleep apnea syndrome: an update for 2007. An American Academy of Sleep Medicine report. Sleep 2008;31(1):141–7.

165. Sawyer AM, Gooneratne NS, Marcus CL, et al. A systematic review of CPAP adherence across age groups: clinical and empiric insights for developing CPAP adherence interventions. Sleep Med Rev 2011;15(6):343–56.

166. Russo-Magno P, O'Brien A, Panciera T, et al. Compliance with CPAP therapy in older men with obstructive sleep apnea. J Am Geriatr Soc 2001;49(9):1205–11.

167. Aarab G, Lobbezoo F, Hamburger HL, et al. Oral appliance therapy versus nasal continuous positive airway pressure in obstructive sleep apnea: a randomized, placebo-controlled trial. Respiration 2011;81(5):411–9.

168. Holley AB, Lettieri CJ, Shah AA. Efficacy of an adjustable oral appliance and comparison with continuous positive airway pressure for the treatment of obstructive sleep apnea syndrome. Chest 2011;140(6):1511–6.

169. Doff MH, Veldhuis SK, Hoekema A, et al. Long-term oral appliance therapy in obstructive sleep apnea syndrome: a controlled study on temporomandibular side effects. Clin Oral Investig 2012;16(3):689–97.

170. Colrain IM, Black J, Siegel LC, et al. A multicenter evaluation of oral pressure therapy for the treatment of obstructive sleep apnea. Sleep Med 2013;14(9):830–7.

171. Kezirian EJ, Weaver EM, Yueh B, et al. Incidence of serious complications after uvulopalatopharyngoplasty. Laryngoscope 2004;114(3):450–3.

172. Jaghagen EL, Berggren D, Dahlqvist A, et al. Prediction and risk of dysphagia after uvulopalatopharyngoplasty and uvulopalatoplasty. Acta Otolaryngol 2004;124(10):1197–203.

173. Loredo JS, Ancoli-Israel S, Kim EJ, et al. Effect of continuous positive airway pressure versus supplemental oxygen on sleep quality in obstructive sleep apnea: a placebo-CPAP-controlled study. Sleep 2006;29(4):564–71.

174. Toyama T, Seki R, Kasama S, et al. Effectiveness of nocturnal home oxygen therapy to improve exercise capacity, cardiac function and cardiac sympathetic nerve activity in patients with chronic heart failure and central sleep apnea. Circ J 2009;73(2):299–304.

175. Curgunlu A, Doventas A, Karadeniz D, et al. Prevalence and characteristics of restless legs syndrome (RLS) in the elderly and the relation of serum ferritin levels with disease severity: hospital-based study from Istanbul, Turkey. Arch Gerontol Geriatr 2012;55(1):73–6.

176. Hornyak M, Trenkwalder C. Restless legs syndrome and periodic limb movement disorder in the elderly. J Psychosom Res 2004;56(5):543–8.

177. Rose KM, Beck C, Tsai PF, et al. Sleep disturbances and nocturnal agitation behaviors in older adults with dementia. Sleep 2011;34(6):779–86.

178. McCarter SJ, St Louis EK, Boeve BF. REM sleep behavior disorder and REM sleep without atonia as an early manifestation of degenerative neurological disease. Curr Neurol Neurosci Rep 2012;12(2):182–92.

179. McCarter SJ, Boswell CL, St Louis EK, et al. Treatment outcomes in REM sleep behavior disorder. Sleep Med 2013;14(3):237–42.

180. Morgenthaler T, Kramer M, Alessi C, et al. Practice parameters for the psychological and behavioral treatment of insomnia: an update. An American Academy of Sleep Medicine report. Sleep 2006;29(11):1415–9.

181. National Institutes of Health Consensus Panel. NIH State-of-the-Science Conference statement on manifestations and management of chronic insomnia in adults. NIH Consens State Sci Statements 2005;22(2):1–30.

182. Ancoli-Israel S, Kripke DF, Klauber MR, et al. Sleep apnea in community-dwelling elderly. Sleep 1991;14(6):486–95.

Substance Abuse Among Older Adults

Alexis Kuerbis, LCSW, PhD[a,*], Paul Sacco, PhD, LCSW[b], Dan G. Blazer, MD, PhD[c],
Alison A. Moore, MD, MPH[d]

KEYWORDS

- Older adults • Alcohol • Prescription medication • Substance use • Assessment
- Assessment tools • Brief interventions • Treatment

KEY POINTS

- Although the current proportions of older adults with substance use disorders remain low compared with the general population, a growing proportion and number of older adults are at risk for hazardous drinking, prescription drug misuse, and illicit substance use and abuse.
- The identification of problematic substance use with older adults can be difficult because of overlapping symptoms with medical disorders that are common in older age.
- The assessment should include a respectful and nonstigmatizing approach along with direct questions about drinking, prescription medication, and illicit drug use.
- Several brief interventions centered on education about the harms of substance use have been shown to be effective with older adults.
- For older adults with more severe substance use problems, more intensive treatments geared toward a general population have been shown to be effective for older adults; however, treatments tailored for older adults have shown particular promise.

INTRODUCTION

The initial wave of the baby boom generation turned 65 years old in 2011, a generation that comprises 30% of the total US population.[1] The size of this generation and their longer life expectancies[2] led the US Census Bureau to project that the number of older adults will increase from 40.3 million to 72.1 million between 2010 and 2030.[3] Historically, older adults have not demonstrated high rates of alcohol or other drug use

Disclosure: Dr Moore's time to write this paper was supported with funding from the National Institute on Alcohol Abuse and Alcoholism (K24 AA15957).
[a] Department of Mental Health Services and Policy Research, Research Foundation for Mental Hygiene, Inc, Columbia University Medical Center, 3 Columbus Circle, Suite 1404, New York, NY 10019, USA; [b] University of Maryland School of Social Work, 525 West Redwood Street, Baltimore, MD 21201, USA; [c] Department of Psychiatry and Behavioral Sciences, Academic Development, Duke University, DUMC 3003, Durham, NC 27710, USA; [d] Department of Medicine, Division of Geriatrics, David Geffen School of Medicine at UCLA, 10945 Le Conte Avenue, Suite 2339, Los Angeles, CA 90095, USA
* Corresponding author.
E-mail address: alexis.kuerbis@gmail.com

compared with younger adults[4,5] or presented in large numbers to substance abuse treatment programs.[6] These facts have helped to perpetuate a misconception that older adults do not use or abuse mood-altering substances. Indeed, substantial evidence suggests that substance use among older adults has been underidentified[7,8] for decades. The aging of the baby boom generation creates a new urgency to effectively identify and treat substance use among older adults.

Baby boomers are distinct compared with past generations as they came of age during the 1960s and 1970s, a period of changing attitudes toward and rates of drug and alcohol use.[9,10] The prevalence rates of substance use disorder (SUD) have remained high among this group as they age,[5] and both the proportions and actual numbers of older adults needing treatment of SUD are expected to grow substantially. SUD rates among people older than 50 years are projected to increase from about 2.8 million in 2006 to 5.7 million in 2020.[11] There is, therefore, widespread recognition among both generalists and specialists in gerontology and psychiatry,[3,12,13] and health care overall, of the need for more information about assessment and interventions related to problematic substance use among older adults.

PREVALENCE OF SUBSTANCE USE AMONG OLDER ADULTS
Alcohol Use

Despite increasing rates of illicit and prescription drug misuse among adults older than 65 years,[5,6,10] alcohol remains the most commonly used substance among older adults.[6,10] Therefore, most of the research on substance use among and treatment of older adults has centered on alcohol use disorders (AUD). Among the population at large, older adults reduce their alcohol use as they age.[14–17] As of 2002, among individuals aged 65 years and older in the general population, the estimated prevalence is 1.2% for the *Diagnostic and Statistical Manual of Mental Disorders* (Fourth Edition) (*DSM-IV*) alcohol abuse and 0.24% for *DSM-IV* alcohol dependence.[18] Prevalence estimates inclusive of those older than 50 years are higher (2.98% for all AUD). Within heath care settings, the rates of AUD among older adults ranges up to a proportion of 22%.[19–21] Although these rates are lower than for younger adults, they are likely impacted by the underreporting of heavy drinking,[7] difficulties with differential diagnoses of AUDs in older adults, and unidentified comorbidities.[22]

At-risk drinking is more prevalent among older adults than AUD and is likely responsible for a larger share of the harm to the health and well-being of older adults. Guidelines provided by the American Geriatrics Society and the National Institute for Alcohol Abuse and Alcoholism recommend that older adults drink no more than 7 standard drinks (12-oz beer, 4- to 5-oz glass of wine, 1.5 oz of 80-proof liquor) per week.[10,16] Prevalence rates for older-adult at-risk drinking (defined as more than 3 drinks on one occasion or more than 7 drinks per week) are estimated to be 16.0% for men[23,24] and 10.9% for women.[20,21] There is also a substantial proportion of the older-adult population who are binge drinkers (generally defined as 5 or more standard drinks in one drinking episode, though definitions vary for older adults).[25] Rates of older-adult binge drinking are 19.6% for men and 6.3% for women using data from the 2005–2006 National Survey on Drug Use and Health.[20,26] In a study of community-based older adults who reported drinking one or more drinks in the previous 3 months, 67% reported binge drinking in the last year.[25]

Tobacco Use

Tobacco use is quite prevalent among older adults, with about 14% of those aged 65 years and older reporting tobacco use in the last 12 months,[10] and just more than 6% used tobacco and alcohol together in the last 12 months. Clinical trials examining smoking cessation interventions demonstrate that older-adult smokers tend to be long-term, heavy smokers who are also physiologically dependent on nicotine.[27–29]

Illicit Substance Use

Illicit drug use is more prevalent among American older adults than among older adults in almost any other country in the world.[30] Results from the 2012 National Survey on Drug Use and Health revealed that rates of past month use of illicit substances doubled on average (from 1.9%–3.4% to 3.6%–7.2%) among 50 to 65 year olds between 2002 and 2012[5]—a statistically significant increase driven by the baby boom generation.[5,11] Generally, individuals aged 50 to 64 years report more psychoactive drug use than older groups.[24,31,32] For example, in 2012, 19.3% of adults aged 65 years and older reported having ever used illicit drugs in their lifetime, whereas 47.6% of adults between 60 and 64 years of age reported lifetime drug use. Among those that do use illicit substances, 11.7% meet the criteria for past-year SUD.[31] There are no recommendations for safe levels of illicit drug use among older adults.[33]

Cannabis use by older adults is considerably more prevalent than other drugs. Among adults aged 50 years and older in 2012, 4.6 million reported past-year marijuana use, and less than one million reported cocaine, inhalants, hallucinogens, methamphetamine, and/or heroin use in the past year. These rates are consistent with those reported by other studies.[24,31] With the passage of medical marijuana legislation and relaxed enforcement of drug possession related to marijuana, the prevalence rate of use among older adults may increase as they use it to cope with illness-related side effects,[20] potentially facilitating an increase in recreational use.

Prescription, Nonprescription, and Over-the-Counter Medication Use

Older adults take more prescribed and over-the-counter medications than younger adults,[22,34] increasing the risk for harmful drug interactions, misuse, and abuse. A cross-sectional community-based study of 3005 individuals aged 57 to 85 years found that 37.1% of men and 36.0% of women used at least 5 prescription medications concurrently.[35] The study also found that about 1 in 25 of the participants were at risk for a major drug interaction, and half of these situations involved nonprescription medications. In 2012, 2.9 million adults aged 50 years and older reported nonmedical use of psychotherapeutic medications in the past year.[5] Estimates of prescription medication misuse among older women are 11%.[36] Blazer and Wu[32] reported that 1.4% of adults aged 50 years and older used prescription opioids nonmedically in the last year, which was higher than sedatives, tranquilizers, and stimulants (all <1%). Actual prescription opioid use disorder among this same group was 0.13%, yet dependence was more common than abuse.[31] Benzodiazepines are the most commonly prescribed psychiatric medication among all adults. Despite contraindications for use with older adults, they are widely prescribed[37] and are disproportionately prescribed to older adults.[38] Rates of benzodiazepine use among older adults have ranged from 15.2% to 32.0%.[39] It is important to note that the rates of benzodiazepine use may be impacted by overprescription, misdiagnosis, or polypharmacy rather than intentional misuse or abuse.

UNIQUE VULNERABILITIES FOR OLDER ADULTS USING MOOD-ALTERING SUBSTANCES

Although the rates of SUD and use of drugs and alcohol are generally lower among older adults than the general population, aging itself presents specific risks for harm when considering even minimal amounts of substance use among older adults. Risk factors may vary considerably by substance and the specific clinical presentation of a patient (eg, age, medical comorbidities, current medications, and health history). Understanding substance-specific risks can help practitioners to recognize and respond to unhealthy use that does not meet the narrow definition of problem use.

Alcohol

Alcohol has a unique physical impact on the body in late life as compared with adults in young to middle age.[40] As one ages, the percentages of lean body mass and total body water decrease, and the ability of the liver to process alcohol is also diminished; blood-brain barrier permeability and neuronal receptor sensitivity to alcohol in the brain increase.[22] Because of these changes, older adults experience higher blood alcohol concentrations and increased impairment compared with younger adults[40] at equivalent consumption levels and with less awareness of their impairment,[41–43] thus, rendering them more vulnerable to the ill effects of alcohol even in moderate amounts. Compared with moderate drinkers, older-adult at-risk drinkers are more likely to experience alcohol-related problems[14,25] and basic functional impairment, such as impaired instrumental activities of daily living (eg, shopping, cooking, responsibility for medication).[25] The increased rate of comorbid medical and psychiatric conditions and the medications used to treat them create a complicated picture of risk and unique vulnerabilities for older adults.[10] Even healthy drinking levels established in young to middle age and then sustained through older age may be a risk factor for health problems among older adults.[44]

Despite the older person's increased vulnerability to alcohol, moderate alcohol consumption is associated with decreased morbidity and mortality among older adults.[45,46] A large body of research suggests that those older adults who are moderate drinkers (no more than one standard drink per day) experience better health than their heavier drinking and abstinent peers.[47–49] For example, moderate-drinking older adults have been discovered to have fewer falls, greater mobility, and improved physical functioning when compared with nondrinkers.[40]

It is important to note that many of the health benefits of moderate alcohol use for older adults may come with negative trade-offs. For example, moderate drinking may decrease the risk of ischemic stroke but increase the risk of hemorrhagic stroke[50] and have many potential interactions with medications.[51] As with other age groups, it would seem that the benefits of alcohol for older adults varies across individuals and depends on each person's unique biopsychosocial context, including age, comorbid illnesses, sex, and genetics.

Medications and Illicit Drugs

The same biologic changes that increase the effect of alcohol among older adults also increase the effect of medications and illicit drugs, causing an increased vulnerability to drug effects and drug interactions.[22] For example, older adults process benzodiazepines and opiates differently than younger adults; these medications should be prescribed with caution. Benzodiazepines with long half-lives are contraindicated for older adults as they can cause excessive sedation.[36] Benzodiazepines are fat-soluble drugs; as adults have less lean muscle mass and more body fat as they age, these drugs have a longer duration of action. Other risks associated with medication use in older adults occur because they may see multiple doctors, each of who may prescribe them medications that may interact with each other and/or with alcohol or other substances. Alcohol and marijuana increase the sedative effects of drugs such as barbiturates, benzodiazepines, and opiates.[52] Older adults may also unintentionally misuse a medication by borrowing a prescribed medication from another person (eg, taking a dose of another person's lorazepam or zolpidem for sleep), taking more than intended, or confusing pills.

The increasing acceptance of marijuana use, both medicinally and recreationally, may also pose unique risks in an aging population. Marijuana is known to cause impairment of short-term memory; increased heart rate, respiratory rate, elevated blood pressure; and a 4-time increase in the risk for heart attack after the first hour of smoking marijuana.[53] These risks may be pronounced in older adults whose cognitive or cardiovascular systems may already be compromised. Additionally, tobacco use among older adults is associated with greater mortality, risks of coronary events and cardiac deaths, smoking-related cancers, chronic obstructive pulmonary disease, decline in pulmonary function, development of osteoporosis, risk of hip fractures, loss of mobility, and poorer physical functioning.[54,55] Incidentally, smoking also impairs or inhibits effective treatments for these conditions.[56] It is unclear which of these correlates to smoking tobacco also appear for marijuana.[53]

RISK FACTORS FOR OLDER ADULTS USING SUBSTANCES

Most research on the correlates and predictors of substance use in late life has been conducted on alcohol use. Individual, social, and familial factors that contribute to or are associated with late-life unhealthy drinking may also apply to other substances. **Box 1** lists some of the potential risk factors for older adults associated with use of alcohol and, where known, other substances.

Box 1
Risk factors related to substance use in late life

Physical risk factors

    Male sex (for alcohol), female sex (for prescription drug)

    Caucasian ethnicity

    Chronic pain

    Physical disabilities or reduced mobility

    Transitions in care/living situations

    Poor health status

    Chronic physical illness/polymorbidity

    Significant drug burden/polypharmacy

Psychiatric risk factors

    Avoidance coping style

    History of alcohol problems

    Previous and/or concurrent SUD

    Previous and/or concurrent psychiatric illness

Social risk factors

    Affluence

    Bereavement

    Unexpected or forced retirement

    Social isolation (living alone or with nonspousal others)

Demographics

Being male,[23] more affluent,[20,57,58] Caucasian,[23,59] and young-old (those in the early stages of late life)[23] are consistently associated with unhealthy drinking in late life. Among all the demographics that are associated with increased drinking, only one is a predictor of increased drinking in older age: having more financial resources or longer financial horizons.[57,58] Female sex is associated with prescription drug abuse.[36]

Physical and Mental Health

Both current alcohol use and unhealthy drinking in older age are associated with being in better overall health[23,57]; however, this does not imply a causal relationship but rather suggests that those in good health are apt to drink more than their counterparts in poor health. Indeed, drinking has been shown to decrease as hospitalizations, disabilities, or depression increase.[23,60,61] Importantly, across studies, older heavy drinkers demonstrate poorer physical and mental health[23,40,61,62] as compared with their low-risk drinking counterparts. Drinking to reduce pain is a crucial long-term predictor of alcohol use in older adulthood.[58]

Because comorbid psychiatric disorders, such as anxiety, depression, and personality disorders, are common and recognized among younger adults, it is assumed that these comorbidities also continue into late life. Although there is little research about psychiatric comorbidity with substance use among older adults, some evidence suggests there is a high correlation between substance use, specifically alcohol use, and depression[63,64] and other affective disorders[33,65] among older adults.[66,67] The co-occurrence of depression and AUD can greatly complicate the diagnosis and treatment of both. For example, older adults may be more likely to disclose depressive symptoms and present to primary care settings rather than mental health or substance abuse treatment settings.

Sleep disturbance and sleep disorders are common among older adults who use alcohol[68] and who may use alcohol as a sleep aid.[33] Concurrent use of alcohol and medications for insomnia is risky because of drug interaction effects that cause excessive sedation and cross-tolerance. The factors associated with prescription medication abuse in older adults include a history of a SUD or mental health disorder and medical exposure to prescription drugs with abuse potential.[36] There is also evidence to suggest that overall cognitive impairment and several different types of dementia are more prevalent among older adults with comorbid alcohol use disorders[22,25,69,70] and that the differential diagnosis between Alzheimer disease and alcohol-related dementia is difficult.[33]

Among comorbid SUD, alcohol and tobacco are used commonly together among older adults[10]; being a smoker increases the likelihood of being an at-risk drinker.[71] Little else is known about the use patterns among older adults and the use of multiple substances simultaneously.

Coping Style

An individual's coping style for stress or tension may predict the development of a drinking problem in late life. An analysis of the Health and Retirement Study revealed that individuals who relied on avoidance coping to deal with stress or solve problems had a greater likelihood of developing and maintaining a late-life drinking problem than those who coped in other ways.[57] Similarly, a community-based survey of older adults who had contact with an outpatient health care facility found that relying on substances to reduce tension was associated with having a late-life alcohol problem.[72]

History of Alcohol Problems

There are a few studies that identified a history of problem drinking as a risk factor for unhealthy drinking among older adults. Platt and colleagues[57] found there was a significant increase in the likelihood of increasing one's drinking in later life among older adults with a history of drinking problems who did not abstain. Another longitudinal study of a community-based sample found that having drinking problems by 50 years of age significantly increased the likelihood of drinking and/or unhealthy drinking in late life.[58]

Social Factors

Some social factors are consistently associated with late-life drinking. Being divorced, separated, or single is positively associated with increased or unhealthy drinking in late life,[10,23] though this may differ across sexes. Social contact with friends or close family members among residents of retirement communities was found to be associated with increased alcohol use.[73] In this same study, a lack of religious affiliation was also found to be associated with higher categorical levels of drinking, each of which were defined by an increase in quantity and frequency of drinking. Although increased social interaction is associated with drinking among older adults, social isolation is associated with prescription drug abuse.[36]

Certain life events and social transitions common in late life may also heighten the risk of substance use or misuse. For example, bereavement (death of spouse, family, or friends), physical ill health, loneliness, caregiving for an ill spouse, change in living arrangement, and loss of occupation can all be factors in the substance use of older adults.[74–77] A review of the impact of retirement on older-adult drinking revealed that preretirement conditions, such as high job satisfaction or workplace stress, seem to increase the overall use of and problems with alcohol after retirement.[78] In addition, involuntary retirement and broadened social networks after retirement increase the likelihood of increased alcohol consumption or drinking problems.[78,79] Finally, housing status or living situation can facilitate or sustain substance use. For example, homelessness has been found to be a correlate of late-life drinking problems[69,80]; substance use among older adults has also been found to continue and even be enabled in the context of nursing homes.[81–83]

DIAGNOSIS

The formal diagnosis of SUD in the general population generally relies on the criteria outlined by the *DSM*.[84,85] **Table 1** outlines several symptoms of SUD based on physical and/or social factors. Because of particular biologic and social factors unique to late life, these criteria may be less relevant to older adults. This circumstance presents unique challenges for an accurate diagnosis of SUD among older adults.[16] For example, because of the age-associated physiologic changes that increase the effects of alcohol and other substances, older adults generally experience a reduction of tolerance to these substances, thus interfering with one of the hallmarks of SUD, increased tolerance. Furthermore, interruption in social and vocational roles or other consequences of drinking or drug use may be less likely to occur or less noticeable in old age.[44,86] Aging is often associated with a natural departure from these roles, such as through retirement[78] or social isolation caused by mortality of age-group peers.[87] Furthermore, the criterion related to continued use despite persistent or recurrent problems may not apply to many older adults who do not recognize that their problems, such as depression, are related to drinking.[16]

Table 1
SUD (formerly substance abuse or dependence) criteria[a]

DSM-5 Criteria for SUD	Consideration for Older Adult
A substance is often taken in larger amounts or over a longer period than was intended.	Cognitive impairment can prevent adequate self-monitoring. Substances themselves may more greatly impair cognition among older adults than younger adults.
There is a persistent desire or unsuccessful efforts to cut down or control substance use.	It is the same as the general adult population.
A great deal of time is spent in activities necessary to obtain the substance, use the substance, or recover from its effects.	Consequences from substance use can occur from using relatively small amounts.
There is craving or a strong desire to use the substance.	It is the same as the general adult population. Older adults with entrenched habits may not recognize cravings in the same way as the general adult population.
There is recurrent substance use resulting in a failure to fulfill major role obligations at work, school, or at home.	Role obligations may not exist for older adults in the same way as for younger adults because of life-stage transitions, such as retirement. The role obligations more common in late life are caregiving for an ill spouse or family member, such as a grandchild.
There is continued substance use despite having persistent or recurrent social or interpersonal problems caused or exacerbated by the effects of the substance.	Older adults may not realize the problems they experience are from substance use.
Important social, occupational, or recreational activities are given up or reduced because of substance use.	Older adults may engage in fewer activities regardless of substance use, making it difficult to detect.

There is recurrent substance use in situations in which it is physically hazardous.	Older adults may not identify or understand that their use is hazardous, especially when using substances in smaller amounts.
Substance use is continued despite knowledge of having a persistent or recurrent physical or psychological problem that is likely to have been caused or exacerbated by the substance.	Older adults may not realize the problems they experience are from substance use.
Tolerance is developed, as defined by either of the following: 1. A need for markedly increased amounts of the substance to achieve intoxication or the desired effect 2. A markedly diminished effect with continued use of the same amount of the substance	Because of the increased sensitivity to substances as they age, older adults will seem to have lowered rather than increase in tolerance.
Withdrawal, as manifested by either of the following: 1. The characteristic withdrawal syndrome for the substance 2. The substance or a close relative is taken to relieve or avoid withdrawal symptoms	Withdrawal symptoms can manifest in ways that are more "subtle and protracted."[149] Late-onset substance users may not develop physiologic dependence; or nonproblematic users of medications, such as benzodiazepines, may develop physiologic dependence.

[a] SUD is defined as a medical disorder in which 2 or more of the aforementioned listed symptoms are occurring in the last 12 months.[85]

Adapted from Barry KL, Blow FC, Oslin DW. Substance abuse in older adults: review and recommendations for education and practice in medical settings. Subst Abus 2002;23(Suppl 3):105–31; and *Data from* American Psychiatric Association. Diagnostic and statistical manual of mental disorders. 5th edition. Arlington (VA): American Psychiatric Publishing; 2013. p. 491.

Using the Item Response Theory with 2009 National Survey on Drug Use and Health data, one study explored whether there were age-related biases among the criteria for AUD.[86] The findings revealed that there were differential responses among older versus middle-aged adults, such that older adults were half as likely as middle-aged adults to endorse the criteria related to tolerance, activities to obtain alcohol, social/interpersonal problems, and physically hazardous situations. The criteria that were most successful in discriminating AUD among older adults were unsuccessful efforts to cut back, withdrawal, and social and interpersonal problems. With the release and adoption of *DSM-5*, a wider proportion of older adults will likely be classified as having SUD than under the *DSM-IV* criteria; however, a large proportion will likely remain unidentified.[86]

As a result of these diagnostic problems, many who study substance abuse in older adults de-emphasis the reliance on *DSM* criteria to identify problematic substance use requiring intervention. Instead, they use a 2-tier categorical classification: at risk and problem use of substances (**Table 2**).[16] At-risk substance use (also referred to as excessive use or hazardous use)[33] is characterized by those who use substances above the recommended or prescribed levels but who experience few or no physical, mental, emotional, or social problems as a result of use. These individuals may be at high risk for the development of such problems and, therefore, still merit thorough screening and secondary prevention.

Problem substance use is characterized by those individuals who are already experiencing problems in the aforementioned areas as a result of their use. Identification of problem use among older adults does not depend on the quantity and frequency of use but on the context in which substances are used. For example, older adults may experience extreme problems with alcohol even when ingesting it at minimal levels because of medical conditions, such as gout or pancreatitis. Although the terms *at risk* and *problem use* are extremely useful in settings such as primary care, they can pose difficulties in helping older adults access more formal treatment, as third-party

Table 2	
Categorization of substance use among older adults	
Abstinence	No drinking at all and no use of illicit drugs
Low-risk use	Drinking within safety guidelines (7 standard drinks per week, no more than 2 drinks on any one occasion) Only appropriate/prescribed use of prescription or over-the-counter medications No guidelines for low-risk use for illicit drugs
At-risk use (also referred to as unhealthy or hazardous use)	Drinking beyond safety guidelines; drinking while taking medications in which consuming alcohol is contraindicated Intentional or unintentional off-label use of prescription or over-the-counter medications; taking medication, even once in awhile, that is not prescribed directly for that person Any use of illicit substances (primarily because these substance are not quality controlled or standardized)
Problem use	Substance use that results in social, medical, or psychological consequences, regardless of quantity or frequency of substance use[33] Problem user may or may not meet criteria for SUD

payers often require formal SUD diagnoses to justify intensive or more lengthy treatments.

SCREENING AND ASSESSMENT

Historically, older adults are less likely to be screened for substance use.[88,89] For example, in a study of 400 primary care physicians who were provided with a list of symptoms related to problematic substance use by a hypothetical older female patient, only 1% of physicians considered the possibility of a substance use problem.[16] Although there is an increasing acceptance that older adults should be routinely screened for alcohol and other drug use or misuse,[3,12,35] there are several factors that still inhibit screening and subsequent identification of risky alcohol or other drug use, including the limited time clinicians have to screen for several potential problems or illnesses; the potential stigma related to and discomfort assessing for addiction; the similarities of the symptoms of alcohol and other drug use with other illnesses common in later life[69,90]; and the common perception among older adults that symptoms experienced by the use of alcohol or drugs are seen as a part of normal aging rather than resulting from the substance use itself.[91] Furthermore, older adults are known to have difficulty identifying their own risky behaviors around substance use,[42] making the identification of such behavior even more difficult.

Overall Considerations

When assessing or speaking to older adults about substance use, some general considerations should apply. Older adults are known to respond more to a supportive, nonconfrontational approach than more assertive styles of assessment and intervention.[92–94] Older adults are far more likely to provide information about potentially stigmatizing behaviors if they think that the clinician is genuinely interested in their overall health and well-being.[44,90] Discussions of alcohol and other substance use should occur in the context of an overall assessment and in reference to the presenting problem with the goal of health promotion and a complete understanding of their health behaviors. Approaching the assessment with the goal of identifying a drug abuser is likely to stigmatize the older adult, engender defensiveness, and is inconsistent with the idea that any drug or alcohol use has the potential to be problematic.[44] Therefore, in a gentle and respectful manner, detailed questions about quantity and frequency of drinking, medications (prescription and over the counter), and illicit drugs (especially marijuana) should be asked with the assumption that this information is important, whether the older adults' use is a problem or not. This reduces stigma by normalizing the behavior without endorsing it.

Many older adults, and even their families, view alcohol use as being their "one last pleasure,"[83] creating a complex picture of substance use in late life. In a study of alcohol-dependent older adults at a Veteran Affairs medical center, older adults were found to be less strongly motivated to change their drinking than their younger counterparts, as they did not perceive their alcohol use as being particularly severe.[95] For some older adults, a foreshortened sense of future may further inhibit motivation to reduce alcohol use. In addition, self-efficacy to reduce drinking may decline with age,[96] depending on the level of control an older adult perceives in his or her life.[91] In addition, low self-efficacy is related to fewer health-promotion behaviors among older adults because they perceive their physical limitations as an unavoidable component of aging.[91]

Box 2 reviews the potential symptoms or indicators of problematic substance use.

Box 2
Potential indicators of substance misuse and abuse

Physical symptoms or potential indicators

    Falls, bruises, and burns[149]

    Poor hygiene[149] or impaired self-care[69]

    Headaches[149]

    Incontinence[149]

    Increased tolerance to alcohol or medications[149] or unusual response to medications[69]

    Poor nutrition[149]

    Idiopathic seizures[149]

    Dizziness[149]

    Sensory deficits[69]

    Blackouts[69]

    Chronic pain

Cognitive symptoms or potential indicators

    Disorientation[149]

    Memory loss[149]

    Recent difficulties in decision making[149]

    Overall cognitive impairment[69]

Psychiatric symptoms or potential indicators[149]

    Sleep disturbances, problems, or insomnia

    Anxiety

    Depression

    Excessive mood swings

Social symptoms or potential indicators

    Family problems[149]

    Financial problems[149]

    Legal problems[149]

    Social isolation[149]

    Running out of medication early[44]

    Borrowing medication from others[44]

Assessments should start with questions about drinking, medication use, and illicit substances. The focus should be on the facts of substance use rather than questioning the person's judgment (eg, do you have a drinking or drug use problem?).[44] During this discussion, questions about overuse and misuse can be included in a nonjudgmental way.[44] For instance, asking a patient whether they sometimes take an extra pill to fall asleep or to cope with pain, run out of medication early, or borrow medications from others may provide important information and a gateway to further discussion about problematic use of substances.[44] It should be noted that even if the older adult is currently abstinent from alcohol and other drugs, questions about use or misuse in the past are also important, as the answers may indicate increased vulnerability to other psychiatric disorders or cognitive decline.[33]

Screening Tools

Brief screening instruments can assess the level of risk caused by alcohol and drugs. Some screening tools are adaptations of instruments created for younger adults, and others have been designed for older adults. Interview screening tools or global self-report measures are less intrusive or burdensome to the older adult than blood or urine tests. Furthermore, the use of biologic screening (ie, laboratory tests) has limited utility and can be problematic in older adults, as isolating impaired bodily functions (ie, liver function) as the result of alcohol or other substances versus prescribed medications may be difficult. Each of the instruments listed next have strengths and weaknesses related to resources required to implement them or applicability to older adults.

CAGE-Adapted to Include Drugs (CAGE-AID)

The most common screening tool for substance misuse is the CAGE questionnaire, which focuses on the potential for alcohol dependence. The CAGE was later adapted to assess for alcohol *and* other drugs and called the CAGE-AID.[97] The CAGE-AID contains the following 4 questions:

1. Have you ever felt that you should **C**ut down on your drinking or drug use?
2. Have people **A**nnoyed you by criticizing your drinking or drug use?
3. Have you ever felt bad or **G**uilty about your drinking or drug use?
4. Have you ever had a drink or used drugs first thing in the morning to steady your nerves or to get rid of a hangover (**E**ye opener)?

The questions can be adapted to a specific substance, such as a prescription medication, and they can be asked either in the context of an interview or self-administered. One or more positive responses are considered a positive screen. Psychometric properties of the CAGE-AID have not been reported, yet the CAGE has been extensively studied. The CAGE has been validated in an older-adult population, demonstrating as high as 86% sensitivity and 78% specificity for a score of one or more[56,98]; however, the CAGE may identify a different group of drinkers than other measures, such as the Short Michigan Alcoholism Screening Test–Geriatric Version (SMAST-G), and it does poorly in detecting heavy and binge drinkers.[99] Furthermore, it has not performed well in the psychiatric population.[100] A major limitation of the CAGE-AID is that it does not distinguish between current and lifetime use, an especially difficult issue among the aging, who may have a history of problematic use without having a current problem. Because of the brief nature of the CAGE-AID, it can be a useful screening tool; but it should not be a substitute for a more thorough assessment, such as consumption levels, consequences of use, and functional deficits.

The Michigan Alcohol Screening Test-Geriatric Version

The Michigan Alcohol Screening Test-Geriatric Version (MAST-G)[101] is an instrument designed to identify drinking problems and was developed specifically for the elderly by modifying the Michigan Alcohol Screening Test. This screening tool contains 24 questions with yes/no responses; 5 or more positive responses indicate problematic use. The MAST is highly sensitive and specific and generally has strong psychometric properties.[102] It is also administered in a short form, the SMAST-G, which has 10 questions, with 2 positive responses indicating a problem with alcohol. Because of the diagnostic challenges outlined earlier, the MAST-G focuses more on potential stressors and behaviors relevant to alcohol use in late life, as opposed to questions toward family, vocational, and legal consequences of use. This tool has many of the advantages of the CAGE, such as ease of administration and low cost. It is also more specific than the CAGE in identifying problematic use. Although useful as an indicator of lifetime problem use, it lacks information about frequency, quantity, and current problems important for intervention.

The Alcohol Use Disorders Identification Test

Developed by the World Health Organization (WHO), the Alcohol Use Disorders Identification Test (AUDIT) assesses for current alcohol problems.[103] The test consists of 10 questions pertaining to amount and frequency of use, alcohol dependency, and the consequences of alcohol abuse; it can be administered through an interview or self-administered. Each of the 10 questions is scored on a 4-point continuum, with total scores ranging from zero to 40. The AUDIT was validated in older adults to detect problematic or hazardous use.[104] Although the cutoff threshold to indicate AUD among a general population is 8, a cutoff threshold of 5 was identified to indicate AUD among older adults.[100,105] Five items on the AUDIT (items 1, 2, 4, 5, and 10) are particularly sensitive and specific to AUD among older adults and together have outperformed the full AUDIT and the CAGE.[105]

The Alcohol, Smoking, and Substance Involvement Screening Test

The Alcohol, Smoking, and Substance Involvement Screening Test (ASSIST) is another instrument developed by the WHO to screen across substances for potential problem use.[106] It is an interview-based tool that consists of 8 questions that help identify the level of risk to help guide decisions for intervention. The ASSIST has yet to be validated among older adults, and there is at least anecdotal evidence that it underperforms in this population in part because of the same limitations with a formal *DSM* diagnosis; the criteria do not apply in the same way for older adults as they do with younger adults.

The Comorbidity-Alcohol Risk Evaluation Tool

The Comorbidity-Alcohol Risk Evaluation Tool (CARET)[107] is a screening instrument whose precursor is the Short Alcohol Related Problems Survey.[108] It identifies older adults who are at risk because of the quantity and frequency of their alcohol consumption, presence of comorbid diseases, high-risk behaviors (such as drinking and driving), and concomitant use of medications whose efficacy may be diminished or that may interact negatively with alcohol. It has demonstrated good face, content, and criterion validity with older adults.[107–109] One of the strengths of the CARET is that it identifies hazardous alcohol use apart from simply the quantity and frequency of drinking, accounting for a wider spectrum of unhealthy use that could present dangers more common in later life. As a result, the CARET identifies at-risk or problem alcohol use among older adults with more sensitivity than the AUDIT and the MAST-G.[107] Most older adults identified as at-risk drinkers using the CARET are identified as such because of their use of alcohol with medications.[110]

INTERVENTIONS

A continuum of treatment options are available for older adults, depending on the setting and the severity of the problems indicated.[44] Contrary to the assumption that older substance users are stuck in permanent patterns of use, older adults have demonstrated treatment outcomes as good, or better, than those seen in younger groups[111,112]; however, access to specialized services tailored for older adults is limited. A national survey of substance abuse treatment programs found that only about 18% were specifically designed for older adults.[44,113] Even if programs were available to them, overall, mental health utilization rates are lower among older adults than any other age group.[39] Some of the barriers to specialized treatment that older adults face include stigma and shame surrounding substance use and related problems, geographic isolation, inability to pay, or difficulties with transportation.[16,114] Interventions in nontraditional settings, such as emergency rooms, senior centers, and primary care offices,[44,115] have been implemented in an attempt to reach vulnerable older adults outside the formal treatment system.

Because, in part, of the relative invisibility of older-adult substance use and SUD, relatively little published research exists on the efficacy and/or effectiveness of substance abuse treatment of older adults.[112] In a recent review of research on substance abuse treatments for older adults,[112] the researchers found a relative absence of published, rigorous, internally valid research. Therefore, the review of interventions discussed later is of those treatments for which there is some initial evidence of efficacy and/or effectiveness among this population.

Brief Intervention

Effective brief interventions[110,116,117] occur in primary care settings, focus on alcohol and prescription medication misuse or abuse, and vary in length from 15 minutes to five 1-hour sessions.[90,112] Their purpose is to provide education about the substance and how it might be harmful, enhance motivation for change, and connect severe users with more intensive treatments,[42] when necessary. Normative feedback, in which a patient's drinking is compared with his or her peers, combined with brief advice is one of the most common brief interventions used and seems to be highly effective for older-adult drinkers.[19,112,117]

Most brief interventions are described as using aspects of motivational interviewing (MI)[118] or motivational enhancement therapy (MET),[119] which encourages a client-centered, nonjudgmental approach to discussing substance use and encouraging positive, healthy changes to the individual's life. Formal MI and MET aim to reduce ambivalence by assisting the client to identify in his or her own words the perceived pros and cons to making a change versus maintaining the status quo.[44] For the older adult, the reasons for change may include maintaining independence, optimal health, and mental capacity.[90] Although MI and MET are consistent with a nonconfrontational supportive approach, there is little evidence to suggest that formal MI works with older adults in regard to substance use. No studies among those that contributed to establishing MI as an evidenced-based practice included individuals older than 62 years.[120] Some studies demonstrate efficacy of MI with older adults targeting other health behaviors,[121] including smoking cessation[122]; some evidence suggests that it works in the context of case management to engage older adults in more formal treatment.[19] Rigorous controlled trials of older adults and MI, or any other treatment, have yet to be conducted.

Pharmacology

A growing number of pharmacologic treatments can be used for SUD. Most of the research to date with older adults has been done on medications treating smoking cessation and alcohol use. Disulfiram, acamprosate, and naltrexone are medications approved by the Food and Drug Administration that are used to treat SUD; other medications, such as varenicline, are just emerging. Medication options for older adults are more limited than those in the general population, as evidence is lacking still about the efficacy and safety for some of these medications for an older population. Disulfiram is an aversive agent that increases the ill effects of alcohol ingestion by increasing acetaldehyde levels.[123] Although it has been used with adults older than 50 years with some benefit,[124] it has limitations. Disulfiram is only useful with strict adherence to the medication. There is also evidence that it places extra strain on the cardiovascular system within older adults and, thus, may be contraindicated.[123]

Acamprosate is an NMDA and GABA receptor modulator used to reduce craving and the pleasant effects of alcohol.[123,125] No trials have been conducted to examine the efficacy of acamprosate for individuals aged 65 years and older. Because of the few reports of adverse effects across populations, it is considered relatively safe among older adults.[126] In younger adults, 2 to 3 g of acamprosate is the recommended dose[123]; it has been tested in trials of 16 weeks[127] to 1 year in length.[128]

Naltrexone is the most well-studied medication used for SUD treatment among older adults,[112] and it has demonstrated some effectiveness with this population. Naltrexone is an opioid receptor antagonist thought to reduce craving and the pleasurable or stimulating effects of alcohol by blocking alcohol-induced dopamine release in the brain.[123] It can be taken daily or as needed, although only daily treatment of naltrexone has been tested with older adults. The standard dose of naltrexone is 50 mg, but some studies have investigated its effects at larger doses (eg, 100 mg). The major limitation of naltrexone in an older-adult population, many of whom have chronic pain, is that it blocks the effect of opiate-based pain medications. It can also potentiate preexisting major depressive disorder symptoms. Patients with histories of comorbid depression should be closely monitored.

Two randomized controlled trials examined the impact of naltrexone versus placebo on older adults.[129,130] In one study, 44 male veterans aged 50 years and older were randomly assigned to 50 mg/d of naltrexone or placebo and followed for 12 weeks.[129] In addition to the medication, each participant also received weekly group therapy and case management. There were no significant differences between medication conditions on abstinence or relapse rates; however, among those individuals *exposed to alcohol*, older adults on naltrexone were significantly less likely to relapse than those on placebo. In a study of 183 adults,[130] two-thirds of the subjects were randomly assigned to receive 100 mg of naltrexone and one-third to placebo during 3 months of treatment. All participants received a medication management intervention with qualities similar to age-specific treatments, such as a nonconfrontational style.[131] In a post hoc analysis, participants were divided into 2 age groups: 21 to 54 year olds and those 55 years old and older.[130] Older adults demonstrated significantly greater rates of treatment engagement and medication adherence than the younger adults; however, only a trend level difference was found in medication effects between older and younger adults. Small sample sizes of older adults may have impeded the ability to detect significant main effects in both studies.

Varenicline is a nicotinic agonist that is a now widely used to aid smoking cessation.[132,133] It has also recently been applied to alcohol dependence in a similar fashion as naltrexone.[134] Although there are relatively few studies on varenicline with alcohol, existing studies demonstrate a reduction in drinking overall[135] or a reduction in heavy drinking[134] among a general population. No research yet exists on its effect with older adults.

Case Management

Case and care management models, which are offered in primary care settings or community-based agencies, take advantage of nontraditional settings to engage older adults in reducing their use and/or connecting them to treatments.[44] These interventions offer several advantages to an older-adult population. First, they provide a comprehensive approach by addressing the complexity of medical and psychiatric comorbidities common in this population[16,90] while also connecting isolated older adults to needed community resources. Another advantage of these interventions is that substance use interventions are embedded in a broad approach to addressing health, lessening stigma, and also working toward a likely common goal among older adults: overall better health.[16] Program evaluations of this model support the notion that case management is an important tool in working with this population.[136–140] Case management models may be particularly effective at engaging and maintaining older at-risk drinkers in treatment.[138]

Types of Care Available in the Formal Treatment System

As with younger populations, formal substance abuse treatment of older adults is provided on a continuum of intensity depending on problem severity, ranging from detoxification to outpatient treatment or aftercare.[44] All treatment plans should be individualized and flexible according to the specific needs of the client. Because of the unique issues facing older adults, both individual and group treatments are recommended. Although group treatment can reduce isolation and shame related to substance use and is often the preferred method of providing substance abuse treatment, the lack of elder-specific treatment available in the community[113] may actually enhance feelings of isolation and shame in a group context. Older adults may not easily relate to or feel uncomfortable discussing their problems with younger persons. Individual therapy provides a private and confidential forum for older adults to explore their unique issues, without these same risks.

Two psychosocial and psychotherapeutic approaches have been explored specifically in the context of older adults: supportive therapy models (STM)[141] and cognitive-behavioral therapy (CBT).[92–94,142,143] STM represent traditional treatment with age-specific modifications. Twenty-five years ago, STM approaches arose out of a concern about whether older adults could effectively engage in standard treatment.[141] It was observed that confrontational approaches were ill suited and disrespectful to older adults and that the unique issues faced by older individuals, including health conditions, depression comorbidity, and social isolation, went unaddressed.[16] Although it is now widely accepted that confronting denial in any individual about their drug or alcohol use is ineffective in helping individuals modify their behavior to be more healthy,[118] STM were designed to focus on developing a culture of support and successful coping for older-adult substance abusers; supportive therapies concentrate on building social support, improving self-esteem, and taking a global approach to treatment planning through addressing multiple biopsychosocial arenas in the client's life.[44] Although there has been relatively little research on age-specific treatments incorporating these techniques, there is at least some evidence that older adults demonstrate better outcomes in these settings than in nonadapted settings.[112,141,144]

CBT focuses on identifying and altering sequences of thinking, feeling, and behaving that lead to problem drinking or drug use.[145] CBT can be delivered individually or in group settings, and there is strong evidence for positive outcomes across populations and age groups.[146] There is also evidence for the effectiveness of CBT with older adults,[92–94,142,143] and the Substance Abuse and Mental Health Services Association published a CBT treatment manual specific to substance-using older adults.[16] The highly structured, didactic approach taken in CBT may be particularly helpful to older adults because of the tendency to present with memory difficulties.[16] Finally, CBT interventions have outperformed nicotine replacement therapies among older adults participating in a smoking cessation program.[27]

SELF-HELP GROUPS

Alcoholics or Narcotics Anonymous and their related groups can be useful to older adults in reducing isolation, shame, and stigma,[44] though there have been no systematic studies on the effects of these groups on older adults.[147] Older adults may encounter the same barriers to participation in self-help groups as they do with formal treatment: primarily stigma and shame of needing to attend to these issues in late life in the presence of a younger generation. Older generations of older adults whose primary substance is alcohol may also experience more discomfort in attending meetings that include younger polysubstance users,[147] though this may be less of an issue for baby boomers. Furthermore, specific meetings may be more or less suited to older adults given the variation in the pace of meetings and the general focus of the group. Some experts have recommended traditional self-help groups be modified for older adults, such as slowing the pace of the meeting to reflect cognitive changes in aging and devoting attention to handling losses and extending social support.[148] Being aware of elder-friendly meetings in the geographic area may be helpful for intervening with older adults. When referring to self-help groups, it is also important to encourage older adults to try more than one meeting before deciding whether it is a good fit because each meeting has a unique tone and feel.

SUMMARY

The myth that older adults do not use substances and/or do not use substances problematically has been dispelled. Older-adult substance users may not present with the same symptoms as their younger counterparts and, therefore, may be more difficult to identify. Treatment options remain generally limited, as few programs or health care settings offer tailored interventions for older adults. Health care professionals need to continue to do as thorough of assessments as possible and enlist the help of formal measures, Web-based assessment, and build in the questions outlined earlier as routine. As the baby boom generation ages, the health care system will be challenged to provide culturally competent services to this group, as they are a unique generation of older adults. Knowledge about older-adult substance use and the issues that contribute to late onset or maintained addiction in late life will need to be continually updated as we learn how and why this generation of adults uses substances. Furthermore, the advancement and development of interventions that may be more useful for, effective for, and desired by this incoming generation of older adults than previous generation, such as mobile interventions, will be crucial to alleviating the projected pressures on the health care system.

REFERENCES

1. U.S. Census Bureau. Population profile of the United States. 2010. Available at: http://www.census.gov/population/www/pop-profile/natproj.html. Accessed April 11, 2011.
2. World Health Organization. Life expectancy: Life expectancy data by country. 2012. Available at: http://apps.who.int/gho/data/node.main.688?lang=en. Accessed May 13, 2013.
3. Institute of Medicine. The mental health and substance use workforce for older adults: in whose hands? Washington, DC: The National Academies Press; 2012.
4. Cummings SM, Bride B, Rawlins-Shaw AM. Alcohol abuse treatment for older adults: a review of recent empirical research. J Evid Based Soc Work 2006; 3(1):79–99.

5. Substance Abuse and Mental Health Services Administration. Results from the 2012 National Survey on Drug Use and Health: summary of national findings. NSDUH Series H-46, HHS Publication No. (SMA) 13–4795. Rockville (MD): Substance Abuse and Mental Health Services Administration; 2013.

6. Arndt S, Clayton R, Schultz S. Trends in substance abuse treatment 1998-2008: increasing older adult first time admissions for illicit drugs. Am J Geriatr Psychiatry 2011;19:704–11.

7. Atkinson RM. Aging and alcohol use disorders: diagnostic issues in the elderly. Int Psychogeriatr 1990;2(1):55–72.

8. Atkinson RM, Ganzini L. Substance abuse. In: Coffey CE, Cummings JL, editors. Textbook of geriatric neuropsychiatry. Washington, DC: American Psychiatric Press; 1994. p. 297–321.

9. Ekerdt DJ, De Labry LO, Glynn RJ, et al. Change in drinking behaviors with retirement: findings from the Normative Aging Study. J Stud Alcohol 1989; 50(4):347–53.

10. Moore AA, Karno MP, Grella CE, et al. Alcohol, tobacco, and nonmedical drug use in older U.S. adults: data from the 2001/02 National Epidemiologic Survey of Alcohol and Related Conditions. J Am Geriatr Soc 2009;57(12):2275–81.

11. Han B, Gfroerer JC, Colliver JD, et al. Substance use disorder among older adults in the United States in 2020. Addiction 2009;104:88–96.

12. Institute of Medicine. Retooling for an aging America: building the health care workforce. Washington, DC: The National Academies Press; 2008.

13. Jeste DV, Alexopoulos GS, Bartels SJ, et al. Consensus statement on the upcoming crisis in geriatric mental health: research agenda for the next two decades. Arch Gen Psychiatry 1999;56(9):848–53.

14. Moos RH, Schutte KK, Brennan PL, et al. Older adults' alcohol consumption and late-life drinking problems: a 20-year perspective. Addiction 2009;104: 1293–302.

15. Kirchner J, Zubritsky C, Cody M, et al. Alcohol consumption among older adults in primary care. J Gen Intern Med 2007;22:92–7.

16. Center for Substance Abuse Treatment. Substance abuse among older adults: Treatment Improvement Protocol (TIP) Series 26. Rockville (MD): Substance Abuse and Mental Health Services Administration; 1998.

17. Moore AA, Gould R, Reuben DB, et al. Longitudinal patterns and predictors of alcohol consumption in the United States. Am J Public Health 2005;95(3):458–65.

18. Grant BF, Dawson DA, Stinson FS, et al. The 12-month prevalence and trends in DSM-IV alcohol abuse and dependence: United States, 1991–1992 and 2001–2002. Drug Alcohol Depend 2004;74:223–34.

19. Conigliaro J, Kraemer KL, McNeil M. Screening and identification of older adults with alcohol problems in primary care. J Geriatr Psychiatry Neurol 2000;13:106–14.

20. Blazer DG, Wu L. The epidemiology of at risk and binge drinking among middle-aged and elderly community adults: national survey on drug use and health. Am J Psychiatry 2009;166:1162–9.

21. Holroyd S, Duryee JJ. Substance use disorders in a geriatric psychiatry outpatient clinic: prevalence and epidemiologic characteristics. J Nerv Ment Dis 1997;185:627–32.

22. Kennedy GJ, Efremova I, Frazier A, et al. The emerging problems of alcohol and substance abuse in late life. J Soc Distress Homel 1999;8(4):227–39.

23. Merrick EL, Horgan CM, Hodgkin D, et al. Unhealthy drinking patterns in older adults: prevalence and associated characteristics. J Am Geriatr Soc 2008;56: 214–23.

24. Blazer DG, Wu L. The epidemiology of substance use and disorders among middle aged and elderly community adults: national survey on drug use and health. Am J Geriatr Psychiatry 2009;17:237–45.

25. Moore AA, Endo JO, Carter MK. Is there a functional relationship between excessive drinking and functional impairment in older persons? J Am Geriatr Soc 2003;51:44–9.

26. Sorocco KH, Ferrell SW. Alcohol use among older adults. J Genet Psychol 2006; 133(4):453–67.

27. Hall SM, Humfleet GL, Munoz RF, et al. Extended treatment of older cigarette smokers. Addiction 2009;104:1043–52.

28. Rimer B, Orleans CT, Fleisher L, et al. Does tailoring matter? The impact of a tailored guide on ratings and short-term smoking-related outcomes for older adult smokers. Health Educ Res 1994;9:69–84.

29. Blazer DG, Wu LT. Patterns of tobacco use and tobacco-related psychiatric morbidity and substance use among middle-aged and older adults in the United States. Aging Ment Health 2012;16:296–304.

30. Degenhardt L, Dierker L, Chiu WT, et al. Evaluating the drug use "gateway" theory using cross-national data: consistency and associations of the order of initiation of drug use among participants in the WHO World Mental Health Surveys. Drug Alcohol Depend 2010;108(1–2):84–97.

31. Wu LT, Blazer DG. Illicit and nonmedical drug use among older adults: a review. J Aging Health 2011;23:481–504.

32. Blazer DG, Wu L. Nonprescription use of pain relievers by middle-aged and elderly community-living adults: national survey on drug use and health. J Am Geriatr Soc 2009;57:1252–7.

33. Oslin DW, Mavandadi S. Alcohol and drug problems. In: Blazer DG, Steffens DC, editors. Textbook of geriatric psychiatry. Arlington (VA): American Psychiatric Publishing; 2009. p. 1–17.

34. Golden AG, Preston RA, Barnett SD, et al. Inappropriate medication prescribing in homebound older adults. J Am Geriatr Soc 1999;47(8):948–53.

35. Qato DM, Alexander GC, Conti RM, et al. Use of prescription and over-the-counter medications and dietary supplements among older adults in the United States. JAMA 2008;300(24):2867–78.

36. Simoni-Wastila L, Yang HK. Psychoactive drug abuse in older adults. Am J Geriatr Pharmacother 2006;4(4):380–94.

37. Achildi O, Leong SH, Maust DT, et al. Patterns of newly-prescribed benzodiazepines in late life. Am J Geriatr Psychiatry 2013;21(3 Suppl 1):S90–1.

38. Llorente M, David D, Golden AG, et al. Defining patterns of benzodiazepine use in older adults. J Geriatr Psychiatry Neurol 2000;13:150–60.

39. Bartels SJ, Coakley EH, Zubritsky C, et al. Improving access to geriatric mental health services: a randomized trial comparing treatment engagement with integrated versus enhanced referral care for depression, anxiety, and at-risk alcohol use. Am J Psychiatry 2004;161:1455–62.

40. Oslin DW. Alcohol use in late life: disability and comorbidity. J Geriatr Psychiatry Neurol 2000;13:134–40.

41. Gilbertson R, Ceballos NA, Prather R, et al. Effects of acute alcohol consumption in older and younger adults: perceived impairment versus psychomotor performance. J Stud Alcohol Drugs 2009;70(2):242–52.

42. Blow FC, Barry KL. Older patients with at-risk and problem drinking patterns: new developments in brief interventions. J Geriatr Psychiatry Neurol 2000;13: 115–23.

43. Sklar AR, Gilbertson R, Boissoneault J, et al. Differential effects of moderate alcohol consumption on performance among older and younger adults. Alcohol Clin Exp Res 2012;36(12):2150–6.

44. Sacco P, Kuerbis A. Older adults. In: Vaughn MG, Perron BE, editors. Social work practice in the addictions. New York: Springer; 2013. p. 213–29.

45. Thun MJ, Peto R, Lopez AD, et al. Alcohol consumption and mortality among middle-aged and elderly U.S. adults. N Engl J Med 1997;337(24): 1705–14.

46. Mukamal KJ, Kuller LH, Fitzpatrick AL, et al. Prospective study of alcohol consumption and risk of dementia in older adults. JAMA 2003;289(11): 1405–13.

47. Chen LY, Hardy CL. Alcohol consumption and health status in older adults. J Aging Health 2009;21(6):824–47.

48. Kaplan MS, Huguet N, Feeny D, et al. Alcohol use patterns and trajectories of health-related quality of life in middle-aged and older adults: a 14-year population-based study. J Stud Alcohol Drugs 2012;73:581–90.

49. Maraldi C, Harris TB, Newman AB, et al. Moderate alcohol intake and risk of functional decline: the Health, Aging, and Body Composition study. J Am Geriatr Soc 2009;57(10):1767–75.

50. Saitz R. Unhealthy alcohol use. N Engl J Med 2005;352(6):596–607.

51. Moore AA, Whiteman EJ, Ward KT. Risks of combined alcohol/medication use in older adults. Am J Geriatr Pharmacother 2007;5:64–74.

52. Doweiko HE. Concepts of chemical dependency. 6th edition. Pacific Grove (CA): Brooks/Cole; 2006.

53. National Institute on Drug Abuse. Marijuana abuse. Bethesda (MD): National Institute on Drug Abuse; 2012.

54. LaCroix AZ, Guralnik JM, Berkman LF, et al. Maintaining mobility in late life. II. Smoking, alcohol consumption, physical activity and body mass index. Am J Epidemiol 1993;137(8):858–69.

55. LaCroix AZ, Omenn GS. Older adults and smoking. Clin Geriatr Med 1992;8(1): 69–87.

56. Stewart D, Oslin DW. Recognition and treatment of late-life addictions in medical settings. Journal of Clinical Geropsychology 2001;7(2):145–58.

57. Platt A, Sloan FA, Costanzo P. Alcohol-consumption trajectories and associated characteristics among adults older than age 50. J Stud Alcohol Drugs 2010;71: 169–79.

58. Moos RH, Brennan PL, Schutte KK, et al. Older adults' health and late-life drinking patterns: a 20-year perspective. Aging Ment Health 2010;14(1):33–43.

59. Collins PM, Kayser K, Platt S. Conjoint marital therapy: a practitioner's approach to single-system evaluation. Fam Soc 1994;75:131–41.

60. Perriera KM, Sloan FA. Life events and alcohol consumption among mature adults: a longitudinal analysis. J Stud Alcohol 2001;62:501–8.

61. Sacco P, Bucholz KK, Spitznagel EL. Alcohol use among older adults in the National Epidemiologic Survey on Alcohol and Related Conditions. J Stud Alcohol Drugs 2009;70(6):829–38.

62. Balsa AI, Homer JF, Fleming MF, et al. Alcohol consumption and health among elders. Gerontologist 2008;48(5):622–36.

63. Speer DC, Bates K. Comorbid mental and substance disorders among older psychiatric patients. J Am Geriatr Soc 1992;40:886–90.

64. Oslin DW. Treatment of late-life depression complicated by alcohol dependence. Am J Geriatr Psychiatry 2005;13(6):491–500.

65. Blow FC, Cook CL, Booth BM, et al. Age-related psychiatric comorbidities and level of functioning in alcoholic veterans seeking outpatient treatment. Hosp Community Psychiatry 1992;43:990–5.

66. Lin JC, Karno MP, Grella CE, et al. Psychiatric correlates of alcohol and tobacco use disorders in U.S. adults aged 65 years and older: results from the 2001-2002 National Epidemiologic Survey of Alcohol and Related Conditions. Am J Geriatr Pharmacology 2013. Epub ahead of print.

67. Wu LT, Blazer DG. Substance use disorders and psychiatric comorbidity in mid and later life: a review. Int J Epidemiol 2014;43(2):304–17.

68. Adlaf EM, Smart RG. Alcohol use, drug use, and well-being in older adults in Toronto. Int J Addict 1995;30(13–14):1985–2016.

69. Dar K. Alcohol use disorders in elderly people: fact or fiction? Adv Psychiatr Treat 2006;12:173–81.

70. Thomas VS, Rockwood KJ. Alcohol abuse, cognitive impairment, and mortality among older people. J Am Geriatr Soc 2001;49:415–20.

71. Moore AA, Giuli L, Gould R, et al. Alcohol use, comorbidity, and mortality. J Am Geriatr Soc 2006;54:757–62.

72. Moos RH, Schutte KK, Brennan PL, et al. Late-life and life history predictors of older adults' high risk consumption and drinking problems. Drug Alcohol Depend 2010;108:13–20.

73. Adams WL. Alcohol use in the retirement communities. J Am Geriatr Soc 1996; 44:1082–5.

74. Brennan PL, Schutte KK, Moos RH. Reciprocal relations between stressors and drinking behavior: a three-wave panel study of late middle-aged and older women and men. Addiction 1999;94(5):737–49.

75. Center for Substance Abuse Treatment. Substance abuse relapse prevention for older adults: a group treatment approach. Rockville (MD): Substance Abuse and Mental Health Services Administration; 2005.

76. Myers JE, Harper MC. Evidence-based effective practices with older adults. J Couns Dev 2004;82:207–18.

77. Laidlaw K, Pachana NA. Aging, mental health, and demographic change: challenges for psychotherapists. PrPsychol Res Pract 2009;40(6):601–8.

78. Kuerbis A, Sacco P. The impact of retirement on the drinking patterns of older adults: a review. Addict Behav 2012;37:587–95.

79. Bacharach SB, Bamberger PA, Cohen A, et al. Retirement, social support, and drinking behavior: a cohort analysis of males with a baseline history of problem drinking. J Drug Issues 2007;37(3):525–48.

80. Stergiopoulos V, Herrmann N. Old and homeless: a review and survey of older adults who use shelters in an urban setting. Can J Psychiatry 2003;48(6): 374–80.

81. Joseph CL. Alcohol and drug misuse in the nursing home. Int J Addict 1995; 30(13–14):1953–84.

82. Joseph CL, Atkinson RM, Ganzini L. Problem drinking among residents of a VA nursing home. Int J Geriatr Psychiatry 1995;10(3):243–8.

83. Klein WC, Jess C. One last pleasure? Alcohol use among elderly people in nursing homes. Health Soc Work 2002;27(3):193–203.

84. American Psychiatric Association. Diagnostic and statistical manual of mental disorders. 4th edition. Washington, DC: Author; 2000.

85. American Psychiatric Association. Diagnostic and statistical manual of mental disorders. 5th edition. Arlington (VA): American Psychiatric Publishing; 2013.

86. Kuerbis A, Hagman BT, Sacco P. Functioning of alcohol use disorders criteria among middle-aged and older adults: implications for DSM-5. Subst Use Misuse 2013;48(4):309–22.

87. Moody HR. Aging: concepts and controversies. 5th edition. Thousand Oaks (CA): Pine Forge; 2006.

88. Duru OK, Xu H, Tseng CH, et al. Correlates of alcohol-related discussions between older adults and their physicians. J Am Geriatr Soc 2010;58(12): 2369–74.

89. D'Amico EJ, Paddock SM, Burnam A, et al. Identification of and guidance for problem drinking by general medical providers: results from a national survey. Med Care 2005;43(3):229–36.

90. Barry KL, Oslin DW, Blow FC. Alcohol problems in older adults. New York: Springer Publishing Company; 2001.

91. Rodin J. Aging and health: effects of the sense of control. Science 1986;233: 1271–6.

92. Dupree LW, Broskowski H, Schonfeld L. The Gerontology Alcohol Project: a behavioral treatment program for elderly alcohol abusers. Gerontologist 1984; 24:510–6.

93. Schonfeld L, Dupree LW. Treatment approaches for older problem drinkers. Int J Addict 1995;30(13–14):1819–42.

94. Schonfeld L, Dupree LW, Dickson-Fuhrman E, et al. Cognitive-behavioral treatment of older veterans with substance abuse problems. J Geriatr Psychiatry Neurol 2000;13:124–8.

95. Lemke S, Moos RH. Prognoses of older patients in mixed-age alcoholism treatment programs. J Subst Abuse Treat 2002;22:33–4.

96. Gecas V. The social psychology of self-efficacy. Am Rev Sociol 1989;15: 291–316.

97. Brown RL, Rounds LA. Conjoint screening questionnaires for alcohol and other drug abuse. Wis Med J 1995;94(3):135–40.

98. Buchsbaum DG, Buchanan R, Welsh J, et al. Screening for drinking disorders in the elderly using the CAGE questionnaire. J Am Geriatr Soc 1992;40:662–5.

99. Adams W, Barry KL, Fleming MF. Screening for problem drinking in older primary care patients. JAMA 1996;276:1964–7.

100. O'Connell H, Chin AV, Hamilton F, et al. A systematic review of the utility of self-report alcohol screening instruments in the elderly. Int J Geriatr Psychiatry 2004; 19:1074–86.

101. Blow FC, Brower KJ, Schulenberg JE, et al. The Michigan Alcohol Screening Test: Geriatric Version (MAST-G): a new elderly specific screening instrument. Alcohol Clin Exp Res 1992;16:172.

102. Barry KL, Blow FC. Screening, assessing and intervening for alcohol and medication misuse in older adults. In: Lichtenberg PA, editor. Handbook of assessment in clinical gerontology. Burlington (MA): Elsevier; 2010. p. 307–30.

103. Babor TF, Higgins-Biddle JC, Saunders JB, et al. The Alcohol Use Disorders Identification Test (AUDIT): guidelines for use in primary care. 2nd edition. Geneva (Switzerland): Department of Mental Health and Substance Dependence, World Health Organization; 2001.

104. Beullens J, Aertgeerts B. Screening for alcohol abuse and dependence in older people using DSM criteria: a review. Aging Ment Health 2004;8(1):76–82.

105. Piccinelli M, Tessari E, Bortolomasi M, et al. Efficacy of the alcohol use disorders identification test as a screening tool for hazardous alcohol intake and related disorders in primary care: a validity study. BMJ 1997;314(8):420–4.

106. Humeniuk R, Henry-Edwards S, Ali R, et al. The alcohol, smoking, and substance involvement screening test (ASSIST). Geneva (Switzerland): World Health Organization; 2010.

107. Moore AA, Beck JC, Babor TF, et al. Beyond alcoholism: identifying older, at-risk drinkers in primary care. J Stud Alcohol 2002;63(3):316–24.

108. Fink A, Morton SC, Beck JC, et al. The Alcohol-Related Problems Survey: identifying hazardous and harmful drinking in older primary care patients. J Am Geriatr Soc 2002;50:1717–22.

109. Barnes AJ, Moore AA, Xu H, et al. Prevalence and correlates of at-risk drinking among older adults: the project SHARE study. J Gen Intern Med 2010;25(8): 840–6.

110. Moore AA, Blow FC, Hoffing M, et al. Primary care-based intervention to reduce at-risk drinking in older adults: a randomized controlled trial. Addiction 2011; 106(1):111–20.

111. Brennan PL, Nichol AC, Moos RH. Older and younger patients with substance use disorders: outpatient mental health service use and functioning over a 12-month interval. Psychol Addict Behav 2003;17(1):42–8.

112. Kuerbis AN, Sacco P. A review of existing treatments for substance abuse among the elderly and recommendations for future directions. Subst Abuse 2013;7:13–37.

113. Schultz SK, Arndt S, Liesveld J. Locations of facilities with special programs for older substance abuse clients in the US. Int J Geriatr Psychiatry 2003;18(9): 839–43.

114. Fortney JC, Booth BM, Blow FC, et al. The effects of travel barriers and age on utilization of alcoholism treatment aftercare. Am J Drug Alcohol Abuse 1995; 21(3):391–407.

115. Schonfeld L, King-Kallimanis BL, Duchene DM, et al. Screening and brief intervention for substance misuse among older adults: the Florida BRITE project. Am J Public Health 2010;100(1):108–14.

116. Fleming MF, Manwell LB, Barry KL, et al. Brief physician advice for alcohol problems in older adults: a randomized community-based trial. J Fam Pract 1999; 48(5):378–84.

117. Fink A, Elliot MN, Tsai M, et al. An evaluation of an intervention to assist primary care physicians in screening and educating older patients who use alcohol. J Am Geriatr Soc 2005;53:1937–43.

118. Miller WR, Rollnick S. Motivational interviewing: preparing people for change. 2nd edition. New York: The Guilford Press; 2002.

119. Miller WR, Zweben A, DiClemente CC, et al. Motivational enhancement therapy manual: a clinical research guide for therapists treating individuals with alcohol abuse and dependence. Rockville (MD): National Institute on Alcohol Abuse and Alcoholism; 1992.

120. Hettema J, Steele J, Miller WR. Motivational interviewing. Annu Rev Clin Psychol 2005;1:91–111.

121. Cummings SM, Cooper RL, Cassie KM. Motivational interviewing to affect behavioral change in older adults. Res Soc Work Pract 2009;19(2):195–204.

122. Hokanson JM, Anderson RL, Hennrikus DJ, et al. Integrated tobacco cessation counseling in a diabetes self-management training program: a randomized trial of diabetes and reduction of tobacco. Diabetes Educ 2006;32: 562–70.

123. Barrick C, Connors GD. Relapse prevention and maintaining abstinence in older adults with alcohol-use disorders. Drugs Aging 2002;19(8):583–94.

124. Garbutt JC, West SL, Carey TS, et al. Pharmacological treatment of alcohol dependence: a review of the evidence. JAMA 1999;281(14):1318–25.

125. Tempesta E, Janiri L, Bignamini A, et al. Acamprosate and relapse prevention in the treatment of alcohol dependence: a placebo controlled trial. Pharmacopsychiatry 2000;29:27–9.

126. U.S. National Library of Congress. DailyMed. 2013. Available at: http://dailymed.nlm.nih.gov/dailymed/about.cfm. Accessed May 4, 2013.

127. Anton R, O'Malley SS, Ciraulo DA, et al. Combined pharmacotherapies and behavioral interventions for alcohol dependence. The COMBINE study: a randomized controlled trial. JAMA 2006;295:2003–17.

128. Rubio G, Jimenez-Arriero MA, Ponce G, et al. Naltrexone versus acamprosate: one year follow up of alcohol dependence treatment. Alcohol Alcohol 2001; 36(5):419–25.

129. Oslin DW, Liberto JG, O'Brien J, et al. Naltrexone as an adjunctive treatment for older patients with alcohol dependence. Am J Geriatr Psychiatry 1997;5(4):324–32.

130. Oslin DW, Pettinati H, Volpicelli JR. Alcoholism treatment adherence: older age predicts better adherence and drinking outcomes. Am J Geriatr Psychiatry 2002;10(6):740–7.

131. Volpicelli JR, Pettinati HM, McLellan AT, et al. Combining medication and psychosocial treatment for addiction: the BRENDA approach. New York (NY): Guilford Press; 2001.

132. Keating GM, Lyseng-Williamson KA. Varenicline: a pharmacoeconomic review of its use as an aid to smoking cessation. Pharmacoeconomics 2010;28(3): 231–54.

133. Garrison GD, Dugan SE. Varenicline: a first-line treatment option for smoking cessation. Clin Ther 2009;31(3):463–91.

134. Plebani JG, Lynch KG, Rennert L, et al. Results from a pilot clinical trial of varenicline for the treatment of alcohol dependence. Drug Alcohol Depend 2013;133(2):754–8.

135. Litten RZ, Ryan ML, Fertig JB, et al. A double-blind, placebo-controlled trial assessing the efficacy of varenicline tartrate for alcohol dependence. J Addict Med 2013;7(4):277–86.

136. Lee HS, Mericle AA, Ayalon L, et al. Harm reduction among at-risk elderly drinkers: a site-specific analysis from the multi-site primary care research in substance abuse and mental health for elderly (PRISM-E) study. Int J Geriatr Psychiatry 2009;24(1):54–60.

137. Levkoff SE, Chen H, Coakley E, et al. Design and sample characteristics of the PRISM-E multisite randomized trial to improve behavioral health care for the elderly. J Aging Health 2004;16:3–27.

138. Oslin DW, Grantham S, Coakley E, et al. PRISM-E: comparison of integrated care and enhanced specialty referral in managing at-risk alcohol use. Psychiatr Serv 2006;57(7):954–8.

139. Zanjani F, Mavandadi S, TenHave T, et al. Longitudinal course of substance treatment benefits in older male veteran at-risk drinkers. J Gerontol A Biol Sci Med Sci 2008;63A(1):98–106.

140. D'Agostino CS, Barry KL, Blow FC, et al. Community interventions for older adults with comorbid substance use: the Geriatrics Addiction Program (GAP). J Dual Diagn 2006;2(3):31–43.

141. Kofoed LL, Tolson RL, Atkinson RM, et al. Treatment compliance of older alcoholics: an elder-specific approach is superior to "mainstreaming". J Stud Alcohol 1987;48:47–51.

142. Rice C, Longabaugh R, Beattie M, et al. Age group differences in response to treatment for problematic alcohol use. Addiction 1993;88:1369–75.

143. Schonfeld L, Dupree LW. Age-specific cognitive behavioral and self-management treatment approaches. In: Gurnack AM, Atkinson RM, Osgood NJ, editors. Treating alcohol and drug abuse in the elderly. New York: Springer Publishing Company; 2002. p. 109–30.

144. Kashner M, Rodell DE, Ogden SR, et al. Outcomes and costs of two VA inpatient treatment programs for older adult alcoholic patients. Hosp Community Psychiatry 1992;43:985–9.

145. Rotgers F. Cognitive-behavioral theories of substance abuse. In: Rotgers F, Morgenstern J, Walters ST, editors. Treating substance abuse: theory and technique. 2nd edition. New York: The Guilford Press; 2003. p. 166–89.

146. Morgenstern J, McKay J. Rethinking the paradigms that inform behavioral treatment research for substance use disorders. Addiction 2007;102:1377–89.

147. Atkinson RM, Misra S. Further strategies in the treatment of aging alcoholics. In: Gurnack AM, Atkinson RM, Osgood NJ, editors. Treating alcohol and drug abuse in the elderly. New York: Springer; 2002. p. 131–51.

148. Schonfeld L, Dupree LW. Treatment alternatives for older adults. In: Gurnack AM, editor. Older adults' misuse of alcohol, medicine, and other drugs. New York: Springer; 1997. p. 113–31.

149. Barry KL, Blow FC, Oslin DW. Substance abuse in older adults: review and recommendations for education and practice in medical settings. Subst Abus 2002;23(Suppl 3):105–31.

Community Treatment of Older Adults

Principles and Evidence Supporting Mental Health Service Interventions

Whitney L. Carlson, MD*, Mark Snowden, MD, MPH

KEYWORDS

- Depression • Older adult • Mental health services • Nursing home

KEY POINTS

- Effective models of evidence-based treatment for depression and severe and persistent mental illness exist, but access has been limited by slow implementation and application in real-world settings.
- Despite evidence-based treatment for these conditions, many individuals do not respond to such treatment or have been excluded from research studies.
- A recent focus of qualitative research has been to investigate the barriers to engaging difficult-to-reach populations.
- Training and supervising those who work with the geriatric population to use and develop interventions in nontraditional research settings could help leverage the expertise of limited geriatric psychiatry specialists.

INTRODUCTION

The Institute of Medicine Committee on the Mental Health Workforce for Geriatric Populations noted that while precise prevalence rates are not known, reasonable estimates based on available data suggest that 14% to 20% of the overall elderly population of the United States has one of the 27 Diagnostic and Statistical Manual (DSM) and other conditions it identified as significant mental health- or substance use-related disorders.[1] Depressive disorders are the most common, followed by dementia-related psychiatric and behavioral symptoms. Depression broadly impacts quality of life, medical costs, mortality, and functional independence of older adults. Prevalence estimates for major depression in older adults range from 1% to 4%.[2] Rates of minor depression range from 8% to 16% of older age population-based samples and occur

Department of Psychiatry and Behavioral Sciences, University of Washington School of Medicine, 325 Ninth Avenue, Seattle, WA 98104-2499, USA
* Corresponding author.
E-mail address: cwhitney@u.washington.edu

Clin Geriatr Med 30 (2014) 655–661
http://dx.doi.org/10.1016/j.cger.2014.04.010   geriatric.theclinics.com

in twice as many home-bound elders.[2–6] Those with minor depression are 5 times more likely than nondepressed individuals to develop major depression and develop similar rates of hopelessness and death or suicidal ideation even though they have fewer depressive symptoms.[7–9]

Antidepressants and several forms of psychotherapy have been shown to effectively treat depression in older adults; yet system gaps result in inadequate treatment for many patients. The high prevalence of depression in older people, good evidence for treatment efficacy, widely recognized problems of underdiagnosis and undertreatment, and the limited supply of psychiatrists have spurred development and testing of new models of depression care that extend access to individuals who would not otherwise be treated. Health services research has focused on ways to structure and implement existing depression treatments into system-based interventions that improve outcomes compared with usual care approaches. These models increasingly rely on interventionists employed by community agencies, and redefine the role of psychiatrists as expert caseload supervisors rather than providers of direct care. Depression care management interventions in clinic and community settings are discussed here in terms of quantitative outcomes and qualitative studies of ongoing implementation challenges.

Community-based organizations serve large numbers of depressed older adults. For example, in an analysis of 2005 Washington statewide data for clients 60 years and older (N = 16,032) being evaluated for receipt of home- and community-based services by Aging and Disability Services Administration case workers using the Centers for Epidemiological Studies Depression Scale 10-item version, 27% had scores of 10 or greater, suggesting major depression, and 35% had scores between 6 to 10 felt to be consistent with minor or subsyndromal depression. In nursing homes, rates of clinically significant depression are estimated to be between 27% and 34%.[10,11] Like major depression, minor depression is linked to impaired functional status, increased service use, and poorer physical, social, and mental health[12] and impacts performance of activities of daily living needed for maintaining independence.[13] Depression can increase mortality unrelated to suicide.[14] Ambulatory medical costs in depressed older adults have been shown to be 43% to 51% higher and inpatient ambulatory total costs 47% to 51% higher in older adults with depression.[15] Reducing the number of adults with major depressive disorder is a major objective of Healthy People 2020.[16]

More severe and persistent mental illnesses such as schizophrenia, although much more rare than depression, with estimates of 0.2%–0.8% of all elderly, have significantly greater negative impact on function.[1] Because of their greater care needs, individuals with these illnesses continue to experience higher rates of institutional care, with nursing home prevalence rates exceeding 10%.[10]

HEALTH SERVICE INTERVENTIONS
Home-Based Care for Depression

Effective treatment for depression in older adults through collaborative care depression care management models in primary care has been demonstrated in several randomized controlled trials such as Improving Mood-Promoting Access to Collaborative Treatment (IMPACT)[17] and Prevention of Suicide in Primary Care: Collaborative Treatment (PROSPECT).[18] However, many depressed older adults are socially isolated, have significant medical comorbidity and impaired physical functioning, and may be homebound. These groups are less able to seek appropriate care for depression via clinic-based models even where collaborative care has been implemented. The

Program for Enhancing Active Rewarding Lives for Seniors (PEARLS) program is a home-based depression care management intervention that was designed in partnership with an Area Agency on Aging home and community services case management program for homebound, frail older adults aged 60 and older with chronic medical conditions who were identified as having symptoms of depression. PEARLS has been shown in 2 randomized controlled trials (RCTs), one involving adults aged 60 and older[19] and one involving all age adults with epilepsy,[20,21] to effectively reduce symptoms of depression and increase rates of remission of symptoms over usual care for minor depression, dysthymia, and major depression. Home health agencies represent another means of providing community-based depression treatment for homebound elders. The program, Training in Assessment of Depression (TRIAD), was shown to effectively train home health nurses to assess depression and increase appropriate referrals for treatment.[22] Patients referred in this manner experienced improved depression outcomes as measured with 24-item Hamilton Depression Rating scale.

Barriers to Effectiveness of Mental Health Services Interventions

Even with these evidence-based approaches to organizing care, significant numbers of patients do not respond as hoped, with estimates that half of subjects do not achieve the target of 50% reduction in depression scale score. What is to be done with these patients in real-world settings, or those who do not meet the typical eligibility requirements of the research study conditions (eg, those with coexisting moderate or more severe dementia)? Current integrated care models are increasingly using the psychiatric supervisor of the care manager to provide step-up direct patient care of these difficult-to-treat patients.

Recent qualitative studies have been conducted to identify benefits and barriers to implementation of PEARLS and strategies to overcome the barriers.[23,24] Barriers to program implementation have included enrollment criteria, carried over from effectiveness trials, which exclude clients who do not speak English, have comorbid psychiatric conditions or substance abuse disorders, and are younger-aged yet homebound, depressed, and often disabled. Focus groups identified the need to broaden eligibility criteria to address such barriers. A second study worked with 3 social service agencies to identify hard-to-reach populations, barriers to reaching them, and strategies for improving recruitment to the PEARLS program.[24] This study identified veterans, African Americans, Filipino men, other immigrants and non-English speaking clients, older-old adults (75 years of age and older), those residing in rural communities, people with limited education, recent retirees, people in assisted living and retirement communities, members of the lesbian, gay, bisexual, transgender community, and caregivers as hard-to-reach populations. Issues around trust and culturally appropriate treatment approaches, starting from a point acceptable to the client in terms of overall acceptance of depression, and strategies to address it in a flexible way were identified as barriers to participation and ways to overcome these barriers. Partnering with trusted organizations and leaders who work with these communities (such as religious leaders, veterans' organizations, community and senior centers, senior housing units, and other health care and social service agencies) was 1 potential strategy identified to reach and engage these populations.

Effective programs for treatment of substance use conditions (Screening, Brief Interventions and Referral for Treatment [SBIRT]) and programs for persons with severe and persistent mental disorders such as schizophrenia (Helping Older Persons Experience Success [HOPES]) exist and are highlighted in the Institute of Medicine report.[1] Each of them share the common, real-world implementation challenges of depression care management programs highlighted in detail previously, involving slowness of program dissemination and diffusion that ultimately hinder reaching clients in need of service and adoption by organizations capable of offering the intervention, as well as challenges regarding treatment of those with less than robust or ideal responses. The solutions to these challenges will differ based on the individual program and locales, but in broad terms will require: (1) balancing program fidelity with flexibility; (2) mainstream maintenance funding for services versus pilot development mechanisms; and (3) creation of next-step referral and treatment options. Increasingly, the role for the limited supply of geriatric psychiatrists will be to provide treatment for patients who have not fully benefitted from initial treatment by other providers.

A Special Population: Residents of Long-term Care Facilities

Older adults residing in adult family homes, assisted living facilities, and nursing homes are also vulnerable to depression; however, evidence-based treatment intervention studies are significantly lacking among these populations. Rates of depression range from 15% to 50% depending on study methodology.[1] Despite high rates of antidepressant use in nursing home residents, 20% of residents prescribed an antidepressant have clinically significant symptoms of depression, suggesting a need for increased monitoring and stepped care treatment algorithms and protocols and evidence-based studies of outcomes.[25] Current federal and state regulations do not require the availability of specialized mental health personnel or that nursing home staff demonstrate minimum competency in the care of geriatric mental health issues. Survey statistics indicate that only 25% of nursing homes have mental health providers on staff, and only 24% use on-call providers.[26] These findings point to a serious gap in mental health services for the significant numbers of nursing home residents who have symptoms of depression and other chronic mental illness.

Patients with severe and persistent mental illness such as bipolar disorder, schizophrenia, and schizoaffective disorder frequently reside in nursing homes, with some estimates of the prevalence rate of schizophrenia reaching as high as 17% of residents.[10] Nursing home placement of these patients is typically related to consequences of physical health problems, which develop in part as a result of poor engagement in primary and preventive care, as well as poorly sustained treatment of their chronic mental disorders.

Proposed Collaborative Care Management for Depression in Nursing Homes

The use of a care management intervention, based on models used successfully in primary care, has been proposed as 1 way to improve identification and treatment for residents in the nursing home setting. Because of limitations on access to specialty psychiatric care on site at nursing homes, the identification and training of a nursing home staff member, possibly a nurse, in the role of a depression care manager who could be supervised by a psychiatrist has been proposed. Although nursing homes are essentially alternative primary care settings for most residents—suggesting that the principles of collaborative care should apply—the frailty and high rates of cognitive impairment in nursing home residents have made research in this setting extremely difficult.[27]

Therefore, existing approaches to the care of depressed (as well as severely mentally ill) patients in nursing homes center upon continued revision and modification of care approaches defined in the 1987 Nursing Home Reform Act. The latest iteration of the Minimum Data Set (MDS 3.0) includes more evidence-based approaches to screening and identification of depression, with the incorporation of the PHQ-9 (Patient Health Questionnaire) and Geriatric Depression Scale and the Brief Interview for Mental Status (BIMS). However, as has been noted in prior research and incorporated into the recommendations of the US Preventive Services Task Force recommendations, screening for depression without organized systems for accurate diagnosis and effective treatment has not been shown to improve outcomes.[28] Nursing homes have improved management of decubitus ulcers by combining MDS assessment approaches with wound care team intervention, and the possibility exists for doing the same for depression. An identified care manager would need to manage the initiation and adjustment of antidepressant medications when these are recommended. This model would most likely be more accepted by primary care providers if they and the facility medical director were directly involved in establishing the antidepressant algorithms, perhaps with psychiatric consultation to develop such protocols.

Nursing Homes and Management of Severe and Persistent Mental Illness

Among the challenges of caring for nursing home residents with disorders such as schizophrenia or bipolar mood disorder are federally mandated nursing home regulations that require systematic evaluation of the use of psychotropic medications and recommendations for gradual dose reductions at specified intervals over time. Dose reductions in medications such as antipsychotics, antidepressants, and mood stabilizers in those with persistent mental illness impose risks of psychiatric decompensation if applied universally without regard to the longitudinal history of an individual resident's psychiatric history and response to such medications. Regulatory requirements, combined with the limited education and training staff of nursing homes receive in the recognition and management of symptoms of psychiatric illness and decompensation, impede the ongoing care of such patients. Recent changes in nursing home regulations that allow for continuation of antipsychotics, antidepressants, and mood stabilizers, when used in accordance to standard of care practice, are a substantial improvement, but presume knowledge of the standard treatment of these conditions that may be beyond the expertise of many primary care providers working in nursing homes. The consultative model of care from a psychiatric specialist remains the most evidence-based approach to care for nursing home residents with severe and persistent mental illness; yet shortages of geriatric psychiatry specialists threatens the viability of this model. Some have proposed more aggressive evaluation for community placement of patients with psychotic disorders.[29] Evidence from prior evaluation of the Preadmission Screening program (PASRR) also indicates that significant numbers of mentally ill nursing home residents were felt appropriate for discharge to less restrictive alternate dispositions. However, a significant limitation of the legislation is that screening programs like PASRR have little ability to follow up or assure compliance with recommendations.[30]

SUMMARY

The increased numbers of people in the geriatric demographic increases the urgency of implementing and disseminating effective models of mental health treatment that have already been developed. Research on strategies to overcome existing barriers to their use, and to extend their reach to new populations and health care settings, is necessary, but limited by funding for such research and models of care. Implementation is limited by the need for significant education and training of primary care providers and health systems, caregivers, families, and administrators of long-term care settings in the importance of identifying and fully treating identified mental health disorders such as depression, as well as the need to develop more effective models for the use of limited specialty mental health resources.

REFERENCES

1. Institute of Medicine (IOM). The mental health and substance use workforce for older adults: in whose hands? Washington, DC: The National Academies Press; 2012.
2. Blazer DG. Depression in late life: review and commentary. J Gerontol A Biol Sci Med Sci 2004;58(3):249–65.
3. Ell K, Unutzer J, Aranda M, et al. Routine PHQ-9 depression screening in home health care: depression, prevalence, clinical and treatment characteristics and screening implementation. Home Health Care Serv Q 2005;24(4):1–19.
4. Banerjee S, Macdonald AJ. Mental disorder in an elderly home care population: associations with health and social service use. Br J Psychiatry 1996;168:750–6.
5. Raue PJ, Meyers BS, Rowe JL, et al. Suicidal ideation among elderly homecare patients. Int J Geriatr Psychiatry 2007;22(1):32–7.
6. Bruce ML, McNamara R. Psychiatric status among the homebound elderly: an epidemiologic perspective. J Am Geriatr Soc 1992;40(6):561–6.
7. Lyness JM, Heo M, Datto CJ, et al. Outcomes of minor and subsyndromal depression among elderly patients in primary care settings. Ann Intern Med 2006;144(7):496–504.
8. Geiselmann B, Bauer M. Subthreshold depression in the elderly: qualitative or quantitative distinction? Compr Psychiatry 2000;41(2 Suppl 1):32–8.
9. Chopra MP, Zubritsky C, Knott K, et al. Importance of subsyndromal symptoms of depression in elderly patients. Am J Geriatr Psychiatry 2005;13(7):597–606.
10. Lemke SP, Schaefer JA. Recent changes in the prevalence of psychiatric disorders among VA nursing home residents. Psychiatr Serv 2010;61(4):356–63.
11. Jones A. The National Nursing Home survey: 1999 summary. Vital Health Stat 2002;13(152):1–116.
12. Wagner HR, Burns BJ, Broadhead WE, et al. Minor depression in family practice: functional morbidity, co-morbidity, service utilization and outcomes. Psychol Med 2000;30(6):1377–90.
13. Bruce ML. The association between depression and disability. Am J Geriatr Psychiatry 1999;7:8–11.
14. Katon WJ, Rutter C, Simon G, et al. The association of comorbid depression with mortality in patients with type 2 diabetes. Diabetes Care 2005;28(11):2668–72.
15. Katon WJ, Lin E, Russo J, et al. Increased medical costs of a population-based sample of depressed elderly patients. Arch Gen Psychiatry 2003;60(9):897–903.
16. US Department of Health and Human Services. Office of Disease Prevention and Health Promotion. Healthy People 2020. Washington, DC. Available at: http://www.healthypeople.gov/2020/default.aspx.
17. Unutzer J, Katon W, Callahan CM, et al. Collaborative care management of late-life depression in the primary care setting: a randomized controlled trial. JAMA 2002;288(22):2836–45.
18. Bruce ML, Ten Have TR, Reynolds CF, et al. Reducing suicidal ideation and depressive symptoms in depressed older primary care patients: a randomized controlled trial. JAMA 2004;291:1081–91.
19. Ciechanowski P, Wagner E, Schmaling K, et al. Community-integrated home-based depression treatment in older adults: a randomized controlled trial. JAMA 2004;291(13):1569–77.
20. Ciechanowski P, Chaytor N, Miller J, et al. PEARLS depression treatment for individuals with epilepsy: a randomized controlled trial. Epilepsy Behav 2010;19(3):225–31.

21. Chaytor N, Ciechanowski P, Miller J, et al. Long-term outcomes from the PEARLS randomized trial for the treatment of depression in patients with epilepsy. Epilepsy Behav 2011;20(3):545–9.

22. Bruce ML, Brown EL, Raue PJ, et al. A randomized trial of depression assessment intervention in home health care. J Am Geriatr Soc 2007;55(11): 1793–800.

23. Steinman L, Cristofalo M, Snowden M. Implementation of an evidence-based depression care management program (PEARLS). Prev Chronic Dis 2012;9:E91.

24. Steinman L, Hammerback K, Snowden M. It could be a pearl to you: exploring recruitment and retention of the program to encourage active, rewarding lives (PEARLS) with hard-to-reach populations. Gerontologist 2013. [Epub ahead of print].

25. Datto CJ, Oslin DW, Streim JE, et al. Pharmacologic treatment of depression in nursing home residents: a mental health services perspective. J Geriatr Psychiatry Neurol 2002;15(3):141–6.

26. Jones AL, Dwyer LL, Bercovitz AR, et al. The National Nursing Home Survey: 2004 overview. Vital Health Stat 2009;13(167):1–155.

27. Carlson WL, Snowden M. Improving treatment for depression in the nursing home populations: integrating the model of the depression care manager. Harv Rev Psychiatry 2007;14:128–32.

28. USPSTF (US Preventive Services Task Force). 2009 Recommendations for adults. Available at: http://www.uspreventiveservicestaskforce.org. Accessed February 2, 2014.

29. Andrews AO, Bartels SJ, Xie H, et al. Increased risk of nursing home admission among middle aged and older adults with schizophrenia. Am J Geriatr Psychiatry 2009;17(8):697–705.

30. Snowden M, Piacitelli J, Koepsell T. Compliance with PASARR recommendations for Medicaid recipients in nursing homes. Preadmission screening and annual resident review. J Am Geriatr Soc 1998;46(9):1132–6.

Index

Note: Page numbers of article titles are in **boldface** type.

Clin Geriatr Med 30 (2014) 663–669
http://dx.doi.org/10.1016/S0749-0690(14)00057-3
0749-0690/14/$ – see front matter © 2014 Elsevier Inc. All rights reserved.

geriatric.theclinics.com

Printed and bound by CPI Group (UK) Ltd, Croydon, CR0 4YY

03/10/2024

01040496-0011